The Biological Basis of Clinical Observations

Second edition

William T. Blows

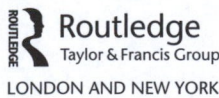
Routledge
Taylor & Francis Group

LONDON AND NEW YORK

First edition published 2001 as *The Biological Basis of Nursing: Clinical Observations*
by Routledge

This edition published 2012
by Routledge
2 Park Square, Milton Park, Abingdon, Oxon, OX14 4RN

Simultaneously published in the USA and Canada
by Routledge
711 Third Avenue, New York, NY 10017

Routledge is an imprint of the Taylor & Francis Group, an informa business

British Library Cataloguing in Publication Data
A catalogue record for this book is available from the British Library

Library of Congress Cataloging-in-Publication Data
Blows, William T., 1947–
    The biological basis of clinical observations / William T. Blows. – 2nd ed.
    p. cm.
    Rev. ed. of: The biological basis of nursing : clinical
    observations / William T. Blows. 2001.
    Includes bibliographical references and index.
    I. Blows, William T., 1947– Biological basis of nursing. II. Title.
    [DNLM: 1. Clinical Medicine–Nurses' Instruction. 2. Physiological
    Phenomena–Nurses' Instruction. 3. Decision Making–Nurses' Instruction. QT 104]
    LCclassification not assigned
    610.73–dc23   2011048812

ISBN13: 978–0–415–67461–4 (hbk)
ISBN13: 978–0–415–67462–1 (pbk)
ISBN13: 978–0–203–11642–5 (ebk)

Typeset in Goudy
by Swales & Willis Ltd, Exeter, Devon

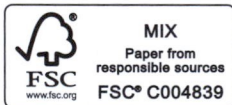

MIX
Paper from
responsible sources
FSC
www.fsc.org   FSC® C004839

Printed and bound in Great Britain by
TJ International Ltd, Padstow, Cornwall

Contents

List of figures

Plates

List of tables

Preface to the second edition

Today, biological studies are a major part of any health care training programme, be it medicine, nursing, midwifery and for other health care professionals, because the sciences are vital for working as an autonomous practitioner. The client's problems will be affecting a biological system, and the treatment will have a biological basis, be it drugs, surgery or other forms of therapy.

In addition, medical sciences have never seen such a remarkable flood of new knowledge as we are seeing today; knowledge which is already changing the way we treat disease. Advances in genetics and neuroscience are two good examples of this. If health care professionals are going to remain at the 'coal face' of this revolution, they must be familiar with the sciences and technologies that underpin the changing face of the care they give.

Clinical specialists therefore need to be taught skills which are themselves based on sound knowledge. One such skill is clinical decision-making, often carried out quickly and under pressure. Decision-making is often based on accurate observations, and involves making the correct choice for your clients. A thorough understanding of the underpinning sciences is essential to broaden the number of choices available, and to facilitate making the correct choice.

This book takes one of the most important care activities carried out by all practitioners, clinical observations, and explores the biology behind them, giving the possible pathological basis for variations in the observed results. The basic observations are usually taught in the early stages of a training programme and are explored here at a fundamental level for students in their first years. However, this book also looks at more advanced observations, for example, neurological observations, which are often taught later in the curriculum. In addition, this book will be of use and interest to educators and trained professionals with students under their leadership.

This second edition has been updated with information on observations related to fluid balance, nutrition, skin, pain and the effects of drugs on the body.

List of abbreviations

α-MSH	alpha-melanocyte-stimulating hormone
ACE	angiotensin-converting enzyme
ADH	antidiuretic hormone
ADP	adenosine diphosphate
AIDS	acquired immune deficiency syndrome
ALS	amyotrophic lateral sclerosis (Lou Gehrig's disease)
ANS	autonomic nervous system
ANV	anticipatory nausea and vomiting
ARP	agouti-related protein
ASD	atrial septal defect
ATP	adenosine triphosphate
AV	atrioventricular
AVR	alveolar ventilation rate
BBB	blood–brain barrier
BIA	bioelectrical impedance analysis
BMI	body mass index
BMR	basal metabolic rate
BP	blood pressure
CAP	community-acquired pneumonia
CART	cocaine- and amphetamine-regulated transcript
CASP	central aortic systolic pressure
CCF	congestive cardiac failure
CFS	cancer fatigue syndrome
CNS	central nervous system
CO	cardiac output
COX	cyclo-oxygenase
CPT	carnitine palmitoyltransferase
CSF	cerebrospinal fluid
CTZ	chemoreceptor trigger zone
CVA	cerebrovascular accident
CVP	central venous pressure
CYP	cytochrome P450 oxidases
DMD	Duchenne muscular dystrophy
DNA	deoxyribonucleic acid
DP	diastolic pressure
DPG	2,3-diphosphoglycerate
DRG	dorsal respiratory group
ECF	extracellular fluid

ECG	electrocardiogram
EEG	electroencephalogram
EGF	epidermal growth factor
ERV	expiratory reserve volume
EWN	Edinger–Westphal nucleus
FAD	flavine adenine dinucleotide
FEV	forced expiratory volume
GABA	gamma-aminobutryic acid
GABA-T	GABA transaminase
GAD	glutamic acid decarboxylase
GFR	glomerular filtration rate
GHP	glomerular hydrostatic pressure
GI	gastrointestinal
hCG	human chorionic gonadotrophin
HLA	human leukocyte antigen
HMD	hyaline membrane disease
HR	heart rate
IBD	inflammatory bowel disease
ICP	intracranial pressure
IOP	intraoccular pressure
IRV	inspiratory reserve volume
IV	intravenous
L2	lumbar vertebra 2
LGN	lateral geniculate nucleus
LMN	lower motor neuron
LP	lumbar puncture
LPS	lipopolysaccharide
LRG	leucine-rich alpha-2-glycoprotein
LVF	left ventricular failure
MAP	mean arterial pressure
MI	myocardial infarction
MLF	medial longitudinal fasciculus
MND	motor neuron disease
MOH	medication overuse headache
MS	multiple sclerosis
NAD	nicotinamide adenine dinucleotide
NAD	nothing abnormal detected
NBM	nil by mouth
NMDA	N-methyl-D-aspartic acid
NNAL	4-(methylnitrosamino)-1-(3-pyridyl)-1-butanol
NNK	4-(methylnitrosamino)-1-(3-pyridyl)-1-butanone
NO	nitric oxide
NPY	neuropeptide Y
NREM	non-rapid eye movement

NSAI	non-steroidal anti-inflammatory
NST	nucleus of the solitary tract
OT	optic tracts
PBP	progressive bulbar palsy
PCA	patient-controlled analgesia
PCO_2	partial pressure of carbon dioxide
PD	Parkinson's disease
PGE	prostaglandin E
PGF	prostaglandin F
PMA	progressive muscular atrophy
PNS	peripheral nervous system
PO_2	partial pressure of oxygen
PR	peripheral resistance
PRG	posterior root ganglion
PT	pretectum
PVR	pulmonary ventilation rate
RAS	reticular activation system
RBCs	red blood cells
RDS	respiratory distress syndrome
REM	rapid eye movement
RF	reticular formation
RICP	raised intracranial pressure
RNA	ribonucleic acid
RR	respiratory rate
RVF	right ventricular failure
SA	sinoatrial
SC	superior colliculus
SMA	supplementary motor area
SOL	space-occupying lesion
SP	systolic pressure
SPM	semi-permeable membrane
SV	stroke volume
TENS	transcutaneous electrical nerve stimulation
TP	transport protein
TPN	total parenteral nutrition
TTM	total temperature management
TV	tidal volume
UMN	upper motor neuron
URTI	upper respiratory tract infection
UTI	urinary tract infection
UVA	ultraviolet A light
UVB	ultraviolet B light
UVL	ultraviolet light
VC	vital capacity

LIST OF ABBREVIATIONS

VLN	ventral lateral nucleus
VMC	vasomotor centre
VOR	vestibulo-ocular reflex
VRG	ventral respiratory group
VSD	ventricular septal defect
WBCs	white blood cells
WHO	World Health Organization

Chapter 1   **Temperature**

Introduction

A great deal of mechanism exists within the body in order to stabilise the internal environment, and this is particularly important with regard to body temperature. At 37°C the human temperature is well balanced to provide the optimum conditions for tissue metabolism. Cooler temperatures would slow down the rate of cellular chemistry, which in turn would reduce cellular function. As it is, most chemical changes require enzymes to speed up the reactions to a level necessary for life. When these temperature-sensitive reactions are cooled, the resultant slowing of metabolism becomes dangerous to health. Hotter temperatures are also problematic, by causing metabolic systems to become inefficient and enzymes to move closer to denaturing. **Denaturing** is a heat-related change in protein structure which again leads to failure of cellular activity.

This essential stabilisation of optimum temperatures must happen despite changes in the external environmental temperature (known as the **ambient temperature**). It is only with help from external factors such as clothes and fires that humans can survive in temperatures that might otherwise be hostile to their cellular chemistry. Survival in the tropics or at the poles is entirely dependent on the body's ability to stabilise the internal environment aided by behaviour designed to retain or lose heat. But extremes of external temperature put great pressures on the body's systems, and they may fail to cope. The resulting dangerous change in a person's internal temperature is the cause of many deaths in very hot or very cold countries, or during very hot or very cold periods occurring in a usually temperate climate.

Measurement of body temperature becomes important for two reasons: it gives insight into the metabolic and homeostatic activity of the body and may also provide information about the possible cause of any abnormal state, contributing to an accurate diagnosis. For the body to balance the temperature, mechanisms must be in place to ensure that the heat gained is equal to the heat lost.

Heat gain

Heat production is part of the energy obtained from the use of the high-energy molecule **ATP (adenosine triphosphate)** in cellular metabolism. All cells use ATP, but some use more than others (e.g. liver and muscle cells) and therefore they liberate more heat. ATP itself is constructed from **ADP (adenosine diphosphate)** using energy from nutrients in the diet. Enzymes within the **mitochondrion**, an organelle at the centre of cellular respiration (i.e. the powerhouse of the cell), produce ATP from the metabolism of glucose and fat.

Glucose

Glucose is the end product of dietary carbohydrate breakdown by the digestive tract and the liver. One gram of glucose can be used by the body to produce about 4 kilocalories of energy, and this is known as the **Atwater** number for glucose. Glucose undergoes glycolysis in the cytoplasm close to the mitochondria. **Glycolysis** is the breakdown of glucose to the substance pyruvate, which can enter the mitochondrial matrix and join the **tricarboxylic (or Krebs or citric acid) cycle.** Pyruvate will first become **acetyl-CoA (acetyl coenzyme A)**, the entry point for substances joining the cycle. Throughout the cycle a series of reactions occurs which results in a return to acetyl-CoA (see Figure 1.1). The purpose of this cycle is twofold.

First, it is a means of shedding excess carbon by combining it with oxygen (O_2) to form the waste gas carbon dioxide (CO_2). Second, it produces hydrogen (H) atoms that are transported to a chain reaction series, the **electron transport system**. The molecules moving the hydrogen from the Krebs cycle to the electron transport system on the inner mitochondrial membrane are **NAD (nicotinamide adenine dinucleotide)** and **FAD (flavine adenine dinucleotide)**, which bind to the hydrogen to form **NADH** and **FADH$_2$** respectively. The hydrogen atoms, at the point of delivery to the first component of the electron transport chain, are split into **ions**, i.e. particles having a positive or negative charge, in this case protons (H^+) and electrons (e^-).

The protons are pumped out of the matrix to a position between the inner and outer mitochondrial membranes, and the electrons are passed down the electron transport system (Figure 1.2). Using enzymes bound to the inner-membrane folds (known as **cristae**) of the mitochondrion (Figure 1.3), this transport system releases electron energy in stages and immediately locks it up by the conversion of ADP and inorganic phosphate (P_i) to ATP.

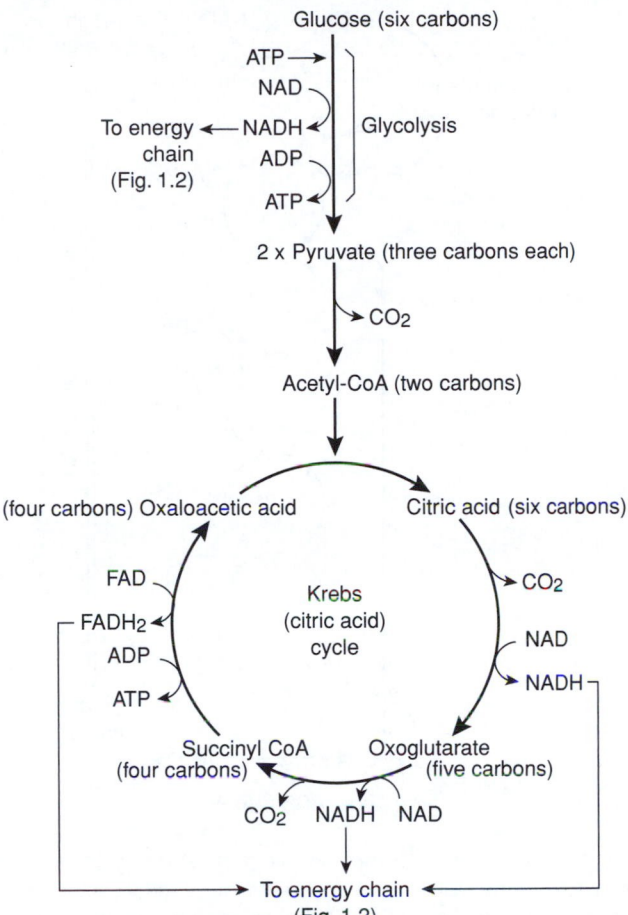

FIGURE 1.1 The Krebs (citric acid, tricarboxylic acid) cycle. Two pyruvates are obtained for each glucose as a result of glycolysis. Some adenosine triphosphate (ATP) is needed to start the process. From pyruvate, acetyl coenzyme A (CoA) feeds into the cycle by binding to oxaloacetic acid to form citric acid. The carbon count of each step is shown, and at various points carbon is lost by combining with oxygen to form CO_2. Nicotinamide adenine dinucleotide (NAD) and flavine adenine dinucleotide (FAD) combine with hydrogen at the points shown to transport this energy-rich hydrogen to the energy chain (Figure 1.2). Adenosine diphosphate (ADP) becomes energy-rich ATP during glycolysis and the cycle.

This generates some heat, but more heat will be liberated later when the ATP is used by the cell for other activities (i.e. the ATP is reduced again to ADP and P_i). Heat is then available for contribution to body temperature. The hydrogen ions that had been previously pumped out return to the matrix, an energy-liberating process driving the enzyme ATPase to further convert ADP and P_i to ATP, and thus store more energy. The reunion of the electron and proton to form hydrogen again at the end of the process is accompanied by the further introduction of oxygen to create water ($2H^+ + 2e^- \rightarrow 2H + O \rightarrow H_2O$).

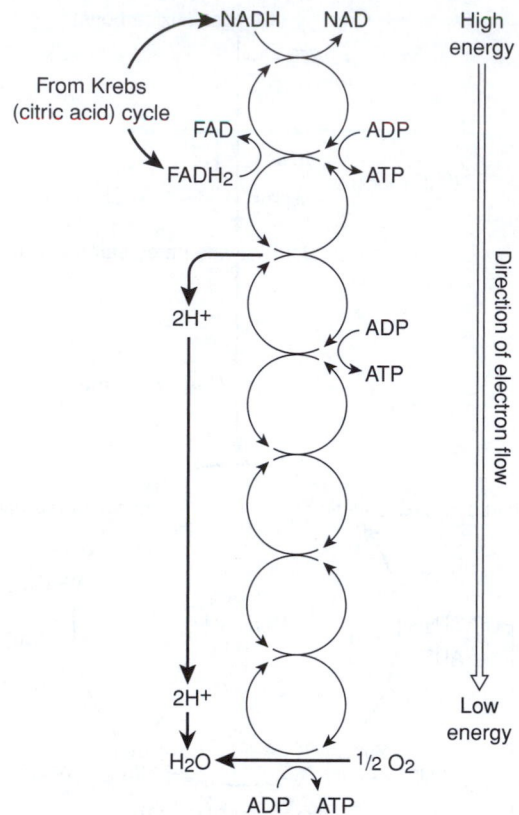

FIGURE 1.2 Electron transport chain. A simplified diagram of the cyclic reactions that electrons pass down from the high-energy end to the low-energy end. Hydrogen ions (H+) and electrons arrive from the Krebs cycle transported by nicotinamide adenine dinucleotide (NAD) and flavine adenine dinucleotide (FAD). As the electrons flow down the chain reactions, they lose energy, which is used to convert adenosine diphosphate (ADP) to adenosine triphosphate (ATP). The hydrogen ions pass directly to the end of the chain reaction, where they join oxygen (half of O_2) to form metabolic water (H_2O). This takes place on the inner membrane cristae of the mitochondrion.

Fats

Whereas glucose enters the Krebs cycle via pyruvate, fats provide energy somewhat differently. The Atwater number for fats is about 9 kilocalories per 1 g, more than twice that of glucose. Fats occur in the diet as **triglycerides**, that is three (hence 'tri-') fatty acids attached to a single glycerol molecule. The molecule takes on the shape of a letter E (Figure 1.4). Fatty acids can be split from the glycerol by the enzyme **lipase**, and free glycerol can be converted to glucose by the liver, a process called **gluconeogenesis** (i.e. genesis = creation, neo = new; the creation of new glucose, or creating glucose from a non-carbohydrate source, as in this case from fats). This new glucose can be used by the liver and the rest of the body in the same way as glucose from carbohydrate. Free fatty acids from the triglyceride

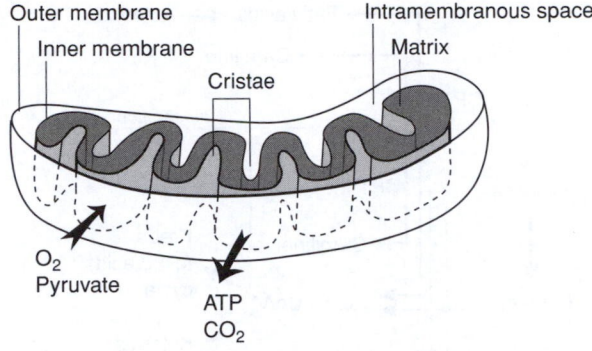

FIGURE 1.3 The mitochondrion. Pyruvate enters the matrix from the outside where glycolysis takes place. The matrix is the site of the Krebs cycle. The energy transport chain occurs on the cristae of the inner membrane. Oxygen (O_2) enters and combines with carbon to form carbon dioxide (CO_2). Adenosine triphosphate (ATP) leaves and passes to all parts of the cell.

molecule can be used by the liver for the Krebs cycle, but they do not form pyruvate first. Instead, they enter the cycle by converting to acetyl-CoA and carrying on around the cycle from there. Thus, fatty acids provide an alternative, more direct input into the cycle other than via pyruvate (Figure 1.5).

Fatty acids arriving at the liver in too large a quantity, as in **diabetes**, cannot all become acetyl-CoA, so they go through a different process leading to **ketone** formation, mostly **acetone**, which is excreted in the urine or breath, having been taken first via the blood to the kidneys or lungs. Normally, muscles are capable of taking up ketones from the blood for use as energy, including heat, but in diabetes this use of ketones may be blocked.

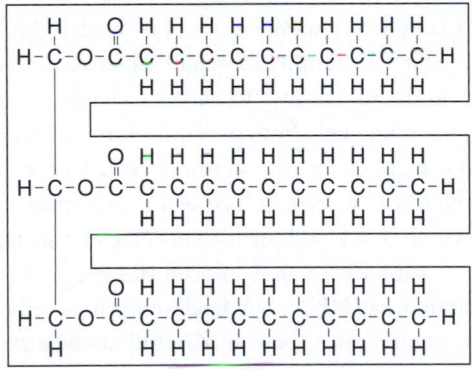

FIGURE 1.4 The E-shaped triglyceride molecule. A glycerol backbone holds together three long carbon (C) chain fatty acids saturated with hydrogen (H) and some oxygen (O).

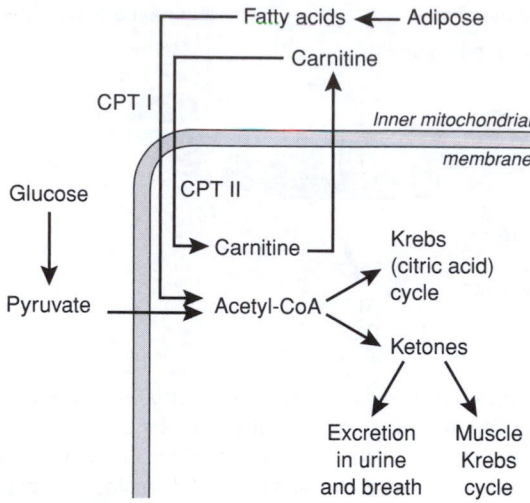

FIGURE 1.5   The entry of fatty acids into the Krebs (citric acid) cycle is an alternative pathway to glucose as an energy source. Movement of fatty acids across the inner mitochondrial membrane is effected by binding with carnitine, which is recycled. Binding with carnitine requires one form of the enzyme carnitine palmitoyltransferase I (CPT I), and removal of carnitine requires the other form, CPT II. Some acetyl-CoA goes on to become ketones, which can be used for muscle energy or excreted.

Protein

Proteins, the body's vital nitrogen source, can also be used for heat production if absolutely necessary. Normally, carbohydrates are the first source of energy, followed by fats if carbohydrates are not available in the diet (e.g. in the case of **starvation**) or cannot be used by the body (e.g. in the case of **diabetes**). If fats are not available either (e.g. because of depletion of stored adipose), protein will be used as a last resort. Whereas fats used for energy causes weight loss, protein used for energy causes **muscle wasting** (see Chapter 6), and usually this means that the patient is in a very serious state of ill-health. Muscle wasting is mostly seen in patients who are dying from a terminal disease, such as cancer, and this state, called **cachexia** (see Chapter 6), results in debility, weakness, emaciation and a mental state of hopelessness. In order to use **amino acids** from proteins as an energy source, the liver must first remove the nitrogenous component, the amine group, a process called **deamination** (Figure 1.6), and convert the rest to glucose (gluconeogenesis again, this time glucose from protein). This glucose can be used as blood sugar to provide energy for cells, giving protein the same Atwater number as carbohydrates, 4 kilocalories per gram. The nitrogen within the amine group becomes **ammonia (NH_3)**, but small quantities only may be released from the liver into the blood, since ammonia is toxic and should not be distributed widely in large amounts. Most of the ammonia is further converted in the liver to **urea** via the **Krebs urea cycle**. Urea is a safer compound to enter the blood and excrete through the kidneys and skin, but it can be toxic if blood levels are constantly raised.

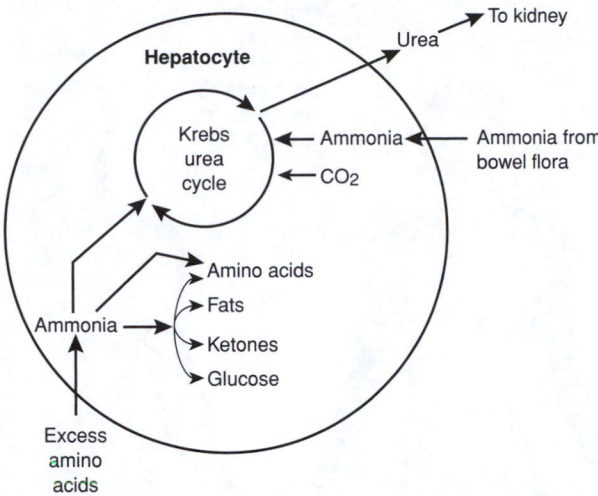

FIGURE 1.6   The Krebs urea cycle in liver cell (hepatocytes). Excess amino acids are split to release ammonia (NH_3). The remaining component can then be converted to glucose, fats or ketones. Some may join with ammonia to form amino acids again. Ammonia from bowel flora joins the cycle with CO_2 to form urea for excretion.

Metabolism

Since **metabolism** is the total of all the chemical reactions in the body that use energy, and therefore liberate heat, it follows that there is a minimum rate of metabolism below which cellular activity may fail, with a subsequent threat to life. Overall, the **basal metabolic rate (BMR)** refers to the minimum total internal energy expenditure when awake but at rest, or the minimum metabolic rate at rest needed to sustain life. As would be expected, more heat energy is produced in areas of the body where cells exist that undergo high metabolic rates (e.g. the liver, but also the brain when active) or undertake movement (e.g. the muscles during exercise). The common factor between these areas is the rapid release of energy, creating heat as an excess product. The body creates an average of about 420 kilojoules (100 calories) of heat per hour, which would raise the body temperature by 2°C per hour if it were not lost at a rate equal to that at which it is produced (Blows 1998). Cells rich in mitochondria are clearly candidates for rapid metabolic rates and therefore high heat production. Areas of the body that house the greater number of cells away from the surface, i.e. the body core (notably the trunk, not the limbs), are sites where heat cannot escape directly into the environment, and are therefore hotter (Figure 1.7). They would be much hotter if heat were not moved away from the core by the blood.

Heat movement and loss

About 1°C difference exists between the **core temperature** and the **peripheral temperature**, but this difference can increase in cold environments to the extent that the hands and feet can be as much as 10°C cooler than the trunk (Figure 1.7). As more heat is produced, it is

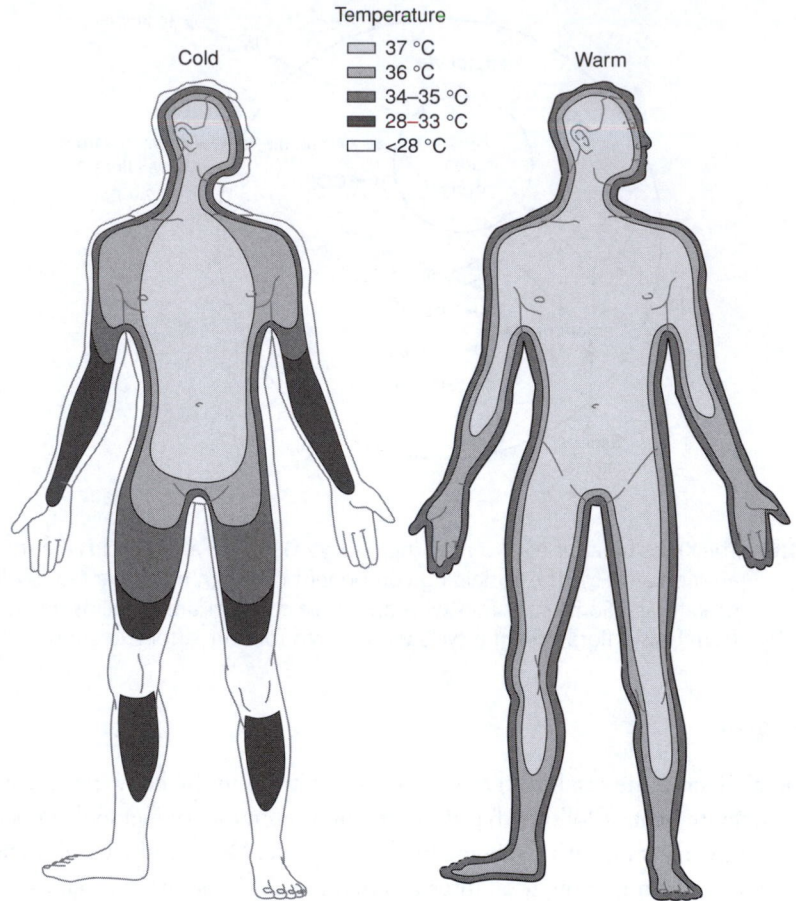

FIGURE 1.7 Temperature profile in a cold and in a warm environment. Notice the restricted core temperature (37°C) in the cold environment, keeping vital organs warm while minimising heat loss from the extremities. Under these conditions, the temperature of the extremities can be as much as 10°C lower than the core.

essential that heat is moved away from the hotter core to the cooler surface tissues by the blood, the main transport system of the body. This is a major role of blood that is often overlooked. Moving heat in this manner is crucial to prevent very active tissues, such as the brain, muscle and liver, from overheating and virtually cooking themselves *in situ*. At the same time, tissues in direct contact with the external environment, mostly the skin and mucous membranes, will not produce enough heat in extreme cold conditions to survive and rely entirely on heat transported into the tissues by the blood. The extremities are a good example of these tissues. Should the blood supply to the extremities fail, as in extreme cold conditions, the tissues can die, causing **gangrene** (an area of dead tissue). Loss of fingers and toes from gangrene in extreme cold conditions is not uncommon.

Removal of heat from the body is achieved mostly through the skin, and to a lesser extent through mucous membrane. Some heat is also lost in faeces and urine, and in exhaled air, since inhaled air is warmed by the nasal and respiratory passages. Sweating is a very important means of heat loss and is a key indicator that the body is too hot. About two million sweat glands exist in a single individual, with greater concentrations in specific areas such as the axillae and palms. Extra body heat is used to convert the sweat from a liquid state at body temperature to a vapour also at body temperature. The heat used for this purpose does not raise the temperature of the sweat, and therefore it is called the **latent (hidden) heat** of evaporation. A similar situation is seen when latent heat is required to convert boiling water at 100°C to steam, which is also at 100°C. Sweat vapour passes into the air taking heat with it. In high-temperature situations, such as a hot day or a high body temperature (e.g. infections or excessive exercise), sweating becomes a vital means of cooling the skin, which can then accept more heat from the core. An environment of high humidity severely reduces the skin's ability to vaporise sweat, which remains as a liquid on the skin, and as the skin temperature rises, so does the core.

Other means of skin heat loss are conduction, convection and radiation. **Conduction** is the passage of heat from the skin into any cooler object touching it. We warm the bed we sleep in, the clothes we wear, the seats we sit on, the pens we hold, and so on, by conduction. It is all heat lost from our cells. However, it constitutes the smallest amount of heat lost during the day unless the body is suddenly immersed in cold water, when rapid conduction can cause quick and severe hypothermia. **Convection** involves the warming of air next to the skin. Since warm air rises, it moves upwards and is replaced by colder air from below. The process is repeated continuously, making humans mobile convector heaters warming any environment they inhabit. This warm air layer is rapidly removed by wind, and if this wind is cold, it causes the body to chill quickly, a phenomenon known as the **wind chill factor**. **Radiation** of heat is also continuous, where heat passes directly out from the skin into any objects it hits, warming that object. Gas or electric fires heat a room, and the sun warms the Earth in the same way. By this means humans warm the walls, floors, ceilings and objects in a room. Much of this heat is in the form of **infrared radiation**, and this is what infrared thermometers use to assess temperature. It is also this form of heat that is picked up by thermal imaging cameras used in rescues from earthquake-damaged buildings and in night vision. With all these mechanisms of heat loss, it is not surprising that a class of students will themselves gradually raise the temperature of a cold classroom!

Heat regulation: gain versus loss

The body must have the ability to switch from increased heat production when it is cold to increased heat loss when it is hot. This is a finely tuned process that is sensitive to small changes in both the internal and the external temperature. Like any homeostatic mechanism, the aim is to stabilise the normal state, often called **normothermia**; in this case to sustain an average 37°C and to try to distribute heat evenly to all the tissues. Like any homeostatic mechanism, it involves sensory feedback to the brain and an output to effector organs. It is a negative feedback mechanism in which the system changes the direction of the original stimulus, i.e. if the temperature goes up, the mechanism drives it down, and vice versa. The area of the brain responsible for this control of temperature is the **hypothalamus**, the body's thermostat. The **preoptic nucleus** of the hypothalamus is rich in both heat- and cold-sensitive neurons able to monitor the temperature of the blood that passes through it and initiate any necessary maintenance action. The heat-sensitive neurons fire impulses faster as the temperature rises, with a similar response from the cold-sensitive neurons to cooler temperatures (Guyton and Hall 2011). Peripheral and ambient temperatures are also monitored by both cold- and heat-sensitive receptors in the skin, and internal temperatures are monitored by sensors within the spinal cord, the abdominal organs and around the major veins. In all these areas cold receptors dominate, indicating the need for the body to avoid low rather than high temperatures. They feed back to the hypothalamus, the brain area that therefore has complete second-by-second information on the total body temperature (Guyton and Hall 2011). The hypothalamus maintains a **set point** of 37.1°C and initiates any changes necessary to stabilise the temperature at this set point. Any situation that causes the body temperature to rise above the set point (i.e. **hyperthermia, pyrexia** or **hyperpyrexia**) results in the hypothalamus activating the **sympathetic nervous system**, which stimulates sweating. At the same time, reduced sympathetic **vasoconstrictor tone** causes vasodilation of the skin vessels coupled with relaxation of the precapillary sphincters. Together these ensure more blood brings more heat to the body surface, causing the skin to be hot and flushed. Skin blood flow can vary from 250 ml to as much as 2500 ml per minute, depending on thermoregulatory needs (Watson 1998). Sympathetic stimulation also results in an associated increase in heart rate, ensuring faster delivery of blood to the skin, and an increase in the respiratory rate to expel more heat in the breath. Behavioural changes also occur; the individual removes clothes or bedding to get comfortable and takes a cold drink or cooling shower.

In **hypothermia** (body temperature below the set point, i.e. 35°C or lower), the hypothalamus initiates sympathetic activity that increases cellular metabolism to generate more heat, and it increases sympathetic **vasoconstrictor tone**, which will constrict the peripheral blood vessels in the skin to reduce the heat loss. Sweating is shut down as much as possible and respirations are reduced. It may seem contradictory that the sympathetic nervous system can be activated in both extremes of body temperature and yet have different effects. This is because the sympathetic nervous system uses the neurotransmitter **noradrenaline** at the termination synapse, and this binds to different receptors with often contradictory results. Hair erector (or **pilomotor**) muscles cause hairs to stand on end, a process that should trap more air next to the skin for improved insulation. Its use is probably limited in humans due to the sparseness of hair compared with animals and because humans wear clothes. It does, however, cause the goose pimples that clearly indicate that the skin is chilled. The **motor nervous system** supplying the skeletal muscle is used to increase muscle tone in a manner that induces shivering, again to boost heat production, as all muscle activity does. The motor system also enhances conscious behavioural responses, like turning on heating systems, exercise, and dressing warmly.

Temperature scales and normal temperature variation

The body temperature is measured in degrees **Celsius** (or **centigrade**, °C) as part of the **International System of Units (SI)**. Strictly speaking, the SI unit for temperature is the **Kelvin (K)**, but this is rather impractical for clinical use since 0K is *minus* 273 degrees centigrade (−273°C, i.e. the lowest, or coldest, possible temperature), making body temperature

310°K. Celcius uses 0°C as the freezing point of water and 100°C as the boiling point of water at one atmosphere air pressure (generally accepted as sea level). This last point is important since boiling point is dependent on the air pressure and water boils at reduced temperatures as air pressure drops, i.e. when ascending away from sea level. In outer space, for example, the freezing and boiling points of water meet: water would instantly freeze due to the very low temperatures and, at the same time, boil due to zero air pressure! The centigrade scale has taken over from the **Fahrenheit** (°F) system, which had the freezing point at 32°F and the boiling point at 212°F. The body temperature at 37°C was previously measured at 98.4°F, a figure that may still be found in older texts. The conversion of Celcius to Fahrenheit uses the formula 1.8 (°C) + 32 = °F, i.e. taking the normal body temperature of 37°C as an example, 1.8 × 37 = 66.6; then 66.6 + 32 = 98.6°F (Figure 1.8).

Normally small local changes in peripheral body temperature are to be expected as a result of variations in the external air temperature or contact with hot or cold surfaces. Such circumstances arise in very hot or very cold weather and in work environments that involve molten metal or refrigeration. These variations can cause thermal injuries if over-exposure occurs. A normal diurnal (24-hour) pattern of fluctuations also occurs, with lowest temperatures in the morning and highest in the evening. The body is also hotter after a warm bath or shower, and the core temperature will be temporarily increased by a hot drink, making oral measurement deceptive.

Taking the body temperature in adults

The traditional means of taking the temperature, i.e. the oral route, is still useful as it measures the temperature of the blood in the carotid artery, blood that is coming directly from the core temperature (Watson 1998). The peripheral and core temperatures are different

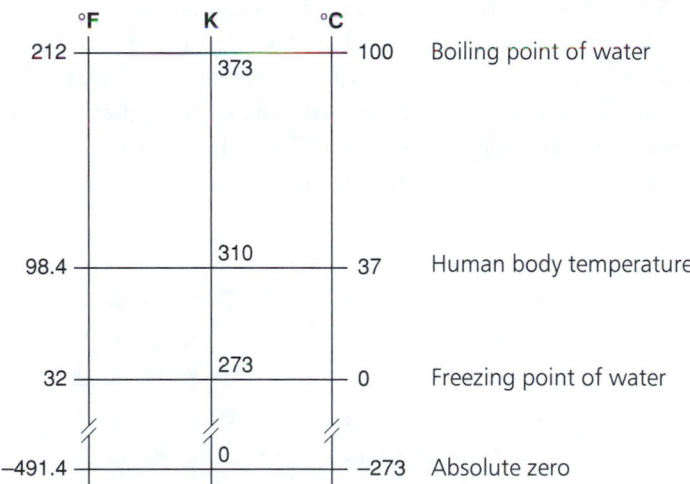

FIGURE 1.8 The Kelvin, Celsius (centigrade) and Fahrenheit temperature scales. The correlation between absolute zero, the freezing point of water, the human body temperature and the boiling point of water is shown.

because the peripheral temperature has the role of losing heat and therefore can fluctuate with the ambient temperature state. The core temperature must remain constant and is therefore the most accurate temperature to measure. It is the only stable temperature available, and it is also the temperature at which the vital organs must exist and function. Other routes such as the axilla, groin, rectum and ear are used, especially in specific client groups or certain situations when oral temperatures are inappropriate. The elderly, the mentally disturbed and very young children are client groups where the oral route is likely to be inadvisable. The clinical thermometer has now been replaced by electronic probes (see p. 13). There is also a need to resolve the problems of the time required for accuracy. O'Toole (1998) gives a good overall assessment of the sites and methods for taking the body temperature. She identified four types of thermometer as mercury-in-glass, disposable, electronic and infrared (the last two with digital readout). Of these, only the mercury-in-glass thermometer is no longer in clinical use.

Disposable thermometers are now available and are as accurate as mercury and electronic thermometers. They are each about one-tenth of the price of the traditional mercury thermometer (O'Toole 1998) but are for single use only. They are individually wrapped and sterilised. A series of temperature-sensitive chemical colour change dots provides an easily read system (Figure 1.9). The dots change from orange/red to blue, and the temperature is read as the highest-valued dot to turn blue. Erickson *et al.* (1996) identified variations in temperature with these chemical-dot skin-recording methods when compared with electronic devices in the same site (oral and axillary) in adults and children. Differences of ±0.4°C occurred frequently, suggesting that skin devices of this kind only allow an approximation of the body temperature (i.e. they record peripheral temperatures). There are also multiuse colour dot strips which are placed on the forehead. These are best read while in contact with the skin because the colour changes reverse if it cools down. They are less accurate than most other thermometers and therefore can only be considered as a guide to the temperature, and their best use is with small children at home.

Electronic devices are available for oral, axillary and rectal use. They take just 1 or 2 minutes to achieve a result in most cases, which is beneficial to both the busy nurse and the patient. Accuracy is generally on a par with the old mercury thermometers and therefore they are found in standard ward situations (O'Toole 1998). They usually display a **digital** result rather than shown on a scale. There are both contact versions, i.e. they need to be in

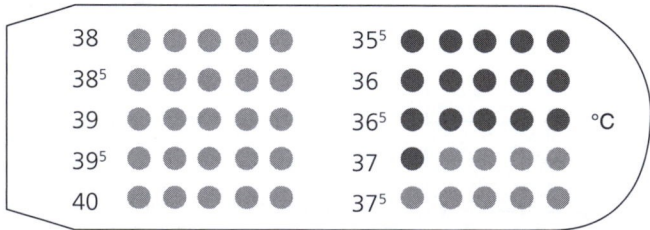

FIGURE 1.9 Tempadot thermometer reading. The dots change from red to blue according to the temperature recorded. Each dot represents 0.1°C. The one illustrated here shows 37°C, i.e. normal body temperature.

contact with the mucous membrane of the mouth or rectum or with axillary skin, and non-contact versions, which use infrared radiation from the skin (see below).

Electronic **infrared** thermometers are primarily for use in the ear, measuring the infrared radiation emitted from the eardrum, but some measure infrared emitted from the skin. The eardrum and the skin emit various levels of infrared radiation according to their temperature. The temperature can be calculated by the thermometer, based on the infrared level detected. The thermometer does this quickly, sometimes in seconds. Using this type of thermometer in the ear is now of growing importance, and it has been recognised that the eardrum shares the same blood supply as the hypothalamus, which makes it very close to core temperature, equating well with pulmonary artery temperature in some studies (O'Toole 1998). It is also easily accessible with a short probe, similar to those on an otoscope that fits into the external canal of the ear. The lens on the tip of the probe must face the membrane and a good seal should be obtained around the probe to ensure that only body heat is sampled. The presence of **cerumen** (ear wax) may give a reading lower than reality. This method has been used on sleeping patients without waking them. The infrared probe is probably better used on adults and older children, who not only have reasonably formed external ear canals but will co-operate better with the procedure.

Why mercury thermometers are a thing of the past

Mercury thermometers have been in use for a long time and are recognised as reasonably accurate (if left in place long enough, usually at least 3 minutes) and they are convenient to use. Several variations are known, including the normal and low-scale range oral versions, and the rectal versions with a blue bulb or a blue dot. A restriction in the mercury (Hg) column traps the mercury in the column and allows the temperature to be read outside the body without the mercury contracting back to the bulb. However, preparation for repeated use requires careful shaking of the instrument to force the mercury back into the bulb. This is when most breakages occur, causing the double hazard of broken glass and released mercury. Mercury is now recognised as a toxic hazard, especially if inhaled as vapour, which can remain in the environment for months after mercury spillage from a glass thermometer. Skin and mucous membrane absorption of mercury is poor, but the vapour is well absorbed through the lungs. Removal of spilt mercury via a vacuum cleaner is not recommended as this vaporises the metal and sprays the vapour around the house. In 1995, a total of 622 calls were made to the National Poisons Information Service about mercury poisoning, mostly concerning broken thermometers, and the majority of these breakages happened in the home. Acute mercury poisoning (within 30 minutes) results in thirst, nausea, vomiting, abdominal pains, diarrhoea with blood, and ultimately renal failure. Chronic mercury toxicity involves irritability, excessive salivation, loose teeth, gum disorders, slurred speech, tremors and unsteady gait. Broken glass causes additional risks with mercury thermometer accidents, e.g. rectal perforations if the thermometer breaks while in rectal use, oral injury if broken in the mouth, and swallowed glass fragments. Where mercury clinical thermometers were in use, special guidelines and mercury spillage kits had to be available for dealing with thermometer breakages. Cross-infection by glass thermometers is another problem that has never been fully resolved, as disinfection is not always convenient, desirable or effective, and disposable plastic covers, called dispotemps, can sometimes break. Organic matter left behind on thermometers after use can contain and grow a variety of organisms, including the influenza virus and *Clostridium*. These problems and hazards caused unacceptable risks in the clinical area, and the traditional mercury thermometer has now been replaced in clinical areas by one of the other electronic/digital types. It is not surprising that with modern technology becoming available the mercury-in-glass thermometer has become a museum piece.

Taking the body temperature in children

There has been a considerable debate in the literature about the route for taking temperatures in children. Some sources suggest that the rectal route, chosen because very young children cannot comply with the oral route and because it was more accurate than the axillary route, was dangerous because of the risk of rectal perforation and other complications. However, Morley (1992) identified multiple reasons for choosing rectal temperature measurements in infants and young children rather than the axillary route, and presented evidence to show the inaccuracy of axillary measurements in the very young. The difference between axillary and rectal temperatures in children can be as much as 3°C, and axillary measurements would miss one-quarter of febrile babies (Morley *et al.* 1992). With regard to using the ear, shape changes in the external canal as a result of different growth stages in children may affect the use of the infrared probe and therefore the accuracy of this type of thermometer. This may be one reason why tympanic measurements of temperature have been reported not to have registered a fever in some children and are probably inappropriate in neonates (Davis 1993). A special infrared probe is designed and available for axillary use in neonates. Currently, the ideal method of taking clinical temperature in children older than 5 years appears to be via the rectal route (NICE 2007; RCN 2007). The exception may be for children younger than 5 years in high dependency or intensive care units, where rectal temperatures may be indicated. Otherwise, children under 5 years but older than 4 weeks should have their temperatures taken by electronic or chemical dot methods. Under 4 weeks, the preferred method is electronic thermometer in the axilla (RCN 2007). However, nurses working with children should always consult and comply with the local policy designated for temperature routes used in children in their clinical areas.

Abnormal high body temperatures

Fevers are high temperatures, i.e. above 38°C (Blumenthal 1998); a **pyrexia** is recognised as a continuous body temperature above 37.5°C up to 39.9°C, and a hyperpyrexia is 40°C or above (Harker and Gibson 1995). Raised temperatures are caused by toxins or drug reactions, infections, prolonged exposure to a hot environment, brain disorders affecting the hypothalamus, neoplasms, autoimmune diseases, or the penguin effect (Blows 1998). Under any of these circumstances the body may fail to control the temperature by the means identified earlier, notably sweating, when the set point is exceeded. The hypothalamic set point is the role of the preoptic nucleus, and it is largely influenced by feedback from the peripheral skin, spinal cord and abdominal visceral temperatures. However, in fevers, first the hypothalamic set point is driven up to a higher level, e.g. 39°C, in a regulated manner, unlike in hyperthermia, in which there is an unregulated temperature rise (Henker *et al.* 1997). In fever, because the control centre has been reset higher, it perceives normal temperature of 37°C as being too low (Figure 1.10). Heat conservation and heat production then drive the temperature up to its new set level. The rise in the set point is due to the action of **pyrogens**, chemical agents that have the ability to readjust the hypothalamus. Pyrogens include various toxins, including proteins or their degraded products, and some endotoxins from bacteria, e.g. the **lipopolysaccharide (LPS)** layer from outside the cell wall of Gram-negative organisms. After death of the organism, the endotoxin is phagocytosed and the phagocyte itself (usually a macrophage) releases the chemical interleukin 1. This agent passes to the brain, where it appears to stimulate the formation of one of the prostaglandins, which in turn acts to reset the set point of the hypothalamus to a higher level. This is a rapid process, the temperature rising within 8–10 minutes of the release of interleukin 1. The endotoxin LPS only needs to cause the production of a few nanograms of interleukin 1 to cause fever. The involvement of prostaglandins is interesting, since this may explain how antipyretics such as aspirin and paracetamol may help to reduce the body temperature. These drugs block prostaglandin production (from a cell wall component called arachidonic acid), and may therefore prevent the effects of interleukin 1 on the hypothalamus.

Hyperthermia is a group of high body temperature disorders that includes **heat stroke** (Edwards 1998; Harker and Gibson 1995). This is a rapid rise in body temperature (to 40°C or more) caused by exposure to a hot environment, and the hypothalamic set point is soon

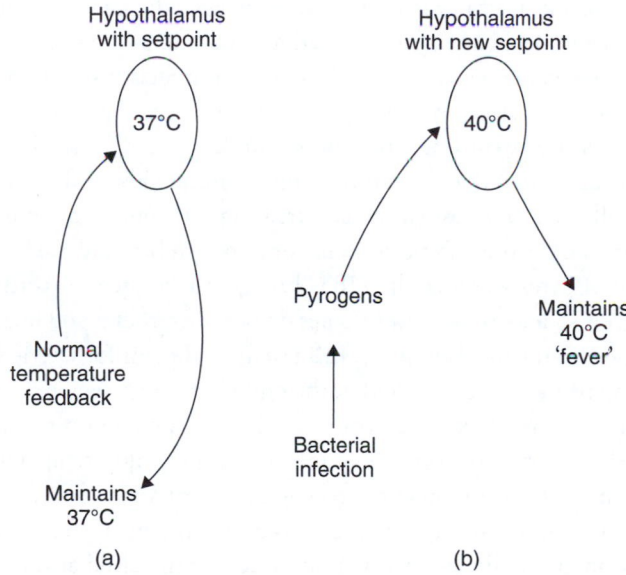

(a) (b)

FIGURE 1.10 The mechanism for fever. (a) The normal body temperature is maintained by the hypothalamus having a set point of 37°C and by feedback from the body indicating any changes to this temperature, which the hypothalamus will correct. (b) In fever, pyrogens released from bacteria re-set the hypothalamic set point to a higher value (here re-set to 40°C but it can be other high figures), and the hypothalamus attempts to maintain that higher temperature.

exceeded. However, sweating fails to control the temperature and the casualty collapses. Symptoms include hot, dry skin, full and bounding pulse, headaches, confusion, dizziness and failing consciousness. The **penguin effect** is a similar heat stroke syndrome caused by a reduced ability to sweat in the centre of a tightly packed crowd. Examples of this occur in crowds at a major event, like a pop music concert, or people packed together in a commuter train on a hot day. It is named after penguins, which crowd together to conserve heat in Antarctica. Emotional excitement, dancing and, possibly, drugs are features at pop concerts that cause excess heat production with reduced ability to sweat. On crowded commuter transport, standing passengers may collapse but remain pinned upright, risking a loss of life. The penguin effect can cause many casualties at once, all suffering from the heat and also from fluid and electrolyte imbalance (Blows 1998). **Heat exhaustion** is associated with exposure to hot environments where the hypothalamus has been able to keep the temperature at relatively normal levels for most of the time by sweating. However, continued heat exposure and profuse sweating result in excessive fluid and electrolyte losses, which eventually lead to collapse with headaches, weak and rapid pulse, confusion, nausea, cramps and pallor. **Malignant hyperthermia** is a complication associated with an inherited muscular disorder triggered by administration of inhalant anaesthetics and muscle-relaxing drugs, mostly in the young. The muscles maintain a state of contraction soon after induction of anaesthesia, and this muscle activity generates heat which can raise the body temperature by as much as 1°C every 5 minutes. About 20% of sufferers can die from the effects as it also induces acidosis, tachycardia and hypotension.

Febrile convulsions in children under 7 years of age indicate two things: a pyrexia usually caused by an infection and a hypothalamus that is too immature to cope with the high temperature. The most common causes are chest and ear infections, both of which will require investigation, but any infection can trigger a fit at this age. The mechanism that responds to a high temperature by causing a fit is poorly understood. Clearly, however, the management is two-pronged: treating and terminating the fit quickly, which involves reducing the temperature, followed by investigating and treating the underlying infection. Preventative measures carried out by the parents at home or nurses in hospital are beneficial and require early detection of pyrexia and cooling the child gently before a fit is triggered. Here, thermometers are not so important. Most homes do not have them, and many parents probably do not know how to use them properly. It is usually sufficient for worried parents to feel the child's head and trunk and recognise that the child has a high temperature. It then becomes more important to remove excess clothing, cool down the environment if it is too hot and get medical help rather than worry about measuring the child's temperature. In the clinical environment, accurate measurement becomes important and is easily achieved. In all cases of febrile convulsion, reassuring the parents is as much part of the treatment as is managing the fit, and includes allowing the parents access to the child at the earliest opportunity and for as long as possible to allay any fears raised about epilepsy, which is only a very rare complication.

In any of the cases of excessive heat disorder, treatment has traditionally involved cooling along with fluid and electrolyte replacement where necessary. Reducing the high temperature is problematic since cooling too rapidly can induce shock and shivering, which would cause more heat production. It has been generally accepted for years that the temperature should be reduced gradually, i.e. at a rate no faster than 1°C per hour, although in practice this has often been difficult to achieve and record. Tepid sponging is most often adopted on the understanding that adding water to the skin promotes heat loss by evaporation. Recent evidence on this, however, is that sponging to reduce fever, especially in children, is probably counterproductive since it causes the body to generate heat through shivering and is uncomfortable for the child (Anon. 1999; Blumenthal 1998). Given that fever is a normal body response to infection or inflammation, there is a growing volume of literature indicating that aggressive (or rapid) efforts to reduce the temperature may not be beneficial and could cause unwanted difficulties (Edwards 1998; Harker and Gibson 1995). This creates a vacuum in terms of what to do for a febrile child or adult. This question becomes critical to parents faced with a febrile child at night. Biologically, there are some basic principles that may help us. In general, provided they are sweating, adults cope with high temperatures better than children because of the maturity of the hypothalamus. Sweating is a sign that the hypothalamus is still doing its job. Children below 7 years of age are the most likely to suffer convulsions, so it may be prudent to try and prevent the temperature from going very high in this age group. Removal of all unnecessary clothing and providing a cool environment to promote natural heat loss is a useful approach. Cool drinks are of value because they reach the core temperature quickly and replace lost fluids. For this, however, it is vital that the child is conscious and able to swallow. Be aware of the risk of shivering and try to prevent this since shivering is an indication that the body has lost heat too quickly and is trying to generate more heat to combat the loss. A controlled environmental temperature is critical. Electric fans help to cool the environment if this is hot but should never be aimed directly at the sufferer since this would cool the periphery and send impulses of cold sensation from thermal receptors in the skin to the brain. These impulses may be misleading to the hypothalamus, which then tries to prevent heat loss from the body and generate more heat. Also, cold air from a fan could cause peripheral vasoconstriction, which then prevents heat transfer by blood from the core to the skin. Although tepid sponging is not generally recommended, it is probably a valid technique when applied to the hyperpyrexic patient who has lost the ability to sweat, i.e. the patient is hot and dry. Failure to sweat suggests that the hypothalamus has failed to respond, probably because the set point has been adjusted to a much higher level than normal. Antipyretic drugs, e.g. paracetamol, have a role to play in the management of elevated temperatures in persons who are capable of taking oral medication, especially children. They block the formation of prostaglandins, which promote elevation of the temperature, as noted earlier. Aspirin is a useful antipyretic, but it should never be given to children below the age of 12 years as this can induce Reye's syndrome, a severe neurological disorder that is known to follow viral illnesses, such as influenza, colds or chicken pox, which have been treated with this drug. Antipyretics alone are unlikely to prevent febrile convulsions, and other measures are required.

Abnormal low body temperatures

Exposure to cold leads to a general loss of body heat, known as **hypothermia**, or a local heat loss, called **frostbite**. Hypothermia can happen in anyone, but the majority of cases occur in the extremes of age: the very young and the very old. This is due again to problems with the hypothalamus. In the very young it is still immature and cannot fully control temperature balance. Below the age at which they crawl, babies can lose heat rapidly without the benefit of the major muscles generating heat by activity. Lying or sitting, without the ability to move or change position, does not allow much production of muscle heat energy. Babies compensate for this with **brown fat** that can generate heat, particularly when stimulated by melatonin, a hormone produced from serotonin in the pineal gland of the brain. Brown fat is largely lost with increasing age as the child becomes a lot more physically active. Very young children may not have developed the ability to shiver, and they cannot therefore gain heat from this mechanism. Despite the warming effect of brown fat, children exposed to prolonged or excessive cold will suffer from hypothermia. They feel cold to the touch and they may shiver, especially older children. They may also appear limp and quiet, and may have cyanosed lips and extremities. They can collapse and possibly die from respiratory or cardiac failure if they are not protected against both the external cold and their own heat loss. Wet children are especially vulnerable after swimming or playing in water. Because of poor insulation caused by very little body hair, the human baby is very vulnerable and is dependent on warm environments and the insulation provided by clothing. **Incubators** have saved the lives of many newborn babies who are unable to sustain normothermia by their own volition, e.g. such babies as **preterm** or **failure to thrive**. Incubation maintains the infants' environmental temperature usually a few degrees higher than average body temperature until it is mature enough to stabilise its own homeostatic control of heat loss. Since incubators must be opened occasionally to allow essential access, the room temperature must also be warm enough to prevent sudden chilling of the infant.

The elderly undergo age-related changes to many body systems, including the brain, and the hypothalamus gradually declines in function as neurons are lost. The temperature control centre becomes less able to respond to body temperature changes quickly and cannot always provide comprehensive heat regulation when environmental temperatures are above or below average for prolonged periods of time. Although hot environments can be harmful to the elderly, who can die in a heat wave, it is the cold that causes the most problems and the most deaths. Cold weather kills many elderly people annually, and special consideration must be given during winter months to older people who live alone in poorly heated homes. It is worse for those with limited mobility and those who are vulnerable to falling. An old person lying injured on a floor will lose heat quickly from his/her large surface area and may die from hypothermia before being found. Of the two age groups, it is probably true to say that children will suffer from the effects of cold quickly, whereas elderly people gradually deteriorate as a result of prolonged cold exposure.

An important cause of hypothermia is surgery: during the **perioperative period** patients are exposed to cool environments and suffer a significant body temperature loss. Intensive care may also put some patients at risk of hypothermia, mainly because patients are inactive (thus not generating much heat), they may be exposed for medical and nursing procedures and their total energy input for the day may be considerably less than what their body is used to. In these specialised clinical areas many units carry out **total temperature management (TTM)**, as a means of preventing hypothermia. This involves continual monitoring of the patient's core temperature by electronic probes placed inside the body, in sites such as the pulmonary artery, oesophagus, rectum or urinary bladder. The temperature can be read at any time as a digital figure on a screen that shows other physiological readings. TTM also involves maintenance of normothermia in the patient during lengthy exposure or surgery using specialised electrically warmed blankets. It also involves very strict control of the environmental temperature, often at a higher than average level, and re-warming of fluids or blood before, or during, intravenous infusion, again with specialised equipment designed with fluid re-warming systems. Because body temperature is linked to metabolism, and metabolism is linked to healing, it becomes obvious that the healing process itself relies on maintaining the correct body temperature.

Clearly the hypothermia sufferer needs to be warmer, but the problems associated with the treatment of hypothermia are about the process of re-warming. The danger lies with the low core temperature at which the vital organs must try to function. Any attempt to re-warm the person by applying heat to the periphery, i.e. warming up the skin, can be counterproductive and dangerous. The use of heat close to the skin, e.g. hot water bottles or the close proximity of heaters, will make the person look better and feel warmer to touch, but they only serve to dilate peripheral blood vessels, which then take vital blood, and therefore heat, away from the core, cooling the core temperature further. This is not the same as using the specialised heated blankets identified in TTM, when the core temperature is essentially normal and the emphasis is on preventing hypothermia, not treating it. The main points about re-warming the established hypothermia are that the person involved must first be urgently removed to a warmer environment to prevent further heat loss. Trying to re-warm someone in a very cold environment is an uphill struggle that the patient may lose. In addition, any wet clothing must be removed and the skin dried. Water on the skin acts like sweating in removing further heat quickly. The body should then be covered in dry clothing and the person preferably put to bed. Warm drinks with sugar given to the conscious person who is still able to swallow would be beneficial. Monitoring of the temperature by an electronic thermometer may be better achieved via a route other than the oral or axillary routes. The oral route may be dangerous in a patient who is in an altered state of consciousness, and axillary routes will only give peripheral temperature results. Re-warming, like cooling of pyrexia, should be gradual: often quoted as 1°C rise per hour. Rapid re-warming, like rapid cooling, is harmful as it can induce shock. It is not possible to raise the core temperature quickly, and any attempts to do so, like using warm or hot baths, will only raise the peripheral temperature, causing dilation of the skin vessels, which in turn causes cardiovascular collapse. Once cooled, the core temperature is only raised by heat produced from tissue metabolism, and this will take time to be effective.

Thermal injury

Frostbite is a local thermal injury, and as such it is akin to burns because tissue is destroyed by an extreme temperature abnormality. The intense local cold causes vasoconstriction to the point of occlusion of blood flow, with resultant anoxia of dependent tissues. All cellular metabolism stops when oxygen delivery and nutrient delivery are shut down, wastes accumulate in the cells and enzymic reactions can no longer function. Apart from cold, early signs of frostbite can include paraesthesia (tingling sensations) and numbness, and pallor of the affected tissues, which may turn blue (cyanosis) and ultimately black. This is when the tissues are dead (**necrosis** or **gangrene**) and may slough off. An infection of the area involved can then follow, with life-threatening results. If the tissues involved survive and recover, they become red, blistered and painful. Emergency treatment involves prevention of the condition worsening by removal to a warmer environment as soon as possible and gentle re-warming by placing the affected parts against warmer areas of the body. Removal of any tight clothing or restrictive jewellery is essential to promote good blood flow and to avoid rubbing the injury, which can cause tissue trauma. Light dressings may help, and medical treatment is usually essential. Frostbite will mostly affect toes and fingers because these parts are at the distal extremes of the cardiovascular system, i.e. they are at the point of lowest tissue perfusion pressure (the **mean arterial pressure**, or **MAP**) and therefore will suffer more damaging vasoconstriction for less environmental temperature drop than those parts closer to the heart. Also, distal extremities are thinner than central parts (compare the thickness of a toe with that of the thigh or the trunk) and therefore cold can penetrate extremities faster, i.e. they have less body mass per unit of surface area than thicker parts of the body. Since it is the surface area that is exposed to the cold, it has less mass of tissue below it to chill than the same surface area of, for example, the thigh. This smaller mass of tissue is not capable of heat production to counteract the cold on the same scale as bulkier parts. The distal extremities are more dependent on heat delivered by the blood than any other parts of the body. This is why feet can get cold quickly and hot water bottles are used by some people to warm their feet in bed. It is also the reason why the temperature of extremities is a good indication of the status of the circulation in that limb. The warm hand or foot has a good circulation, whereas cold extremities indicate poor circulation. This is a useful observation on limbs encased in plaster casts or where an injury or vascular complication may disturb blood flow to that extremity. Using hand or foot temperature to assess the circulation on the unaffected side will identify what the normal circulatory state is at that time, and given both limbs are normally equal, this will indicate what the circulatory state should be in the affected limb. Such a comparison made between the good limb and the affected limb may identify a serious problem that requires urgent attention, e.g. possibly the plaster or bandages are too tight.

Key points

- Body temperature is generally stabilised at 37°C, with a homeostatic negative feedback mechanism in place to ensure this.
- The hypothalamus in the base of the brain is the central control of this mechanism, with input from temperature-sensitive sensory nerve endings in the skin and around vital organs.
- Normally the body gains heat by cellular metabolism from energy-rich food and loses heat by evaporation of sweat, elimination, conduction, convection and radiation.
- Sweating is often a cardinal sign of overheating (pyrexia).
- Shivering is a cardinal sign of the body being too cold (hypothermia).
- The core temperature is the most accurate to record since this is the temperature at which the vital organs must function.
- The peripheral temperature is usually lower than the core temperature since it responds more to the ambient temperature and humidity.

- Disposable, electronic and infrared thermometers have now replaced mercury thermometers in clinical use.
- Younger children are more vulnerable to temperature changes and may suffer febrile convulsions.
- Nurses should check their local protocol concerning routes for taking temperatures in small children.
- Electric fans are useful for cooling the environment but must not be directed at the patient.
- Tepid sponging may be uncomfortable for the patient and may be of little value except in those circumstances of rapid body temperature rise where sweating has failed to control body temperature.
- Re-warming in hypothermia, like cooling in pyrexia, should be gradual, often quoted as 1°C rise per hour. Rapid re-warming, like rapid cooling, is harmful as it can induce shock.
- The temperature of the extremities is a good indication of the status of the circulation in that limb. The warm hand or foot has a good circulation, whereas cold extremities indicate a poorer circulation.

References

Anon. (1999) Fever analysis remains a burning issue. *Nursing Times*, **95**(9): 47.

Blows W. T. (1998) Crowd physiology: the 'penguin effect'. *Accident and Emergency Nursing*, 6: 126–129.

Blumenthal I. (1998) What parents think of fever. *Family Practice*, **15**(6): 513–518.

Davis K. (1993) The accuracy of tympanic temperature measurement in children. *Pediatric Nursing*, **19**(3): 267–272.

Edwards S. L. (1998) High temperature. *Professional Nurse*, **13**(8): 521–526.

Erickson R. S., Meyer L. T. and Woo T. M. (1996) Accuracy of chemical dot thermometers in critically ill adults and young children. *Image: Journal of Nursing Scholarship*, **28**(1): 23–28.

Guyton A. and Hall J. (2011) *Textbook of Medical Physiology*, 12th edition. W.B. Saunders, Elsevier, Philadelphia.

Harker J. and Gibson P. (1995) Heat-stroke: a review of rapid cooling techniques. *Intensive and Critical Care Nursing*, **11**: 198–202.

Henker R., Kramer D. and Rogers S. (1997) Fever. *AACN Clinical Issues*, **8**(3): 351–367.

Morley C. (1992) Why taking temperatures rectally is right. *Paediatric Nursing*, **4**(6): 7.

Morley C. J., Hewson P. H., Thornton A. J. and Cole T. J. (1992) Axillary and rectal temperature measurements in infants. *Archives of Disease in Childhood*, **67**: 122–125.

National Institute for Health and Clinical Excellence (2007) *Feverish Illness in Children*. NICE, London.

O'Toole S. (1998) Temperature measuring devices. *Professional Nurse*, **13**(11): 779–786.

Royal College of Nursing (2007) *Standards for Assessing, Measuring and Monitoring Vital Signs in Infants, Children and Young People*. RCN, London.

Watson R. (1998) Controlling body temperature in adults. *Nursing Standard*, **12**(20): 49–55.

Chapter 2 **Cardiovascular observations (I)**

The pulse and electrocardiogram (ECG)

- Introduction
- Blood physiology
- Heart physiology
- Observations of the pulse, apex beat, electrocardiogram and heart sounds
- The effects of cardiovascular drugs
- The pulse in children
- Key points
- References

Introduction

The need to move many substances from one part of the body to another is vital to the very existence of the individual. The blood has the task of transporting:

- water and nutrients from the digestive system to the cells;
- oxygen from the lungs to the cells;
- carbon dioxide from the cells to the lungs;
- wastes from the cells to the kidneys;
- defensive cells from the bone marrow to sites of infection;
- hormones from the glands to the cells;
- antibodies from lymphocytes to antigens;
- proteins from the liver to all parts of the circulatory system,
- heat (see Chapter 1), and much more.

Moving a liquid like blood requires a pump; and so we have a heart. The heart cycle creates two parameters that we can measure: (1) the number of times it beats per minute, recorded as a pulse; and (2) the pressure of blood leaving the heart, known simply as blood pressure. These are inseparably linked; the pulse is dependent on blood pressure since it is the pressure of blood exerted against the arterial wall in waves corresponding to heart contraction.

Similarly, the pulse varies with the blood pressure, i.e. if the blood pressure falls, the pulse rate rises to compensate, since too low a pressure will deliver inadequate blood to the tissues, and the heart will try to speed up the delivery. Measuring these two parameters alone will give great insight into the system that delivers life to the tissues and therefore provides an understanding of the basic state of the body.

Blood physiology

Blood cells

Blood is a liquid tissue, having a water-based extracellular component (the plasma) housing cells which themselves contain water. The cells are red (**red blood cells** or **RBCs**, also called **erythrocytes**), white (**white blood cells** or **WBCs**, also called **leucocytes**) and small cell fragments called **platelets** (or **thrombocytes**) (Figure 2.1).

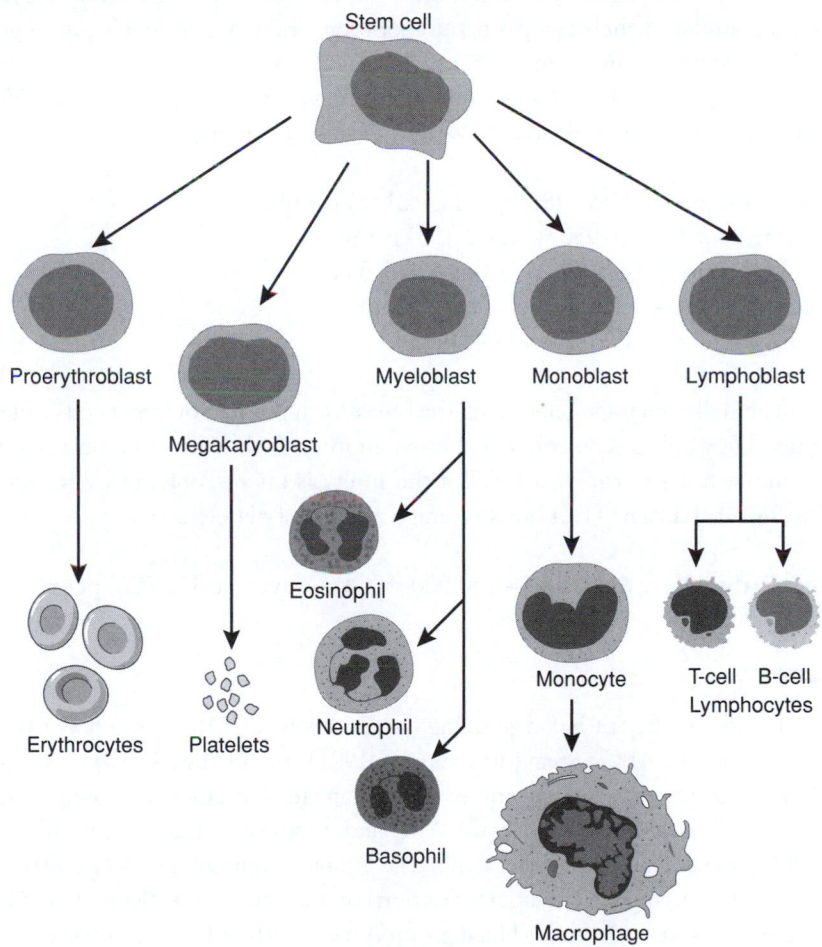

FIGURE 2.1 Blood cells derived from bone marrow stem cells.

Red cells are biconcave discs that give blood its red colour. They carry **haemoglobin (Hb)** which accounts for about 33% of the cell weight. Haemoglobin binds the respiratory gases oxygen and carbon dioxide (see Chapter 4). Like all blood cells, erythrocytes develop in bone marrow, but as mature cells they have no nucleus and therefore their survival in circulation is limited to about 120 days. They are continually being replaced by new ones from the bone marrow. The normal average number of red blood cells varies between the sexes:

- male RBC count = 5.1–5.8 (average 5.4) million per μl
- female RBC count = 4.3–5.2 (average 4.8) million per μl.

White cells last longer, and their role is to fight infection: part of the body's defence strategy. Several kinds of WBCs exist: **lymphocytes**, which use various mechanisms to kill invading organisms (foreign organisms are known as antigens, i.e. the word antigen means anything that provokes an immune reaction); and monocytes, which are **phagocytic**, i.e. they engulf and destroy antigens. Lymphocytes and monocytes are also known as **agranulocytes** (i.e. there are no granules in their cytoplasm). In addition, there are various types of **granulocytes** (i.e. they do have granules in their cytoplasm). The types are neutrophils, eosinophils and basophils, and these release important chemicals as part of the defensive role. The normal average number of white blood cells varies between the different types:

- lymphocyte count = 1000–4800 (average 2185) per μl
- monocyte count = 200–950 (average 456) per μl
- neutrophil count = 1800–7300 (average 4150) per μl
- eosinophil count = 0–700 (average 165) per μl
- basophil count = 0–200 (average 44) per μl.

Platelets are actually cell fragments, being the breakdown product of larger cells called **megakaryocytes**. They help to control blood loss when injury to blood vessels occurs, either by blocking minute holes in the vessel wall if the injury is microscopic, or by triggering the blood-clotting mechanism. The normal average number of platelets is:

- platelets (thrombocytes) count = 150,000–500,000 (average 350,000) per μl.

Blood groups

There are at least 14 different blood grouping systems known. Of these, the only two used in clinical practice are the ABO system (discovered in 1901) and the rhesus (Rh) system (discovered in 1940). The other systems are ignored because any reaction they cause is mild and transient. However, the reactions caused by the ABO and rhesus systems are potentially fatal.

The ABO system is based on the fact that red cells have a combination of two **antigens** (i.e. proteins capable of provoking an immune reaction) on their surface: **antigens A** and **B**. If the red cells have only antigen A, this is **blood group A**; cells with only antigen B produce **blood group B**; antigens A and B together create **blood group AB**, and no A or B antigen present is **blood group O**. **Antibodies** are present in the plasma (antibodies are immune proteins that react with antigens), but clearly individuals cannot have the antibodies that react with their own antigen; instead, they have antibodies that react with *other* antigens (see Table 2.1).

The rhesus system involves another RBC surface antigen called the **D-factor** (the **rhesus factor**). If the D-factor is present, the blood is **rhesus (Rh) positive**, and the plasma has no **anti-D antibody**. If the D-factor is absent, the blood is **rhesus (Rh) negative**, and the plasma has got **anti-D antibody**. Any of the four ABO groups can be either Rh positive or Rh negative, i.e. there are eight blood groups in all. In all these cases the plasma antigens cannot react with their own red cells, but **transfusion** of blood from one person to another creates the conditions that could cause a reaction, and this must be avoided. **Haemolysis** (haemo = blood; lysis = break down) is one type of reaction where red cells are destroyed, **haemoglobin** is released and the patient can suffer severe **anaemia** with **jaundice**. **Agglutination** is another type of reaction where red cells clump together in large lumps that can block smaller vessels, such as the arterioles within the kidneys, causing kidney failure. These happen due to **mismatched** transfusions, and careful checking is required to prevent this (Figure 2.2).

TABLE 2.1 Blood groups and antigens

Blood group	Antigen on RBC	Antibodies in plasma
A	A	Anti-B (reacts with B antigen)
B	B	Anti-A (reacts with A antigen)
AB	A + B	No antibodies
O	No antigens	Anti-A + anti-B (reacts with both)

FIGURE 2.2 The ABO blood groups compatibility grid. The donor's red cells (A and B antigens) are matched with the recipient's plasma (anti-A and anti-B antibodies) to identify any dangerous reaction (×) or no reaction (✓). Recipient AB can take blood from any group (universal recipient) and donor O can give blood to any group (universal donor) provided the rhesus factor (not shown) is compatible.

Blood plasma

Of the nine transported substances listed in the introduction, oxygen and carbon dioxide are mostly carried by the haemoglobin of the RBCs. All the remaining substances are carried in the **plasma**: some dissolved and some in suspension. Plasma consists of 92% water with 7% plasma proteins and 1% dissolved solutes. The end products of digestion and inhaled oxygen are transported to the tissues, while the waste products and carbon dioxide are carried to the excretory organs for elimination. Whole proteins, called **plasma proteins**, remain in the blood. **Albumin** is the most common protein in plasma (60% of all the proteins present) with **globulins** (which include antibodies) being the next most common (35%). The remaining 5% includes the clotting factor **fibrinogen**, various hormones and others.

Plasma proteins have many functions, for example, as **antibodies** (produced by lymphocytes and known as **immunoglobulins**, or Ig), which help to fight infections, and albumin, which aids the return of tissue fluid to the plasma. Clotting factors, which are also proteins, are essential for blood clot formation to prevent bleeding.

Heart physiology

The heart is a muscular pump divided vertically by a wall, the **septum**, into separate left and right sides (Figure 2.3) (Vickers 1999a). Each side has a smaller upper chamber, the **atrium** (plural **atria**), and a larger lower chamber, the **ventricle**. Valves exist between the atria and ventricles, the **atrioventricular (AV)** valves, which close to prevent backflow of blood during heart (ventricular) contraction. These are the **bicuspid** (bi = two, cuspid = cusps or flaps) valve on the left and the **tricuspid** (tri = three) valve on the right. Blood is received into the right atrium from the **vena cavae**, the major veins returning blood from

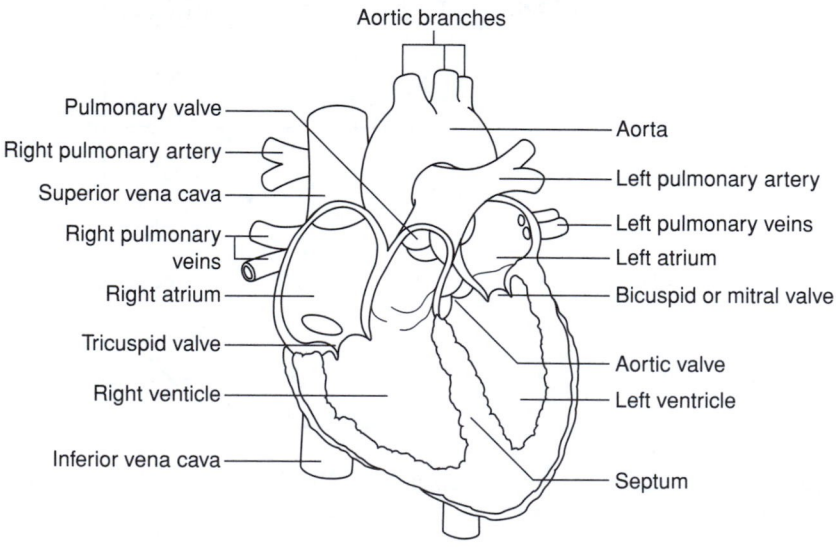

FIGURE 2.3   Cross-section through the heart (viewed anteriorly).

the body to the right side of the heart. On the left side, the atrium receives blood from the **pulmonary veins** returning blood from the lungs. From both the atria, blood passes through the AV valves and fills the ventricles. Contraction of these ventricles pushes blood through **semi-lunar valves**, which prevent backflow to the ventricles: the **aortic valve** on the left and **pulmonary valve** on the right. The **aorta** is the main artery taking blood from the left side of the heart for distribution around the body.

The first branches of the aorta are the **coronary arteries**, which supply the heart wall itself with blood. Partial or complete blockage of these arteries deprives the myocardium of blood, leading to angina or myocardial infarction (both forms of heart attack). The **pulmonary artery** carries blood from the right side of the heart to the lungs for oxygenation. The result is a double circulation, i.e. a **systemic** circulation from the left side of the heart to the tissues and back to the right heart, and a **pulmonary** circulation from the right side of the heart to the lungs and back to the left heart (Figure 2.4). The systemic circulation is much larger, involving all the systems of the body, and is sustained at a high pressure of blood. The much smaller pulmonary system operates at lower pressures because blood has only to pass from the heart to the lungs and back, entirely within the chest.

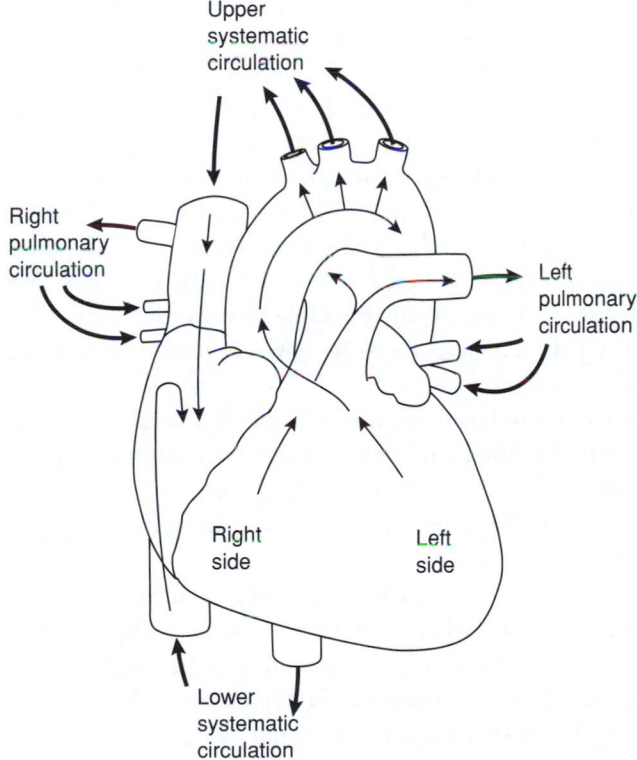

FIGURE 2.4   Double circulation of the blood from the heart. The systemic circulation passes from the aorta to the upper and lower parts of the body. The pulmonary circulation passes from the pulmonary arteries to the left and right lungs.

The heart wall consists of a muscle layer, the **myocardium**, an inner smooth lining of **epithelium**, called the **endocardium**, and an outer membrane, called the **pericardium**. The myocardium has specialised cells that are linked by branches, and this allows them to contract simultaneously, acting as a single unit, known as a **functional syncytium**. Myocardial cells contract during stimulation by nerve impulses that pass through the heart from the **sinoatrial (SA)** node, the pacemaker of the heart. The SA node is capable of triggering regular cardiac contractions without outside control (called an *inherent power of rhythmic contraction*). Despite this, the SA node does have external regulation by the **autonomic nervous system (ANS)**, which maintains the heart rate at an average level (about 72 beats per minute). The **sympathetic** component of the ANS increases the heart rate, whereas the **parasympathetic** component (via the **vagus nerve**) decreases the heart rate (Vickers 1999b). They work together to stabilise the heart rate, but at the same time the presence of both sympathetic and parasympathetic components allows the heart rate to be increased or decreased as the tissues demand for blood changes. During activity, limb muscles in particular force an increase in heart rate to supply more blood, and the sympathetic component will be dominant. At rest, especially during sleep, the parasympathetic component dominates to slow the heart rate down.

The **cardiac cycle** (Vickers 1999c) is the sequence of events the heart goes through from one beat to the next. Contraction of the ventricles is **systole**, when blood is pushed out of both sides of the heart, followed by ventricular relaxation, or **diastole**, the ventricular refilling phase. These events are linked to the electrical conduction activity that starts at the SA node and passes through the myocardium. As it crosses the **atria**, they contract and push some blood downwards to top up the ventricles. The impulse arrives at the level of the AV valves, but it does not progress through the muscle any further downwards beyond this point. At this level, the next node, the **AV node**, comes in to play. This node picks up the impulse and transmits it down the ventricular septum via conduction tissue called the **bundle of His**, which divides into the left and right **bundle branches**. From the lower end of the septum, the impulse passes via the **Purkinje fibres** at the end of the bundle branches to the ventricular muscle. The impulse passes upwards across the ventricles, causing them to contract (Figure 2.5).

So the heart beats in two directions, the atria contract downwards forcing blood downwards into the ventricles, then the ventricles contract upwards forcing blood upwards towards the ventricular escape valves (aortic and pulmonary valves). This creates a repeated cycle: down–up, down–up, down–up, and so on. Each down (atrial contraction) is followed by an up (ventricular contraction).

Regulation of the heart is maintained by the **cardiac centre**, one of the *vital centres* in a part of the brain called the **medulla** within the **brain stem**. If any injury or disorder were to affect the cardiac centre, the heart would stop beating immediately.

The **cardiac output (CO)** is the **heart rate (HR)** multiplied by the **stroke volume (SV)**, i.e. $CO = HR \times SV$. This formula is the volume of blood pumped out of a single ventricle in 1 minute. Each time a ventricle contracts, about 70 ml of blood is pushed into the arteries (the stroke volume). The ventricles contract on average 72 times per minute (the heart rate); so the cardiac output per ventricle is 70 ml multiplied by 72 beats per minute, i.e. 5040 ml per minute. The cardiac output per ventricle is just over 5000 ml (5 litres).

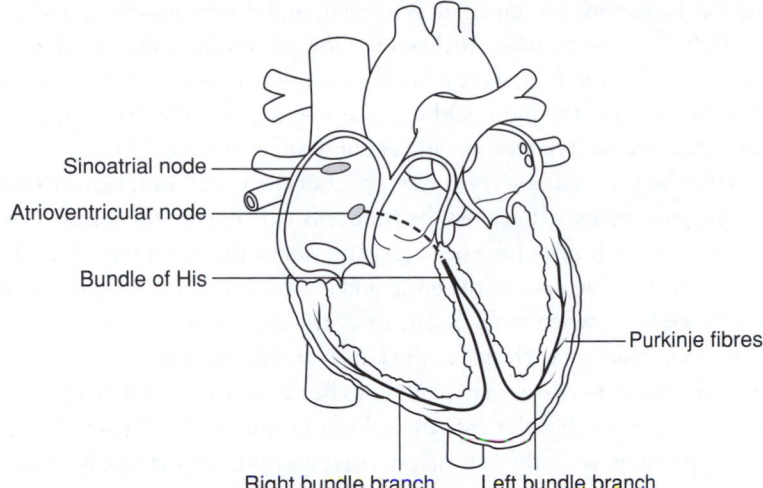

FIGURE 2.5 The cardiac conduction system. Impulses arise from the sinoatrial node and pass across the atria to the atrioventricular node. From here impulses pass down from the bundle of His (also called the atrioventricular bundle) and into the left bundle branch and right bundle branch. The Purkinje fibres are wide terminal branch cells that distribute the impulses to the myocardial cells.

Considering the total blood volume in circulation is on average about 5000 ml, this means that each ventricle pushes out the entire blood volume every minute, and does this for 70+ years. This makes the heart one of the best pumps ever to have evolved, but it also makes it very difficult to build an artificial replacement heart.

Observations of the pulse, apex beat, electrocardiogram and heart sounds

The pulse rate and strength

The **pulse** is caused by pressure exerted on the arterial wall causing expansion of the vessel for the brief moment that the wave of pressure passes. The pressure wave is caused by contraction of the ventricles on the left side of the heart forcing blood into the systemic arteries. The artery swells, stretching the muscular wall as the wave of blood from the heart passes by, then contracts back due to the muscular wall returning to its former state. The heart beats about 72 times per minute at rest, and so this becomes the average adult pulse rate. *All* arteries demonstrate a pulse, but they are not all accessible for observation. For clinical purposes, the **radial** pulse is mostly used. This is found on the inner aspect of the wrist, on the thumb (= radial) side of a ridge (created by a tendon) that runs almost centrally down the distal end of the arm into the wrist. Pulses are normally taken by the observer's middle three fingers, not the thumb, to avoid the observer from feeling their own pulse which is more prominent in the thumb. Taking the radial pulse is acceptable because it is non-invasive, not embarrassing for the patient (as some pulses may be) and for the most part accurate. It only loses accuracy when the blood pressure drops too low, when there are circulatory constrictions placed around the arm (e.g. during blood pressure cuff inflation), or if the arm is too obese to allow palpation of the pulse. Other pulse sites are possible, but they are associated with difficulties and are reserved for specific circumstances (Figure 2.6).

The **brachial** pulse occurs along the inner aspect of the upper arm, beneath the brachial muscle, with the pulse being felt against the **humerus** (the upper arm bone). The **temporal** pulse can be found on each side of the head just anterior to the upper margin of the ear. The **femoral** pulse is about midway across the groin and is used sometimes as a pulse check during cardiac arrest procedures, when embarrassment of the patient is not an issue. The **carotid** pulse lies in the soft tissues on each side of the larynx and is also used in cardiac arrest. Using this pulse on conscious patients, as may sometimes be necessary if the radial pulse is obscure, requires an explanation so that the patient will not be concerned. This pulse must be felt with only gentle pressure, since the carotid artery is part of the blood supply to the brain and must not be obstructed.

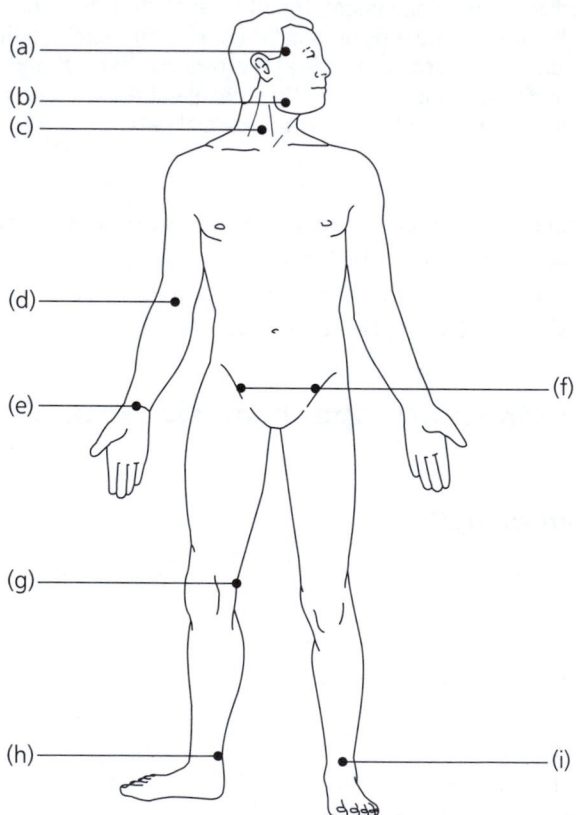

FIGURE 2.6 Arterial pulse sites on the body. (a) temporal; (b) facial (on jaw); (c) common carotid; (d) brachial; (e) radial (thumb side, the usual pulse for clinical practice); (f) right and left femoral; (g) popliteal (behind the knee); (h) posterior tibial; (i) dorsalis pedis (see Figure 2.7 for (h) and (i)).

(a)   (b)

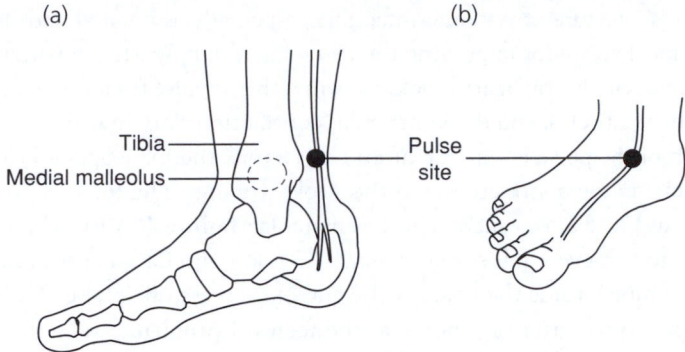

Figure 2.7 Pedal (foot) pulses. (a) post-tibial artery (immediately behind the medial malleolus on the tibia); (b) dorsalis pedis (on the top of the foot midway between the lateral and medial malleolli).

The **pedal** (= foot) pulses, mainly the **posterior tibial** and the **dorsalis pedis** (Figure 2.7), are important for assessing the blood supply to the leg and foot and should be used in any limb vascular disease or during the management of all lower limb injuries and during surgery. They are also essential after any application of potentially restrictive treatments, such as support bandages or splintage material, especially if limb swelling is still likely. Pedal pulses and the radial pulse are considered to be peripheral pulses, i.e. they are on the extremities of the body. The femoral and carotid pulses are considered to be central pulses (i.e. nearer to, and in direct line with, the heart). In everyday clinical use, peripheral pulses are excellent, but they tend to diminish and even disappear when the cardiac output is low (e.g. in shock and cardiac arrest), and central pulses are then more useful.

The pulse rate is normally elevated during exercise and hard physical labour, and a fast rate is also part of the response to fear and excitement. **Tachycardia** is a fast pulse rate, e.g. 100 beats per minute or more, and **bradycardia** is a slow rate, usually below 50 beats per minute. The normal maximum heart rate is about 180 beats per minute, i.e. the maximum above which normal filling of the heart cannot take place. At this rate the entire cardiac cycle lasts just 0.33 seconds. The differences in the systolic and diastolic phases at heart rates of 67 and 180 beats per minute (bpm) are shown in Table 2.2.

To achieve adequate ventricular filling during diastole requires a minimum diastolic phase of about 0.12 seconds, so heart rates above 180 beats per minute would reduce the diastolic phase below this minimum, and the cardiac output would be reduced and the heart is then functioning below optimum efficiency.

Table 2.2 Differences in the systolic and diastolic phases at heart rates of 67 bpm and 180 bpm

	Heart rate 67 bpm	*Heart rate 180 bpm*
Systole	0.35 seconds	0.2 seconds
Diastole	0.58 seconds	0.13 seconds

Tachycardia is a feature of systemic infections, especially associated with fever, and is a compensatory mechanism for improving the tissue blood supply when a patient is in shock. Bradycardia can occur during **heart block**, i.e. when the impulse from the SA node does not always reach the ventricles, and the ventricular contraction rate slows down.

The strength of the pulse is dependent on two factors: the force applied to the blood by the left ventricle during contraction and the stroke volume. The force of contraction can vary normally and in diseases such as **left ventricular failure (LVF)**, where the myocardium is unable to achieve a full stroke volume (Gordon and Child 2000a, 2000b). Excess blood may be retained inside the heart at the end of each systolic phase. This can result in a reduced output to the arteries (known as the **forward problem**) and a backlog of blood unable to enter the ventricles because they are partly filled already and can only accept a limited blood volume from the veins (known as the **backward problem**). The stroke volume will decline in **hypovolaemic shock** (hypo = below normal, vol = volume, aemic = blood), where the blood volume in circulation is less than normal as a result of bleeding or burns. A weak, rapid pulse is characteristic of shock: weak due to a low stroke volume, and rapid because the heart tries to compensate by pumping faster, which is part of the sympathetic response. **Thyrotoxicosis** (raised blood levels of **thyroxin**) and heart block can increase the force of contraction. **Palpitations** are heart beats felt by the patient on the chest wall. They may be associated with arrhythmias but are often normal, being caused by extreme exercise or occasional extra beats.

Apex beat

The radial pulse rate taken at the wrist is a record of the number of times the left ventricle contracts per minute. So another way to measure this would be to listen through the chest wall, via a stethoscope, to the heart itself, counting the heart sounds per minute. It is important to listen to the ventricle (usually the left) at the outermost and lowest point of the heart (the apex of the heart); this is known as the **apex beat**. The radial pulse and heart (apex beat) sounds should be equal in number, but sometimes the ventricular contraction is so weak (i.e. low cardiac output) that the force is insufficient to create a pulse at the wrist (see peripheral pulses above). The difference between the radial and apex beats can be measured by two nurses working together. One takes the radial pulse in the usual way while the other listens to the apex beat. This is found by placing the diaphragm of a stethoscope over the space between the left fifth and sixth ribs close to the **midclavicular line**, an imaginary line drawn down the chest from a point midway along the left clavicle. Using the same watch and counting over the same 60 seconds, both the radial and the apex beats are recorded. Any deficit may show an apex beat higher than the radial beat, and subtracting the later from the former the deficit can be calculated. In an example of an apex beat of 84 and a radial pulse of 74 the difference is 10 beats, i.e. the ventricles have had ten contractions during that minute that were not strong enough to create a radial pulse. Sometimes the radial count is recorded as higher than the apex beat, but this is not possible since the radial pulse depends on ventricular contractions. Such a result is clearly an error and the observation should be repeated.

The electrocardiogram (ECG)

Willem Einthoven (1860–1927), a Dutch physiologist, was awarded the 1924 Nobel Prize in Physiology or Medicine for pioneering **electrocardiography**. In 1909, Augustus Waller demonstrated to the Royal Society in London the recording of an **electrocardiogram** (ECG) from a pet dog called Jimmie (Levick 2010). This procedure is an important, fast, accurate, non-invasive means of diagnosis of cardiac disease that can be carried out almost anywhere. The ECG records the electrical activity of the heart muscle as it occurs at skin level having passed through the extracellular fluid between the heart and the body surface. Electrical activity (called **depolarisation**) at the SA and AV nodes is too small to create recordable changes at the skin surface, but the electrical activity within the larger myocardial muscle bulk can be recorded throughout repeated heart cycles. The tracing represents different views of the heart, similar to seeing different aspects of the same object when viewed from varying angles. The leads attached to the patient provide these different views of the heart (Figure 2.8).

The recording is a measure of the electrical difference between one electrode and another (i.e. bipolar = two leads used) in leads I, II, III, aVR, aVL and aVF (Figure 2.8). The V leads use a free-moving electrode placed at specific sites on the chest wall that measure the electrical activity at each site (i.e. unipolar = one roving lead). The main direction of electrical flow through the heart, called the **electrical axis**, runs down the heart from the SA node to the ventricles. This varies between individuals in positions between the direction of leads I and aVF. The chest leads, therefore, are snapshots of this axis seen differently from these various views. The baseline of the tracing is **isoelectric**, i.e. zero voltage. Any deflection above this line indicates a view looking in the direction of the axis, i.e. positive (+), and a deflection below the baseline indicates a view that is more than 90° away from the axis, i.e.

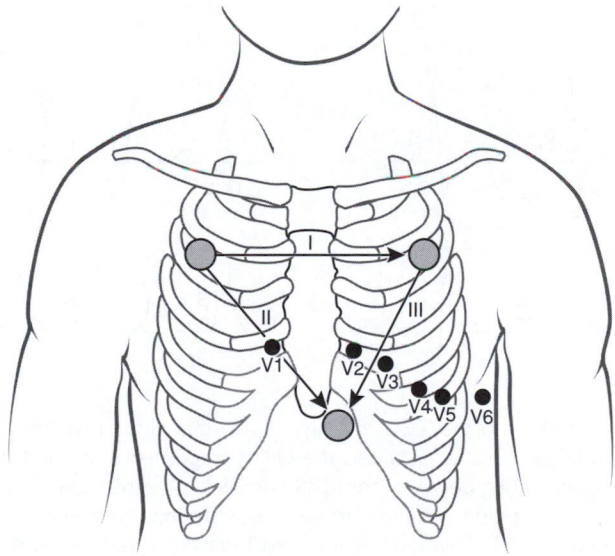

Figure 2.8   ECG lead positions I, II, III and V1 to V6.

negative (–). The normal pattern of activity is known and abnormalities of the tracing can be detected and identified as specific heart disorders (Figure 2.9).

Atrial depolarisation (normally accompanied by atrial contraction) is recorded on the ECG as the P wave, followed by the PQ interval, an isoelectric event as the impulse passes down the bundle of His. The QRS complex is the depolarisation event of the ventricles (ventricular contraction, or systole), followed by ventricular repolarisation, identified as the T wave (ventricular relaxation) (Vickers 1999b). **Sinus rhythm** is the term given to a normal ECG pattern. **Arrhythmias** are deviations of the ECG pattern seen in various cardiac disorders and are used to aid the diagnosis, e.g. **ectopic beats**, which are extra systoles generated within the damaged ventricular myocardium after a myocardial infarction (Figure 2.9) (Hatchett *et al.* 1999).

Heart sounds

Auscultation (listening through a **stethoscope**) has traditionally been part of the doctor's examination of the patient, but now specialist cardiac nurses may train to observe for

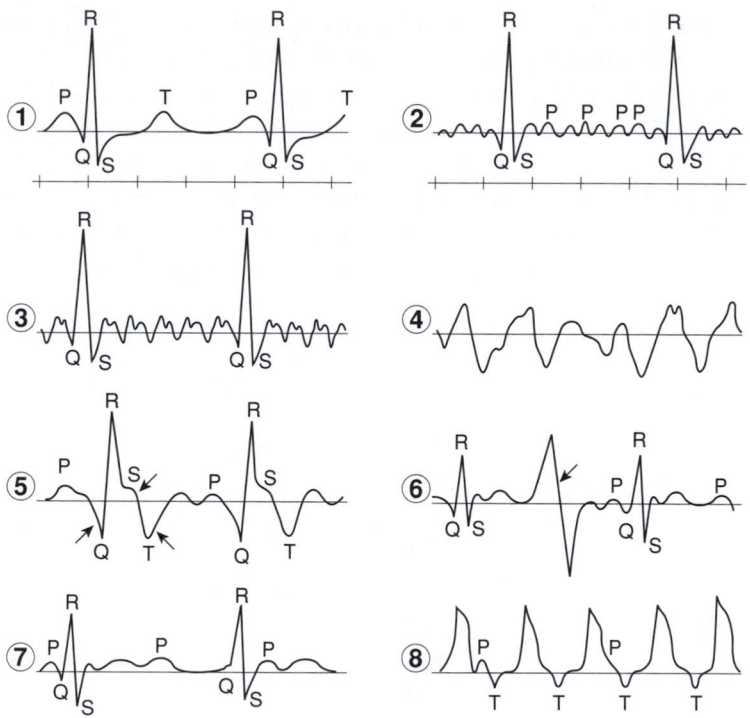

FIGURE 2.9   Normal and abnormal ECG tracings. 1, Normal sinus rhythm; 2, atrial fibrillation with multiple P waves between the QRS complexes; 3, atrial flutter with the saw-tooth appearance between the QRS complex; 4, ventricular fibrillation, causes no cardiac output and requires urgent resuscitation; 5, myocardial infarction with large Q waves, ST elevation and inverted T waves; 6, ventricular extrasystole (ectopic beat); 7, heart block with P waves occurring at any point; 8, ventricular tachycardia with closer packed QRS complexes.

normal and abnormal heart sounds, and their identification is important. The closure (*not* opening) of the heart valves causes normal heart sounds as the valve cusps vibrate. Several heart sounds are recognised: the first (said to sound similar to 'lubb . . .') is the closure of the AV valves (tri- and bicuspid valves), and the second (said to sound similar to 'dubb . . .') is the closure of the semi-lunar valves (aortic and pulmonary). If the aortic valve closes just before the pulmonary valve, the second sound can be split into two sounds, as is common in healthy young people during inspiration. Breathing in causes increased filling of the right ventricle and therefore a raised right ventricular stroke volume. This takes longer to eject during systole and the pulmonary valve closure is delayed. A third sound caused by the entry of blood into the relaxed ventricles at the start of diastole is also common in young people. A fourth sound is audible just before the first and is due to the atrial systole.

Valvular disorders create turbulence in the blood flow through the valve, and this disturbed flow causes extra sounds known as **murmurs**. **Stenosis** is a narrowing of the valve openings because the flaps will not part sufficiently to allow all the blood through. **Incompetence** occurs when a valve will not close properly and it allows backflow of blood, i.e. the valve is *leaky*. Since there are four valves and each is capable of either stenosis or incompetence, a total of eight disorders is possible, resulting in eight murmurs within the heart. But not all murmurs are due to disease. In young people, sometimes during pregnancy or in strenuous exercise, a **benign murmur** can occasionally be heard due to turbulence of the blood leaving the heart, and this is not a problem.

The effects of cardiovascular drugs

Various cardiovascular drugs affect the pulse rate and the blood pressure, and knowledge of this is necessary when evaluating a patient's results. **Positive inotropic drugs** (e.g. the **cardiac glycosides**, especially **digoxin**, and the **phosphodiesterase inhibitors**, such as **milrinone**) increase the force of contraction and are therefore used in heart failure. Digoxin particularly causes slowing of the heart rate, and care must be taken not to allow the pulse rate to drop below 60 beats per minute. Bradycardia is a sign of **digoxin toxicity**, and nurses should check the patient's pulse rate before administration of this drug. In addition, patients taking this drug, especially the elderly, should be observed for confusion, nausea and **coupled beats**, i.e. two pulse beats together followed by a pause.

Beta-blocking drugs, such as **propranolol**, reduce the sympathetic stimulation of the heart and therefore slow the heart rate. These are used to treat angina, i.e. chest pain caused by restricted blood flow down the coronary arteries as a result of arterial disease. By slowing the heart rate, the myocardium needs less blood, and this puts less demand on the coronary artery supply, and this reduces the chest pain.

Antiarrhythmic drugs, e.g. **verapamil** and **lidocaine** (**lignocaine**) hydrochloride, suppress the incidence and intensity of cardiac arrhythmias. This is important because both the incidence and intensity of arrhythmias can escalate into potentially fatal consequences, notably cardiac arrest. Specific drugs are used to suppress **supraventricular** (= above the ventricles, i.e. the atria) or **ventricular** arrhythmias.

The pulse in children

The cardiovascular system in children must cope with its own growth while catering for increased demands on it as a result of growth in all other parts of the body. In children the heart rate range falls gradually from 110–160 beats per minute at less than 1 year of age to 60–100 at more than 12 years of age. Breathing causes more pronounced changes in the heart rate in children than in adults, a difference of up to 30 beats per minute, slowing down during inspiration and accelerating during expiration.

It may be recommended in some paediatric units for the nurse to use the brachial or temporal pulse with the younger child, as this may be easier to find in a less than co-operative child, and will therefore be more accurate. For the older child, when co-operation by the child is achieved, the radial pulse can be used. Using the carotid pulse in children is not justified since it carries specific risks regarding the blood supply to the brain, and should not therefore be used in children of any age.

Rapid heart rates can be caused by heart failure, a complication of **congenital heart defects**. These are distortions of the heart anatomy that the child is born with. **Atrial** or **ventricular septal defects** (**ASDs** or **VSDs**, the so-called hole in the heart) abnormally allow blood to pass from one side of the heart to the other. If blood passes from the right ventricle to the left ventricle through a VSD, deoxygenated blood (i.e. lacking oxygen) fails to go to the lungs for oxygenation from the right ventricle and is pumped by the left ventricle back to the body again. Efforts by the heart to improve the oxygen supply to the body result in an increase in the cardiac output, usually by a rise in the heart rate. Ultimately, if this is not corrected, the heart can enlarge and fail.

Key points

- The total blood volume in circulation is 5000 ml.
- The blood cells are erythrocytes (red blood cells), leucocytes (white blood cells) and thrombocytes (platelets).
- Blood group A has antigen A on the RBCs and anti-B antibodies in the plasma. Similarly, blood group B has antigen B with anti-A antibodies; blood group AB has antigens A and B and no anti-A or anti-B antibodies, and blood group O has no A or B antigen and anti-A and anti-B antibodies.
- The rhesus factor (D-factor) is present in rhesus (Rh) positive, the plasma has no anti-D antibody. The D-factor is absent in rhesus (Rh) negative, the plasma has anti-D antibody.
- The heart wall has a muscular myocardium, an inner endocardium, and an outer pericardium.
- The sinoatrial (SA) node can trigger cardiac contractions with external regulation by the sympathetic nervous system (increases the heart rate) and the parasympathetic nervous system (vagus nerve, decreases the heart rate).
- The cardiac cycle consists of systole (ventricular contraction) followed by diastole (ventricular relaxation).
- Electrical conduction starts at the SA node and passes through the atrial myocardium,

which contracts; the AV node picks up the impulse and transmits it down the ventricular septum via the bundle of His, and then the left and right bundle branches to the Purkinje fibres in the ventricular muscle, which then contracts.

- For clinical purposes the radial pulse is mostly used.
- The normal adult pulse rate is 65–72 beats per minute.
- Tachycardia is a fast pulse rate and bradycardia is a slow rate.
- The apex beat is found on the left outermost and lowest point of the heart: the space between the left fifth and sixth ribs close to the midclavicular line.
- A weak rapid pulse is characteristic of shock.
- A cause of cardiogenic shock is myocardial infarction (MI); an area of dead or dying myocardium (the infarct) results from occlusion of the coronary arteries.
- The ECG P wave occurs with depolarisation of the atria (atrial contraction), followed by the PQ interval as the impulse disappears down the bundle of His; the QRS complex is depolarisation of the ventricles (ventricular contraction, or systole) followed by ventricular repolarisation, the T wave (ventricular relaxation).
- Sinus rhythm is a normal ECG pattern; arrhythmias are abnormal deviations from the ECG pattern.
- Valvular disorders create turbulence in the blood flow through the valve causing extra sounds (murmurs), e.g. stenosis, a narrowing of the valve opening, or incompetence, when a valve will not close properly.
- Bradycardia, confusion, nausea and coupled beats are signs of digoxin toxicity, and nurses should check the patient's pulse before administration of this drug.
- The heart rate falls in children from 110–160 per minute below 1 year of age to 60–100 per minute over 12 years old.
- The brachial or temporal pulse should normally be used for younger children and the radial pulse should be used for older children; the carotid pulse should not be used in children.

References

Gordon K. and Child A. (2000a) Systems and diseases: the heart, part 9: heart failure 1. *Nursing Times*, **96**(12): 53–56.

Gordon K. and Child A. (2000b) Systems and diseases: the heart, part 10: heart failure 2. *Nursing Times*, **96**(16): 49–52.

Hatchett R., Arundale K. and Francis-Reme L. (1999) Systems and diseases: the heart, part four: basic cardiac arrhythmias. *Nursing Times*, **95**(43): 44–47.

Levick J.R. (2010) *An Introduction to Cardiovascular Physiology*, 5th edition. Oxford University Press, New York.

Vickers J. (1999a) Systems and diseases: the heart, part one: anatomy and physiology. *Nursing Times*, **95**(30): 42–45.

Vickers J. (1999b) Systems and diseases: the heart, part two: anatomy and physiology. *Nursing Times*, **95**(34): 46–49.

Vickers J. (1999c) Systems and diseases: the heart, part three: anatomy and physiology. *Nursing Times*, **95**(39): 46–49.

Chapter 3 Cardiovascular observations (II)

Blood pressure

- Introduction
- The physiology of blood pressure
- Observations of blood pressure
- Drugs affecting blood pressure
- Blood pressure in children
- Key points
- References

Introduction

One of the problems of adopting an upright posture is the fact that the brain is then placed somewhat higher than the heart. This then requires the heart to sustain sufficient pressure of blood to supply the brain *uphill*, i.e. *against* gravity. Failure to do this would starve the brain of the vital glucose and oxygen it needs for consciousness and mental function. However, blood pressure is fundamental to the perfusion of blood through *all* the body tissues. Good examples are the kidneys, which must have adequate blood pressure to maintain filtration of urine, the lungs, which need a constant flow of blood for gas exchange, and the digestive system, which has a blood flow to collect nutrients from the diet. Any transport system must move, and movement of a fluid requires pressure. Blood pressure is an index of some of the most fundamental physiological processes in the body, and an understanding of arterial blood pressure and its measurement is essential for the accurate determination of physiological processes and disturbances.

The physiology of blood pressure

The systemic arterial **blood pressure (BP)** is caused *partly* by the contraction of the left ventricle. During **systole** (= ventricular contraction), the left ventricular myocardium pushes the **stroke volume (SV)** of blood into the aorta, and this surge of blood causes the aorta to stretch wider. The stroke volume, the amount of blood ejected with each ventricular contraction, is about 70 ml of blood per ventricle. The wave of high pressure generated continues through the arterial system, causing the **systolic pressure** (**SP**), having an average peak of about 120 mmHg (millimetres of mercury) in the major systemic arteries in adults. This pressure falls as blood is distributed through the remaining arterial system and capillary bed, reaching its lowest at close to 0 mmHg in the venous return to the heart (Figure 3.1).

During **diastole**, the left ventricle is relaxing and filling with blood. There is no output to the aorta, and this creates a lower pressure in the systemic arteries, a **diastolic pressure** (**DP**) of about 80–90 mmHg. The human BP in the major systemic arteries is therefore recorded as 120 over 90 mmHg, i.e. alternating between the systolic and diastolic pressures. But if the left ventricle has no output during diastole, the diastolic pressure should theoretically fall to zero. Zero pressure would mean that blood flow has stopped, and this would be disastrous for the many tissues, especially the brain, which demands a constant blood supply (for oxygen and glucose). Without this supply the brain becomes unconscious (i.e. fainting). The heart goes through about 72 systoles and diastoles per minute, so at a theoretical systemic blood pressure of 120 over 0 mmHg, the person would faint 72 times per minute. Clearly this is not the case; therefore, diastolic pressure must be maintained sufficiently to supply the brain (and all the other tissues) during this period of zero cardiac output. To see how this is achieved, go back to the point where the surge of blood causes the aorta to stretch wider. What stretches during systole must recoil during diastole, and it is this aortic recoil that continues to push blood onward to the tissues while the heart relaxes and refills (Figure 3.2). The aorta is effectively a *diastolic pump*, keeping the pressure up during this time. The same occurs with the pulmonary artery from the right side of the heart, where pulmonary recoil continues to push blood through the lungs during right ventricular diastole. However, since

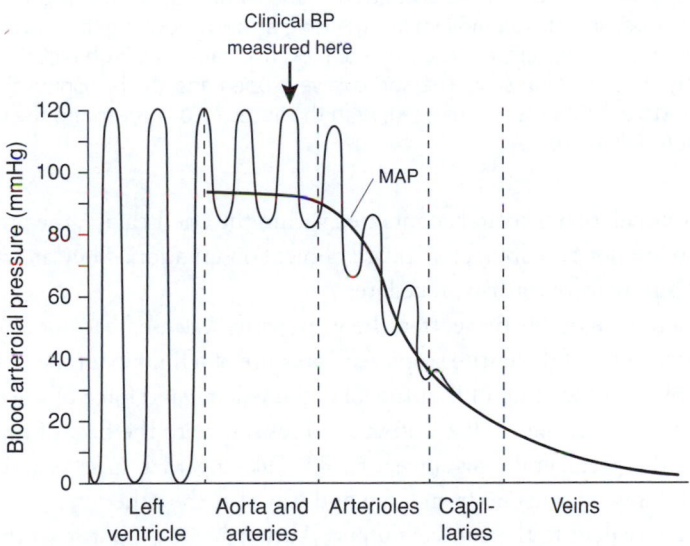

FIGURE 3.1 Blood pressure values through the arterial system. The left ventricle drops to 0 mmHg during diastole and the arterial diastolic pressure is maintained at about 80 mmHg in the arteries. Through the arterioles the mean arterial pressure (MAP) and both the systolic and the diastolic pressures drop with closure of the pulse pressure, i.e. a loss of the pulsatile nature of the flow by the capillaries.

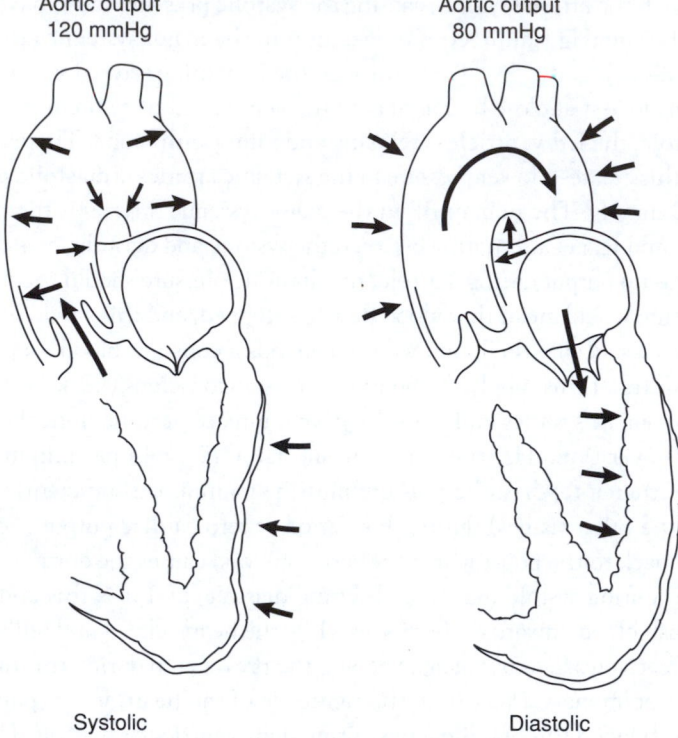

Aortic output
120 mmHg

Aortic output
80 mmHg

Systolic

Diastolic

FIGURE 3.2 The left ventricle and the aorta during the cardiac cycle. The short arrows indicate the direction of wall movement; the long arrows show the direction of blood flow. During systole, ventricular contraction occurs, causing a high blood pressure resulting in aortic expansion. The aortic valve is open and the bicuspid valve is closed. In diastole the events are reversed, with the aortic recoil preventing the blood pressure from falling too low.

the pulmonary circulation is entirely contained within the chest cavity, the pressures within this circulation are not available for standard clinical observation. They are measured only during specialised invasive cardiac procedures.

In the first sentence of this BP section the word *partly* was used because the contraction of the left ventricle is not the entire story. Any pressure of a fluid in a tube is dependent on events taking place at *both* ends of that tube, i.e. the volume and force of the fluid entering the tube at one end (e.g. the cardiac output) and resistance to the flow of that fluid at the other end (e.g. the **peripheral resistance**, or **PR**). Take a garden hose as an example. The water enters the hose at one end from a tap and leaves at the other end. The output from the tap is the equivalent to the cardiac output. Although the output from the hose at the other end is sufficient to reach the nearby plants, those at the back of the flower bed may need a higher pressure to enable the water to reach them. This could be achieved by increasing the output from the tap, but it would probably be easier to place a thumb over the end to narrow the opening and therefore increase the water pressure inside the tube. Water leaving the narrower opening does so at a higher pressure and therefore travels further. Removal of the thumb causes the water pressure to drop and therefore the jet of water returns to normal. In our garden hose the thumb acts as a peripheral resistance, and in the body the arterial peripheral resistance is achieved first by the reduction in size of the **arterioles** into a network of smaller vessels, and then by the **vasoconstriction** or **vasodilation** that these smaller arterioles can achieve. In vasodilation, the arteriole lumen widens and the peripheral resistance is decreased (like the thumb removed from the hose end), allowing the blood pressure to fall. In vasoconstriction, the arteriole lumen narrows and the peripheral resistance is increased (like the thumb placed over the hose end), forcing the blood pressure up (Figure 3.3). Involuntary smooth muscle in the arteriole wall makes the changes to the lumen in response to the **sympathetic nervous system**. This system is influenced by the **vasomotor centre (VMC)**, a series of diffuse nuclei in the medulla that has a profound effect on blood pressure (Figure 3.3).

The VMC can initiate variations in the peripheral resistance by adjusting the sympathetic vasoconstrictor tone, the state of constriction of the smooth muscle wall affecting the lumen of the arterioles. Changes are made in this tone in response to fluctuations in the blood pressure, keeping the BP within normal limits for that individual. To do this, the VMC must have feedback on what the pressure is, and this is achieved via **baroreceptors**, pressure-sensitive receptors found in the aortic arch and carotid arteries that directly measure the arterial BP and send this information to the VMC (Figure 3.4).

When the BP is high, increased baroreceptor activity shuts down the VMC (i.e. **inhibition**), causing vasodilation of the arterioles to lower the pressure. When the BP is low, decreased baroreceptor activity causes increased VMC output, which vasoconstricts the

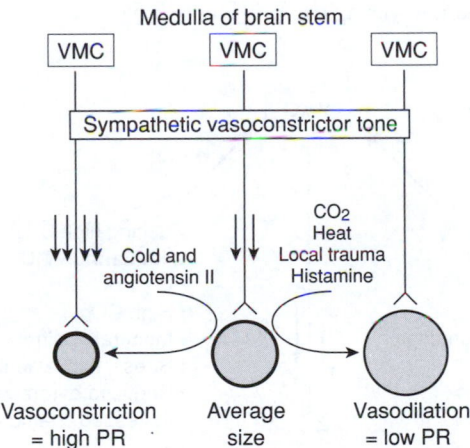

FIGURE 3.3 The vasomotor centre (VMC) and the local factors influencing the peripheral resistance (PR). Vasoconstriction is achieved by increasing the vasoconstrictor tone output from the VMC to the arterioles, or by the local action of cold or angiotensin II, causing the lumen to narrow and raising the PR. Vasodilation is achieved by decreasing the sympathetic vasoconstrictor tone from the VMC or by the local action of heat, trauma, carbon dioxide or histamine, causing the lumen to widen and lowering of the PR. The number of arrows represents the strength of sympathetic stimulation.

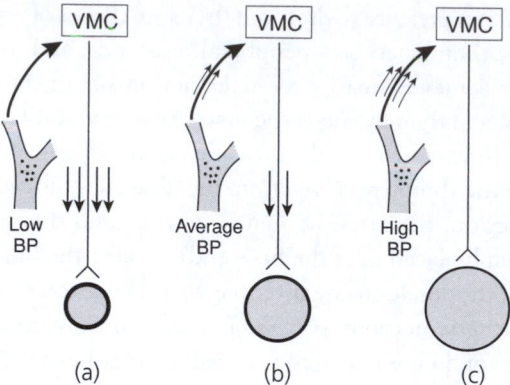

FIGURE 3.4 The effect of the baroreceptors on the VMC. (a) In low blood pressure situations a lack of baroreceptor stimulation allows the VMC to cause vasoconstriction and this raises the blood pressure. (b) Average baroreceptor stimulation allows for normal peripheral resistance. (c) High blood pressure causes considerable baroreceptor stimulation, which inhibits the VMC output and causes vasodilation to lower the blood pressure. The number of arrows in each case represents the degree of stimulation.

arterioles to raise the pressure. The VMC also responds to other factors and adjusts the BP accordingly. A lack of oxygen, an increase in carbon dioxide, mild pain, stress and increased **chemoreceptor** activity all cause more VMC activity and therefore vasoconstriction, raising the BP. Low carbon dioxide, severe pain and emotional shock all cause less VMC activity and therefore vasodilation, lowering the BP (Figure 3.5).

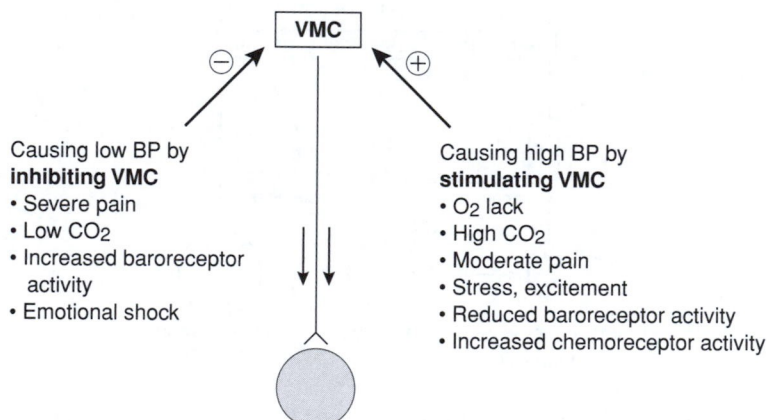

FIGURE 3.5 The factors affecting the VMC. Severe pain, low carbon dioxide, increased baroreceptor stimulation and emotional shock all inhibit the VMC and cause low blood pressure by vasodilation. A lack of oxygen, high carbon dioxide, moderate pain, stress and excitement, reduced baroreceptor stimulation and increased chemoreceptor stimulation all stimulate the VMC causing higher blood pressure by vasoconstriction.

Chemoreceptors detect levels of carbon dioxide in the blood and feed this information back to the brain for blood pressure and respiratory purposes. A sudden drop in the blood pressure is a not uncommon cause of fainting after a sudden emotional shock, such as bad news. Normal BP is maintained by an average vasoconstrictor tone stimulation from the VMC. Local factors influencing the peripheral resistance include cold, causing local vasoconstriction in the affected part, and heat, which will dilate the vessels. **Angiotensin II**, a vasoconstrictive hormone, has much wider effects on increasing the peripheral resistance and therefore also the blood pressure. Angiotensin II is activated under the emergency situation of low blood pressure to the kidneys (Figure 3.6), since blood pressure into the kidneys must be maintained to ensure that filtration continues. The metabolic wastes (metabolites) of muscle activity, such as **carbon dioxide** (see Figure 1.1), and chemical substances associated with **inflammation**, such as **histamine**, cause vasodilation locally. So also does local **trauma** (injury), especially damage to the skin, as seen in **burns**.

Blood pressure can be seen as a *combination* of many effects; the output from the heart (the cardiac output, or CO = heart rate × stroke volume) at the front end of the tube, and the total peripheral resistance (PR) at the distal end of the tube. Thus:

$$BP = CO \times PR \text{ or } (HR \times SV) \times PR$$

Other effects involved include the viscosity (or thickness) of blood, which will vary according to the amount of water obtained from drinking or lost in the urine, and the elasticity of the vessel wall, which will stretch and recoil with the wave of pressure. Reduced elasticity, as seen with increasing age, will resist the pressure wave, which will then remain higher as a result, and if this is a feature throughout the vascular bed, the BP will remain higher than expected.

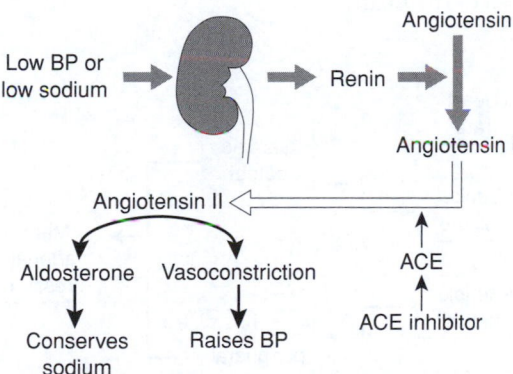

FIGURE 3.6 The renin–angiotensin–aldosterone cycle. Low blood pressure or low blood sodium causes the kidney to release renin. Renin activates angiotensin to angiotensin I, which is then further converted to angiotensin II by angiotensin-converting enzyme (ACE). ACE function can be blocked by ACE inhibitor drugs. Angiotensin II stimulates aldosterone secretion (to conserve sodium) and vasoconstriction (to raise blood pressure), thus correcting the original problem.

The difference between the systolic and diastolic pressures is called the **pulse pressure**, and it is about 30–40 mmHg in the aorta:

pulse pressure = systolic pressure – diastolic pressure, e.g. 120 – 90 = 30 mmHg

The pulse pressure is measured in the larger arteries where standard BP is measured. The normal rapid narrowing and disappearance of the pulse pressure through the smaller arterioles result in a loss of pulsation in the capillary network within the tissues, and therefore blood flows through the tissues continuously (known as **tissue perfusion**). The **mean arterial pressure (MAP)** is the main BP driving force of tissue perfusion. The MAP is influenced by both the cardiac output and the total peripheral resistance, which are themselves influenced by other factors (Figure 3.7). MAP is calculated by adding one-third of the pulse pressure to the diastolic pressure:

MAP = diastolic pressure + one-third pulse pressure, or
MAP = (systolic pressure – diastolic pressure) ÷ 3 + diastolic pressure

and, given our standard BP of 120 over 90 mmHg, the MAP would be:

(120 – 90) ÷ 3 + 90 or (30 ÷ 3) + 90, i.e. 10 + 90

which is 100 mmHg.

Since the heart is in the diastolic period of the cardiac cycle for longer than the systolic period (diastolic = 0.5 seconds, systolic = 0.3 seconds), the mean (= average) arterial pressure must be *closer* to the diastolic pressure, i.e. it is *not* simply the sum of the systolic pressure (SP) and diastolic pressure (DP) halved (i.e. (SP + DP) ÷ 2) as might be expected for an average. The MAP must be closely regulated because if it is too low, the tissues would be deprived of a blood supply, and if it is too high, it would cause vascular damage thereby increasing the work load of the heart.

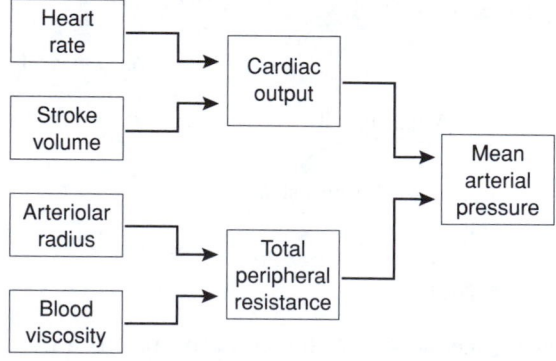

FIGURE 3.7 Factors contributing to the mean arterial pressure (MAP). The cardiac output and the total peripheral resistance are themselves influenced by other factors. The heart rate and stroke volume determine the cardiac output, and the anterior radius and blood viscosity determine the total peripheral resistance.

Observations of blood pressure

Blood pressure measurement

The standard clinical blood pressure is measured in the systemic arteries (i.e. those coming from the left ventricle), usually the **brachial artery** running down the upper arm, using a sphygmomanometer (sphygmo = pulse, manometer = pressure measure: the pulse pressure measure). The sphygmomanometer is used in conjunction with the **stethoscope**, through which the nurse will hear the sounds (= **auscultation**) associated with pressure changes as they occur in the artery. However, nothing is heard if a stethoscope is simply placed over an artery. This is because blood normally passes down arteries in a straight flow without any disturbance, and this movement is silent. It is generally considered that to create sounds that can be heard through a stethoscope, some disturbance to this blood flow is necessary, causing turbulence. Disturbance causes extra currents, so called **eddy currents**, and these disrupt the straightforward flow and cause sounds. To do this, the artery has to be compressed sufficiently to reduce the lumen; this is a job for the sphygmomanometer. It is important to carry out the procedure accurately to avoid false high or low readings as indicated in Table 3.1.

The patient should be lying or seated comfortably with legs uncrossed and should not have changed position for 5 minutes before the procedure. The brachial artery at the point of the **antecubital fossa** (i.e. the *inside* of the elbow) of the patient's right arm should be level with the heart, supported on pillows on a firm surface to relax muscle tension, which may cause a false reading. The left arm should only be used if the right is unavailable, as would be the case if the right had been injured or had been used for an intravenous infusion. A small difference of 5–10 mmHg often exists between the left and right arms of the same individual, and choosing the right arm whenever possible ensures consistency each time the BP is taken. The brachial region above the elbow is exposed, with no clothing restrictions above this. A cuff of the correct dimensions is placed around the upper arm *over* the brachial

TABLE **3.1** Blood pressure measurement errors

Error in technique	False high reading	False low reading
Artery below heart level	✓	
Artery above heart level		✓
Cuff too long		✓
Cuff too short	✓	
Cuff too narrow	✓	
No systolic estimation		✓
Over-inflation of cuff	✓	
Deflation too slow	✓	
Deflation too fast		
Re-inflation without rest	✓	
Crossed legs	✓	
Unsupported arm	✓	
Tight clothing on upper arm	✓	

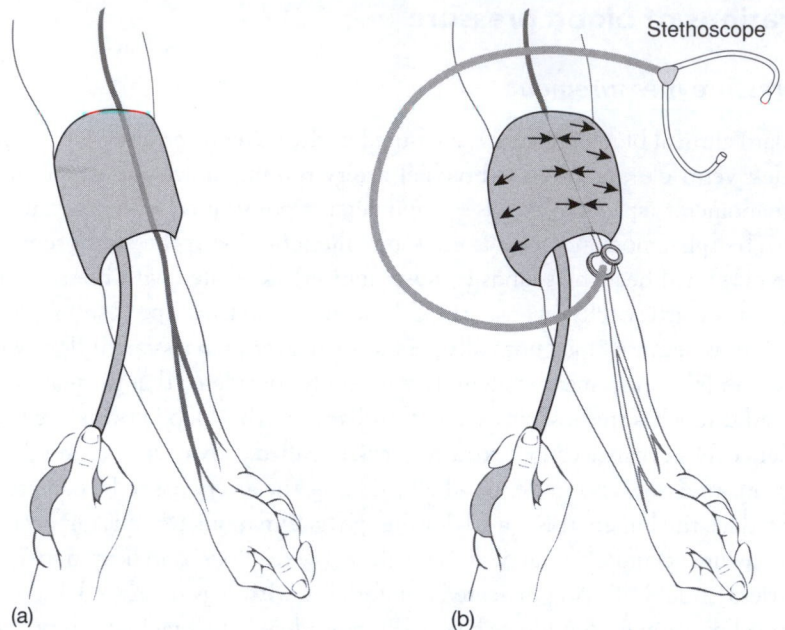

(a) (b)

FIGURE 3.8 Right arm with sphygmomanometer cuff in place. (a) Before inflation of the cuff the artery is fully open and filled with blood (black). (b) After inflation of the cuff the artery is compressed and empty of blood below the compression (i.e. inflated above systolic pressure). No sounds are heard through the stethoscope.

artery. The air bladder of the cuff should cover about two-thirds of the length of the upper arm and at least 80% of the arm circumference (recommended adult width of the bladder is 12–14 cm and the length is 35 cm). Too short an air bladder is more problematic than too long. The centre of the bladder should be in line with the brachial artery, which would be located by palpation (= felt with finger pads, not thumb) at the antecubital fossa (Figure 3.8). As the cuff fills with air, it compresses the arm, and therefore the artery, and the normal flow is disrupted as blood tries to pass the restriction. Sufficient cuff compression causes eddy currents to begin and the sound of blood flow can be heard in five phases (known as Korotkoff sounds, Table 3.2) through a stethoscope.

TABLE 3.2 Korotkoff sounds and phases

Phase	Sounds
I	The appearance of faint, clear tapping sounds that gradually increase in intensity
II	The softening of sounds that may become swishing (possible auscultatory gap here)
III	The return of sharper sounds that become crisper but never fully regain the intensity of phase I
IV	The distinct abrupt muffling of sounds, which become soft and blowing
V	The point at which all sounds cease

The procedure is as follows:

- *Step 1:* The systolic pressure should first be *estimated,* which is achieved by palpation of the brachial pulse during the *rapid* inflation of the cuff until the pulse can no longer be felt. Then, the *slow* deflation of the cuff allows the point to be noted where the brachial pulse returns, followed by rapid complete cuff deflation. Estimation of the systolic pressure prevents over-inflation of the cuff and allows the nurse to miss the **auscultatory gap**, a quiet period (Korotkoff phase II, Table 3.2) occurring between the systolic and diastolic points. If the cuff were inflated to an arbitrary point on the scale, the nurse might then be listening to this gap, which could then be mistaken to be *above* the systolic, and a grossly false systolic pressure would be recorded.
- *Step 2:* One minute is allowed before the full procedure continues; during this time the arm should be momentarily raised above the head to allow maximum drainage of the venous blood.
- *Step 3:* Inflate the cuff to about 30 mmHg above the estimated systolic pressure, the inflation should be rapid to avoid excessive venous congestion.
- *Step 4:* Deflate the cuff slowly, i.e. the recommended deflation rate is about 3 mmHg per second, or per heart beat if the pulse rate is 60 per minute. This rate accommodates most heart rates and prevents venous congestion in the distal vascular bed. During deflation the nurse is listening for the sounds through the stethoscope placed over the brachial artery just distal to, i.e. below, the cuff constriction. Above the systolic there is silence since the artery is fully compressed and all blood flow has stopped. Between the systolic down to the diastolic the sounds of 'thud, thud . . .' with each beat of the heart can be heard. From the diastolic down to 0 mmHg there is silence again (Figure 3.9). While deflating the cuff identify the start of the sounds (the upper point where sound begins, i.e. Korotkoff phase I) and mentally note this point as the systolic pressure. Continue to deflate slowly until the sounds disappear (in adults this is Korotkoff phase V) and mentally note this point as the diastolic pressure, then fully deflate the cuff. Obviously do not keep the cuff inflated too long, especially above systolic pressure, since this cuts off all blood supply to the arm.
- *Step 5:* If the procedure is to be repeated, a brief pause between attempts is necessary to allow blood to flow to and from the arm. Never re-inflate the cuff during or immediately after an attempt as this causes venous congestion and gives a false reading.

It is important to perfect the correct technique, including keeping the arm straight and supported, to maintain accuracy (Campbell *et al.* 1994). Although the sphygmomanometer is measuring the blood pressure, the process is *indirect.* The sphygmomanometer actually measures the pressure of the air in the cuff, but the nurse has skilfully arranged for this air pressure to exactly equal the blood pressure in the artery, first at systolic pressure and then at diastolic pressure.

Accuracy of BP and a new approach to blood pressure technique

The question concerning the accuracy of blood pressure arises because of the possible variability that must occur within the same individual at different times and under circumstances. One study (Powers *et al.* 2011) suggests that five to six separate measurements of

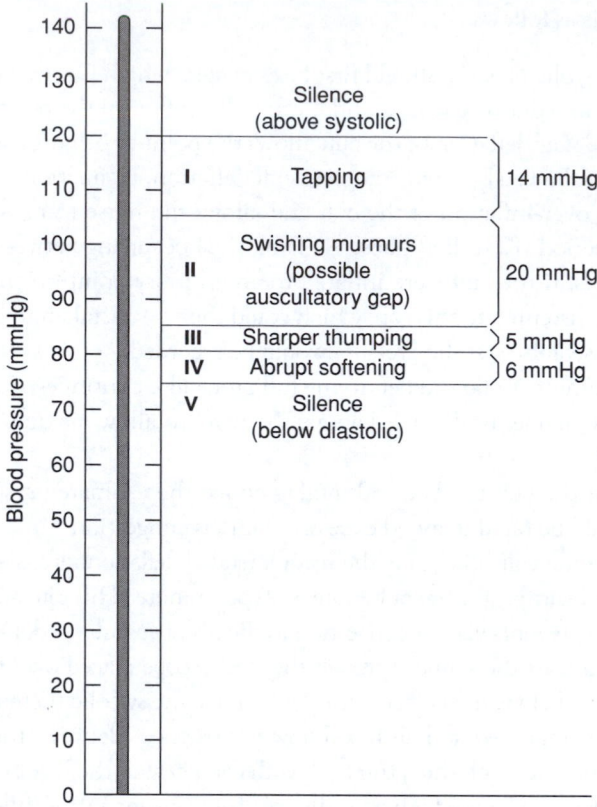

FIGURE 3.9 Korotkoff phases and sounds set against the mercury column (left) with the pressure differences between the phases shown (right).

blood pressure, taken over several days, should be averaged to provide a more accurate reading upon which to make a diagnosis and to base drug prescription.

A 'revolutionary' new approach to taking blood pressure is set to change and improve the traditional method. The new technique still employs a cuff around the upper arm (i.e. to compress the brachial artery), but there is a second wrist strap which measures the pulse wave. Attachments to a monitor allow a computer to calculate the **central aortic systolic pressure (CASP)**, close to the heart, with an accuracy of 99% (compared with aortic pressures measured though an *in situ* catheter). There are clear advantages to measuring this pressure via a non-invasive way rather than the invasive method of catheter insertion. The blood pressure in the central aorta, close to the left ventricle of the heart, is a more relevant pressure to measure than in the brachial artery, and this new technique should give more information about the patient's risk of strokes and heart disease (Hickson *et al.* 2009).

Abnormal blood pressures

Abnormalities of systemic blood pressure mean either the pressure is too high (hypertension) or too low (hypotension). In general, a guide to what is high or low is the pressure

100 mmHg. If the *diastolic* goes *above* 100 mmHg, this suggests hypertension, but if the *systolic* goes *below* 100 mmHg, this suggests hypotension.

Blood pressure rises gradually with age normally, but hypertension produces symptoms resulting from damage to organs and tissues, especially the heart itself and the blood vessels. **Essential hypertension** appears to have no identifiable cause, but whatever the cause, the result is sodium and water retention which drives the BP up. **Secondary hypertension** follows on from another pathology, particularly chronic renal disease, which may be accompanied by renin release (see renin–angiotensin–aldosterone cycle, p. 43) or tumours of the adrenal or pituitary glands. **Malignant hypertension** is regarded as a diastolic pressure exceeding 130 mmHg. It may be irreversible and can cause renal injury leading to kidney failure and death within a few years. The result of persistent hypertension can be any combination of three complications:

1   **cardiac hypertrophy,** or enlargement of the heart, leading ultimately to heart failure (**congestive cardiac failure**, or **CCF**);
2   **arteriosclerosis,** or *hardening of the arteries* due to blood vessel wall changes (which themselves will aggravate the high BP problem); and
3   **cerebrovascular accidents (CVAs)** (see Chapter 10).

The risk of developing hypertension is increased as a result of the following:

*   being male (women suffer less);
*   increasing age;
*   obesity;
*   high levels of salt in the diet;
*   smoking (nicotine is a vasoconstrictor);
*   sometimes a family history of high blood pressure.

It is interesting that 50% of these risk factors are controllable by the individual, meaning that everyone has the opportunity to significantly reduce their risk of hypertension by losing weight, not smoking and reducing salt intake.

Low blood pressure is strongly resisted in the body by **compensatory mechanisms** which drive the BP up. Rapid compensation to increase BP quickly involves the vasoconstriction of distal arterioles to increase the total peripheral resistance, mediated through the sympathetic vasomotor tone and local factors (Figure 3.5), plus increases in heart rate and stroke volume to improve the cardiac output, mediated through sympathetic influences and some hormones, notably **adrenaline** (from the adrenal medulla) and **thyroid hormone** (from the thyroid gland). **Noradrenaline** has the action of selective vasoconstriction (e.g. in the skin), which will increase the PR, and also acts by increasing the **venomotor tone**, which causes a tightening of the veins to improve the venous return of blood to the heart. **Cortisol** is another important hormone that helps in the compensatory mechanisms by preventing water from leaving the circulation into the tissues, thus helping to stabilise the blood volume. Cortisol reduces the permeability of the capillary wall to water and is secreted in higher volumes than normal from the adrenal cortex during stress. In the slightly longer term, water conservation to boost blood volume, and therefore increase BP, can be achieved through greater secretion of **antidiuretic hormone** (**ADH**, from the hypothalamus via the posterior pituitary). ADH conserves water directly by acting on the distal half of the renal tubule. In addition, sodium conservation by **aldosterone** (from the adrenal cortex), also acting on the distal renal tubule, has the effect of conserving water indirectly.

Postural hypotension, a drop in blood pressure on changing position from lying to sitting up or standing, is expected in everyone to some extent, but rapid compensatory adjustments ensure that for most people, particularly the young, it is not a problem. It can become a difficulty experienced with increasing age, and nurses should be aware of this when moving elderly people from one position to another. Getting them up from the bed onto a chair, or from the chair to standing, should be done *slowly* and in stages, allowing time for the BP to adjust after each stage. A drop in BP when *standing up* (often specifically referred to as **orthostatic hypotension**) is of particular concern when standing up elderly people (McCance *et al.* 2010). Communication with the patient is of key importance, allowing the patient to decide the pace of the move and when to rest, and to give the patient the chance to signal any symptoms of low BP that may be experienced, such as feeling faint or dizzy. **Post-operative observations** are critical to the patient's full recovery, and BP checks are paramount among these. Low blood pressure after surgery may indicate blood loss is occurring, either internally or externally, and should be reported and acted on quickly.

The ultimate extreme of profound hypotension occurs as a feature of **shock**, and this represents a stage where the compensatory mechanisms have failed to maintain the BP. Both the stroke volume and the cardiac output fall and therefore so does the blood pressure. Hypovolaemic shock results from **haemorrhage** (haemo = blood, rrhage = bursts forth), which may be internal (within body cavities, or as **bruising** into tissues) or external (into the outside environment). It is difficult to think of bruising as a potential cause of shock, but on an extensive scale it constitutes a considerable amount of blood lost from circulation. Elderly people are at considerable risk of severe shock from bruising, e.g. after a fall downstairs or a brutal assault. Bleeding can be arterial, venous or capillary. Arterial bleeding is far more serious as blood is lost quickly from a high-pressure system in pulses, resulting in a massive and rapid loss from circulation, and speed is essential to control this before the person dies from **exsanguination** (i.e. bleeds to death). Shock, especially hypovolaemic shock, is a major cause of a *narrowing* pulse pressure, i.e. the systolic pressure is falling faster than the diastolic pressure, and the two pressures appear to be converging. If the systolic pressure should fall below 50mmHg, the kidneys are at serious risk of failure.

Other forms of shock occur even when the blood volume remains normal. These are:

- **cardiogenic shock**, i.e. caused by the heart, when the heart as a pump fails to sustain a normal stroke volume;
- **vasogenic shock**, where the cause is the vascular (circulatory) system itself.

A common cause of cardiogenic shock is **myocardial infarction** (**MI**), where an area of *dead or dying myocardium* (known as the **infarct**) results from occlusion of the coronary arteries.

If this occurs in the ventricular myocardium, the force of contraction, and therefore the stroke volume and blood pressure, are greatly and often suddenly reduced.

Vasogenic shock includes several forms depending on the cause. **Neurogenic shock** occurs when the sympathetic nervous system supply to the cardiovascular system is blocked, causing a low cardiac output, reduced peripheral resistance and venous blood pooling. Venous pooling is an important cause of lost circulating blood volume since the veins carry the majority of the blood volume in circulation at any given time, and when this fails to return to the heart, it produces a poor cardiac output. **Anaphylactic shock** is due to a severe allergic reaction, resulting in massive release of the inflammatory chemical **histamine**, which causes a rapid body-wide vasodilation with profound loss of peripheral resistance and collapse of the blood pressure.

Apart from hypotension and tachycardia, shock, whatever the type, will also cause collapse of the individual affected and an altered state of consciousness (e.g. fainting) as the blood supply to the brain is reduced. Other symptoms include pallor (pale skin colour) and cold skin, caused by diversion of blood away from the skin to the vital organs (see noradrenaline), and sweating, caused by sympathetic stimulation of the sweat glands, a side effect of the sympathetic compensatory mechanism.

Central venous pressure (CVP)

The CVP is a measure of the pressure in the major veins returning the blood from the body to the right side of the heart. To understand the importance of this, it is useful to recognise first that the bulk of the blood in circulation at any given time is in the venous system. The total circulatory volume is 5000 ml, and the percentages of this volume for each blood vessel type at any given time are approximately:

- arterial blood = 10% of total volume (500 ml);
- venous blood = 60%–80% of total volume (3000–4000 ml);
- capillary blood = 5% of total blood volume (250 ml).

The remaining blood volume is in the heart and lungs. It is therefore very useful to know the pressure (which is related to volume) in the venous return to the heart. Any reduction in volume will cause changes in the CVP before it affects arterial pressures, which are maintained relatively high by the action of the heart. CVP gives the best indication of the filling pressures on the right side of the heart. CVP is measured through a cannula inserted along a vein towards the heart, the tip arriving in the thoracic vena cava, close to the right atrium (the vena cava and right atrium have almost the same pressures). The cannula is connected to a fluid infusion, e.g. normal saline, and calibrated by aligning the measure with the heart (usually the level of the sternal notch with the patient in a flat position). Measurements are taken manually using a *manometer*. In critical care situations, CVP can be taken electronically. The normal value for CVP is 3–10 mmHg (5–12 cmH_2O). *Low* CVP indicates *hypovolaemia* or dehydration, and *high* CVP may be caused by *hypervolaemia* (possibly due to excessive infusion of fluids or blood) or cardiac failure.

Drugs affecting blood pressure

Since many cardiac drugs have an effect on both the pulse and the blood pressure, they are the same drugs that are mentioned in Chapter 2. Some drugs act to raise the blood pressure but others serve to lower it (Waller *et al* 2009).

Positive inotropic drugs are those that increase the force of contraction and by raising the cardiac output they increase the blood pressure. These include the **cardiac glycosides** (e.g. **digoxin**) and the **phosphodiesterase inhibitors** (see Chapter 2 for details).

Drugs required to lower the BP as a treatment of hypertension include **angiotensin-converting enzyme inhibitors (ACE inhibitors)**, which reduce the blood pressure by blocking the action of angiotensin-converting enzyme (ACE), thereby preventing the formation of angiotensin II, and thus blocking its vasoconstrictive effects (Figure 3.6). The result is a reduction in peripheral resistance, and thus a drop in blood pressure. Beta-blocking drugs also provide a decrease in the cardiac output and a lower BP (see Chapter 2 and Figure 3.10).

The diuretics are a group of drugs that can be used to lower the BP (and are therefore used as a treatment in hypertension) by causing a larger urine output (see Chapter 7). The **thiazides** (e.g. **bendroflumethiazide**) and **loop diuretics** (e.g. **furosemide (frusemide)**) inhibit the re-absorption of sodium in the renal nephron. The extra sodium excreted as a result takes with it extra water, and this water loss reduces the blood volume, one of the influencing factors in BP maintenance. Some diuretic drugs may also have a vasodilatory effect *outside* the kidney, which has some part to play in lowering the BP.

Blood pressure in children

The systolic blood pressure rises normally with age, averaging at about 90 mmHg at 1 year old to about 100 mmHg at 12 years old, although great variation occurs according to growth rate and size. It is important when taking the child's blood pressure to use a cuff of the correct size for their age (see Table 3.3).

The wrong size cuff, especially the use of an adult-size cuff with children, will result in inaccurate results. The procedure also varies in children, with the Korotkoff phase IV sounds (Table 3.2) used to determine diastolic pressure. Children tend to have a higher cardiac output for body size than adults and this causes the fifth-phase Korotkoff sounds, used in adults for determining the diastolic pressure, to be too low for paediatric clinical use.

TABLE 3.3 Blood pressure cuff size in children

Age	Cuff width
Neonate	2–5 cm
1–4 years	6 cm
4–8 years	9 cm

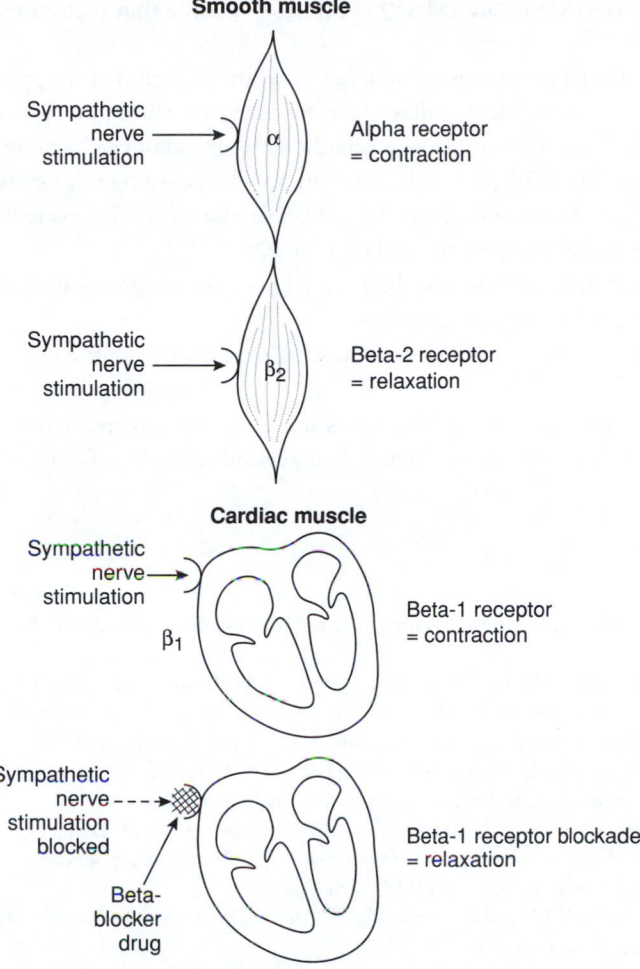

FIGURE 3.10 The action of beta-blocker drugs. Sympathetic stimulation of smooth muscles may cause contraction if the alpha (α) receptor is activated or relaxation if the beta-2 (β_2) receptor is activated. On cardiac muscle, sympathetic stimulation of the beta-1 (β_1) receptor causes the heart to increase the heart rate and force of contraction, unless the receptor is blocked by drugs that prevent sympathetic stimulation and the heart slows down and decreases the force of contraction. Beta-blocking drugs may cause side effects by blocking beta receptors on smooth muscle (e.g. causing bronchoconstriction).

Key points

- Blood pressure = cardiac output × peripheral resistance (BP = CO × PR), where the CO = heart rate × stroke volume (CO = HR × SV).
- The average adult arterial BP is 120 systolic over 80 diastolic measured in mmHg (millimetres of mercury).
- The difference between the systolic and diastolic pressures is called the pulse pressure.

- The mean arterial pressure (MAP) is the driving force that maintains tissue perfusion of blood.
- The mean arterial pressure is calculated by adding one-third of the pulse pressure to the diastolic pressure, i.e. MAP = diastolic pressure + one-third pulse pressure.
- The systolic blood pressure rises normally with age, about 90 mmHg at 1 year old to about 100 mmHg at 12 years old; variation occurs according to growth rate and size.
- It is important to use a cuff that is the correct size for adults and correct for a child's age; the wrong size cuff will give inaccurate results.
- Some 50% of the risk factors for high blood pressure are preventable by losing weight, not smoking and reducing salt intake.
- Nurses should be aware of the risk of postural hypotension in the elderly before moving them.
- Shock is a major cause of low blood pressure and narrowing pulse pressure.
- Systolic blood pressure below 50 mmHg may result in kidney failure.

References

Campbell N. R., McKay D. W., Chockalingam A. and Fodor J. G. (1994) Errors in assessment of blood pressure: blood pressure measuring technique. *Canadian Journal of Public Health*, **85**(Suppl. 2): S18–21.

Hickson S. S., Butlin M., Mir F., Graggaber J., Cheriyan J., Yasmin M., Cockcroft J. R., Wilkinson I. B. and McEniery C. M. (2009) The accuracy of central systolic blood pressure determined from the second systolic peak of the peripheral pressure waveform. *Artery Research*, **3**(4): 162.

McCance K. L., Huether S. E., Brashers V.L. and Rote N.S. (2010) *Pathophysiology: The Biological Basis for Disease in Adults and Children*, 6th edition. Mosby Elsevier, Missouri.

Powers B. J., Olsen M. K., Smith V. A., Woolson R. F., Bosworth H. B. and Oddone E. Z. (2011) Measuring blood pressure for decision making and quality reporting: where and how many measures? *Annals of Internal Medicine*, **154**(12): 781–788.

Waller D. G., Renwick A. G. and Hillier K. (2009) *Medical Pharmacology and Therapeutics*, 3rd edition. W. B. Saunders, New York.

Chapter 4   **Respiratory observations**

- Introduction
- Respiratory physiology
- The neurophysiology of respiration
- Observations of breathing
- Childhood breathing
- Drugs affecting the respiratory system
- Key points
- References

Introduction

We breathe because we need oxygen (O_2) from the air; although this is essentially true, oxygen is, however, not the main driving force of breathing. The primary driving force is carbon dioxide (CO_2), i.e. the need to remove this gas from the body. In Chapter 1 we identified how CO_2 was a by-product of energy production, a means of shedding surplus carbon from the body (see Figure 1.1). The excretory pathway of this gas is via the lungs, having first been transported there by the blood from the tissues. Nursing observations of respiration should be thought of as a means of assessing the efficiency of this process and detecting any abnormalities. Carbon dioxide is both beneficial and harmful, depending on the quantity present. Constant volumes of this gas in both the tissues and the blood are essential to maintain the driving force that keeps us breathing (and thus taking in oxygen), yet too much carbon dioxide will cause congestion of the biochemistry of energy production to the point where this would threaten the very existence of life itself. Compared with this, oxygen has a smaller role in maintaining the respiratory drive, although it is still important, and its complete absence is also incompatible with life.

Air passes from the atmosphere into the lungs through the **airway**, i.e. the passages leading from the nose and mouth to the tiny air sacs deep within the lungs. The airway consists of, in order, the nasal and oral (mouth) openings, the **pharynx**, the **larynx** (often called the *voice box*), the **trachea** (sometimes called the *wind pipe*), both left and right **bronchi**, multiple **bronchioles** and the tiny air sacs (called **alveoli**) at the end. The vast majority of the airway is lined with mucous membrane, which produces **mucin** (mucus). Mucous membrane warms incoming air to body temperature, adds moisture to it so it will not dry out the alveoli, and traps unwanted pollutants, which stick to the mucus. Tiny hair-like cellular extensions (called **cilia**) then beat in an upward motion to 'sweep' the mucus and pollutants out of the lungs towards the throat, where they will be swallowed. This is called the **muco-ciliary escalator**. Beneath the mucus in most of the airway is a smooth muscle layer that can *contract* (causing a narrowing of the airway called **bronchoconstriction**), or *relax* (causing a widening of the airway called **bronchodilation**). The narrowest part of the upper airway is within the larynx, the part known as the **glottis**. This is where the vocal cords are stretched across the airway for the production of sound, as in speech. Some parts of the upper airway wall, especially the trachea and bronchi, are reinforced with stiff cartilage rings to prevent airway collapse, a serious problem which would obstruct airflow into and out of the lungs.

Respiratory physiology

The **alveoli** of the lungs (minute air sacs that make up the bulk of lung tissue) provide the location for gas exchange between the blood and the atmosphere. There are three gas exchange compartments: (1) the *air* within the alveoli (appropriately called **alveolar air**); (2) the *blood*; and (3) the *tissues* of the alveolar wall (Figure 4.1).

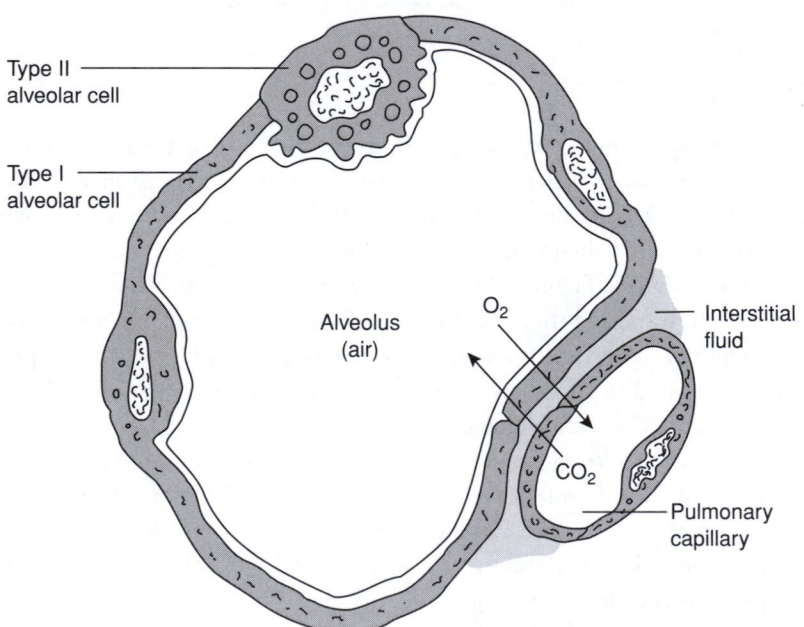

FIGURE 4.1   Microscopic view of the lung, showing an alveolus containing air, with walls of type I and type II cells, a pulmonary capillary containing blood, and interstitial fluid between the capillary and the alveolus. The direction of gas movement is shown.

While the air and blood are constantly being changed, the tissues provide a constant close, yet distinct, barrier between the two. Movement of gases across this barrier uses a fundamental driving force: the **concentration gradient**. Gases, liquids and many elementary particles will flow from a point of high concentration to a point of low concentration if given the opportunity to do so, a movement referred to as **diffusion**. Diffusion is defined as the movement of **solutes** (substances dissolved in a solvent), gas or liquid particles from the point where their concentration is greatest to all other points of lower concentration. In the case of respiration, diffusion refers to the movement of the respiratory gases oxygen and carbon dioxide across the tissues between the alveoli and the blood. The object of diffusion is to equalise the concentrations at both points. However, in the lungs, this equalisation is never achieved, which is just as well since if it were, the gases would stop flowing and we would die from respiratory failure (**asphyxiation**). At the same time, a lack of oxygen, and carbon dioxide poisoning would occur in the tissues. During breathing, oxygen is normally moving into the blood, but is kept in higher concentrations in the lungs than in the blood by the continued addition of new oxygen from the air. Similarly, carbon dioxide is moving into the lungs, but the concentration of this gas in the lungs is kept lower than in the blood by the continued removal of carbon dioxide from the lungs by breathing. In this way, the act of breathing itself ensures that these concentration gradients are maintained and therefore these gases will continue to flow in and out of the lungs and blood.

Mechanics of breathing

The act of breathing is a mechanical process that involves the movement of muscles within the chest wall and diaphragm. Chest wall and diaphragmatic movements govern lung expansion and contraction because the lungs are held tightly against the chest wall by a slight negative pressure (or vacuum, i.e. minus 4 mmHg) which exists between a membrane attached to the outer surface of the lungs (the **visceral layer** of the **pleura**) and a membrane attached to the inner surface of the chest wall (the **parietal layer** of the pleura), causing these two surfaces to stay stuck close together (Figure 4.2).

This suction force is created because the negative intrapleural pressure is 4 mmHg *lower* than the atmospheric pressure, which is both outside the chest wall and inside the lungs at rest. In this sense, it is useful to think of the lungs as being 'vacuum packed', similar to some foods sold at the supermarket. Whatever movements the chest wall makes, the lungs must go along with it, unless the vacuum is broken by the introduction of an abnormal substance between the two pleural layers. If this substance is air, this causes a condition called **pneumothorax**; if it is water, the condition is called **hydrothorax**, the water being derived from the blood plasma; and if it is whole blood, the condition is called **haemothorax**. Any combination can exist, such as **haemopneumothorax**. In any of these cases, the lung will fall away from the inside of the chest wall in varying degrees and fail to respond to chest wall movements, making breathing very difficult and painful.

The muscle movements of the chest wall operate the ribs, which during inspiration are moved upwards and outwards, expanding the volume (or space) within the chest two-dimensionally from front to back and side to side. Contraction of the diaphragm at the same time causes it to flatten, increasing the chest volume in the third dimension, i.e. from

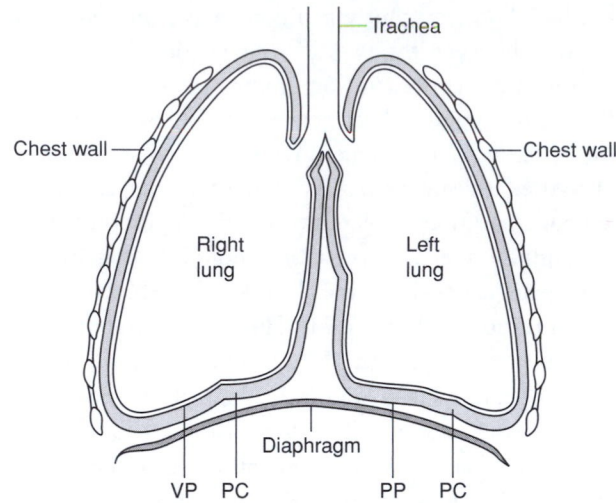

FIGURE 4.2 The lungs and the pleural membrane. PC, pleural cavity containing the negative (suction) pressure; PP, parietal layer of the pleural membrane attached to the chest wall and diaphragm; VP, visceral layer of the pleural membrane attached to the lung surface.

top to bottom. The lungs are stretched outwards in all directions, causing the air pressure inside the lungs to drop below atmospheric pressure, thus creating a partial vacuum within the lungs which must be instantly filled by air taken in from the atmosphere (**inhalation** or **inspiration**). The reverse is also true, when the respiratory muscles relax, allowing the ribs and diaphragm to return to their previous normal position. This squeezes the lungs, increasing the pressure inside the lungs above atmospheric pressure, which then forces the air back out into the atmosphere (**exhalation** or **expiration**) (Figure 4.3).

The cycle of diaphragmatic movements start with contraction of its muscle component, which flattens the normal dome shape. This flattening pushes down on the abdominal contents, notably the liver, which lies immediately below the diaphragm. Relaxation of the diaphragm results in its return to a domed shape, aided by the liver and other abdominal contents pushing back. Thus, pressure from within the abdomen aids expiration, and this is the reason why in some positions abdominal movements can be clearly seen during breathing. The relationship between volume and pressure seen in the lungs is expressed in **Boyle's law**, where the pressure inside the lungs falls if the volume increases at a constant temperature (as in inhalation), or the pressure rises if the volume decreases at a constant temperature (as in exhalation). The muscles used during normal breathing are **primary**, since they act all the time. However, sometimes events require additional effort to be put into the breathing process, for example, immediately after a fast race, and some extra **secondary** (or **accessory**) muscles are used to assist in chest wall movement. These standby muscles of breathing include some of the muscles of the neck and shoulder region. The most efficient position for the use of these muscles is upright, leaning slightly forward, with arms raised to a horizontal position. Severely breathless patients will adopt this position to aid their breathing if they are able to do so.

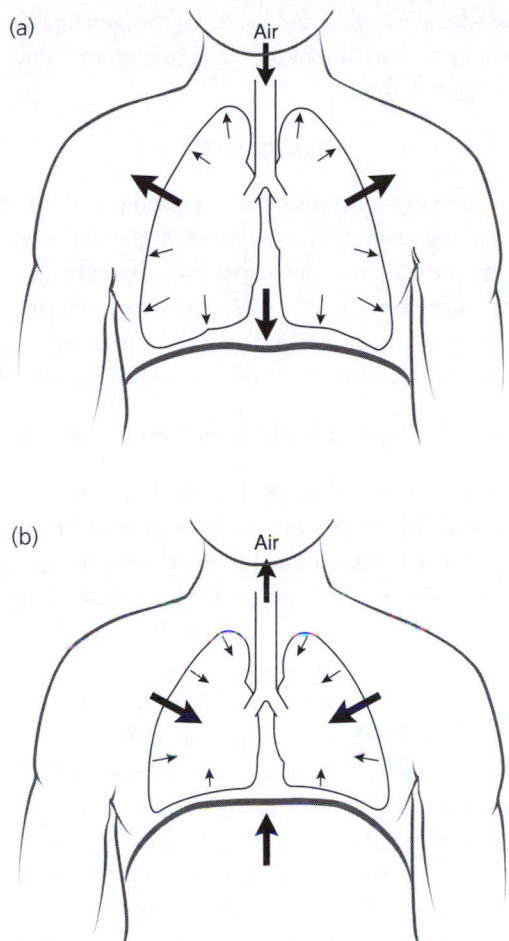

FIGURE 4.3 Inspiration and expiration. (a) During inspiration the chest wall moves upwards and outwards, and the diaphragm flattens, causing the lungs to be stretched in all directions. The resulting increase in the volume inside the lungs causes the pressure to fall and air is drawn in to fill the space. (b) During expiration the return of the lungs and diaphragm decreases the lung space, forcing the pressure up, and air is blown out.

Air volumes

The volume of air we take in with each breath is the **tidal volume**, i.e. air moving in and out of the lungs like water moves with the tides. This volume is about 500 ml of air in adults, depending on the size variation that occurs between different adults. A closer look reveals, however, that this volume can be subdivided into two different volumes based on functional grounds, i.e. a volume that *will* reach the alveoli and exchange gas with the blood (the **alveolar air**) and a volume that *will not* reach the alveoli and thus does not exchange gas (called the **dead space**). Dead space air fills the air passages, the **trachea**, the **bronchi** and the **bronchioles**. Exhaled dead space air contains the same gas mixture as inhaled air, whereas alveolar air has more carbon dioxide and less oxygen in it due to exchange with the blood. So we can state a simple formula:

tidal volume (TV) = alveolar air + dead space air

The dead space remains relatively constant, averaging about 150 ml of air (with some variation between individuals), unless there is any change in the diameter of the bronchi or the bronchioles, the only parts of the air passages capable of changing their diameter (known as bronchoconstriction if the diameter narrows or bronchodilation if the diameter widens). For most purposes, these changes can be ignored and calculations involving tidal volume assume a constant dead space. It therefore becomes easy to calculate the alveolar air volume:

500 ml (TV) − 150 ml (dead space) = 350 ml of alveolar air at rest

These values change during exercise, when we breathe faster and harder. Exercise actually causes us to increase our tidal volume by stretching the lungs further than at rest. A bigger tidal volume means a bigger alveolar air volume rather than dead space volume since the air passages, and therefore the dead space, will increase less. Increases in the alveolar air volume provide more air available for gas exchange with the blood, and respiration becomes more efficient. But respiration also speeds up with exercise, and this can reduce the efficiency if the respiratory rate increases too much. The reason for this is that by squeezing more tidal volumes in per minute, each tidal volume has less time to get in and out, and this results in a smaller tidal volume with each breath taken. Again, assuming a relatively constant dead space, the largest reduction must occur in the alveolar air, making less air available for gas exchange and therefore reducing lung efficiency. Slow, *deep* breathing is more efficient than rapid *shallow* breathing. Here, the words deep and shallow reflect the size of the tidal volume: deep is a *large* tidal volume (mostly alveolar air = efficient) and shallow is a *small* tidal volume (mostly dead space = not efficient). The tidal volume is taken in and out about 18 times per minute at rest (the **respiratory rate** or **RR**). Multiplying the tidal volume by the respiratory rate will give the total volume of air moved in and out of the lungs per minute: the **pulmonary ventilation rate** (**PVR**; thus TV × RR = PVR). It may be important to calculate how much of the PVR is alveolar air, i.e. how much air is exchanging gases with the blood per minute (called the **alveolar ventilation rate**, or **AVR**). This is worked out by deducting the dead space from the tidal volume before multiplying that answer by the respiratory rate, i.e.

(TV − dead space) × RR = AVR

Some patients require a surgical procedure that shortens the airway, a **tracheostomy**, where they breathe through an opening in the throat, directly into the trachea below the larynx. A tracheostomy tube is often in place to maintain the opening. This procedure is done either to relieve or by-pass an obstruction, or to reduce the dead space in those who will be ventilated for some time, thus making ventilation more efficient. Nurses should always check that breathing is normal through a tracheostomy and that no infection or obstruction occurs.

We have a functional **inspiratory reserve volume** (**IRV**), i.e. the maximum inspiration we can possibly take during a deep breath, and a functional **expiratory reserve volume**

(**ERV**), i.e. the maximum expiration we can possibly produce by forced exhalation. The increase in tidal volume during exercise is in fact a widening of the TV to include some of both the IRV and ERV volumes (Figure 4.4).

In other words, we breathe deeper during exercise by using some of our inspiratory and expiratory reserve volumes and adding it to our tidal volume. All the potentially movable air volumes in the lungs add up to create the **vital capacity** (**VC**):

VC = IRV + ERV + TV

The vital capacity can be measured using an instrument called a **spirometer** or a **vitalograph**, which is a portable spirometer. Both require the subject to take a maximum inspiration, followed by a forced maximum expiration into a tube attached to the machine; the output is recorded on a chart. The **forced expiratory volume** in 1 second (**FEV$_1$**) can be directly measured, i.e. the maximum amount of air that can be forcefully expired in 1 second after a maximum inspiration. The use of a constant time period (1 second) enables standardisation between subjects. Most individuals will normally expire about 80% of their vital capacity in 1 second, but reduced patency of the airway (e.g. as in asthma) will delay this process, and the total vital capacity will take several seconds more to expire.

We can never breathe out all the air in our lungs, since to do so would require the lungs to collapse; this remaining volume is called the **residual volume**. The residual volume still exchanges gas with the atmosphere and with the blood. Although it is a volume that remains constant in the lungs, the residual volume is being replaced by new air all the time.

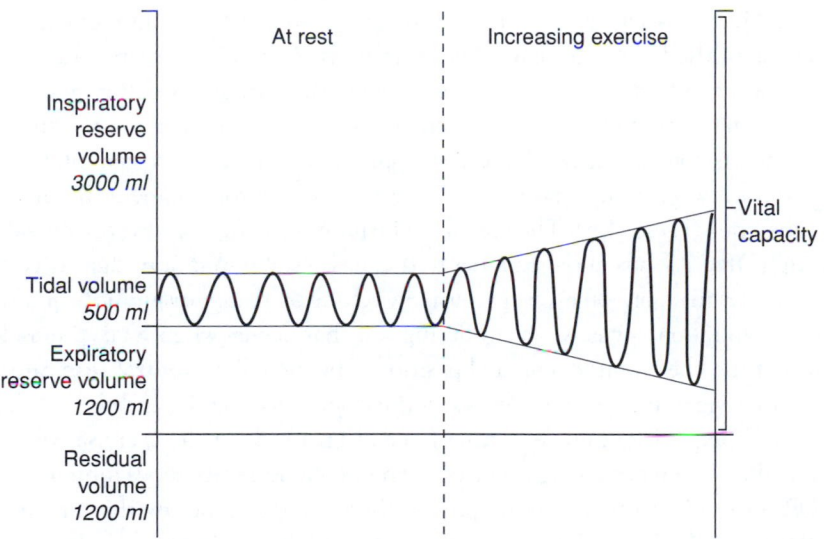

FIGURE 4.4 Breathing volumes at rest and during exercise. The tidal volume (TV) is approximately 500 ml at rest. As exercise begins, the TV increases by incorporating part of the lungs' inspiratory reserve volume (IRV) and expiratory reserve volume (ERV). The residual volume remains in the lungs, preventing lung collapse. The vital capacity (VC) represents the entire movable air in or out of the lungs and is the sum of IRV + ERV + TV.

The neurophysiology of respiration

The control of respiration is dependent on the respiratory centre, a collection of several neuronal groups shared between the **medulla** and the **pons**, both parts of the **brain stem**. The respiratory centre not only makes us breathe by sending nerve impulses to the muscles of the respiratory mechanism but also increases the respiratory rate and depth as required. There are many factors that influence the respiratory centre, but, as we have seen, the most important of these is the CO_2 level in the blood. Rising CO_2 blood level stimulates the centre to increase the rate and depth of breathing, with the effect of increasing the excretion of CO_2, whereas a low CO_2 blood level reduces the stimulus on the respiratory centre and breathing becomes slow and shallow in order to retain CO_2. Complete absence of CO_2 in the blood would cause **apnoea**, i.e. complete cessation of breathing, simply because this would remove any incentive to breathe. This is a typical feedback mechanism, part of the body's homeostatic status designed to regulate the internal environment within defined parameters, in this case, the blood gas concentrations. **Chemoreceptors** in the carotid and aortic arteries and in the medulla itself are sensory nerve endings specialising in detecting the gas composition of the blood and feeding this information back to the respiratory centre. These chemoreceptors are also sensitive to the pH of the blood, i.e. the acid–base balance of the plasma. pH is a measure of the hydrogen ion concentration ($[H^+]$), and a high H^+ concentration causes acidic conditions (i.e. a low pH). Normally blood is about pH 7.4, just on the alkaline side of neutral (pH 7.0), and this blood pH level is critical. A change of just 0.1 in the pH can be hazardous to health. CO_2 is thought of as an acid gas because in combination with water (as in plasma) it forms carbonic acid ($CO_2 + H_2O = H_2CO_3$), and carbonic acid can liberate H^+ (i.e. $H_2CO_3 \rightarrow HCO_3^- + H^+$). For this reason, any CO_2 retention creates a **respiratory acidosis** of the blood. In such acidic conditions of the blood, high concentrations of H^+ (= low pH) can be corrected *in the short term* by stimulating respiration to excrete more CO_2, thus forming less carbonic acid. Alternatively, any oxygen lack mostly stimulates the carotid chemoreceptors, which will increase respiration to improve oxygen intake.

The respiratory centre has several separate groups of neurons, some in the medulla and some in the pons (Figure 4.5). The medullary **inspiratory centre**, called the **dorsal respiratory group (DRG)**, sends nerve impulses to the muscles of respiration, causing contraction of these muscles in an on–off cyclic pattern. Switching on causes inspiration, and switching off permits expiration, a passive event during rest that occurs when relaxed muscles allow the return of the chest wall to a natural position. The medullary **ventral respiratory group (VRG)** helps to maintain the muscle tone of the inspiratory muscles and also actively assists the chest wall expiratory muscles during forceful breathing, as in exercise, when passive expiration alone is not fast enough. The pons **pneumotaxic centre** sends inhibitory impulses to the DRG in order to limit inspiration and therefore fine tune the rhythm and prevent over-inflation of the lungs. The function of the pons **apneustic centre** is less well understood. Impulses from this centre stimulate the DRG and would prolong inspiration if the DRG was not inhibited by the pneumotaxic centre. However, the apneustic centre itself can be directly inhibited by the pneumotaxic centre (Hickey 1997; see also Figure 4.5). Feedback to the DRG on inspiration comes also from the lungs themselves, via stretch receptors located in the bronchi and bronchioles throughout the lungs.

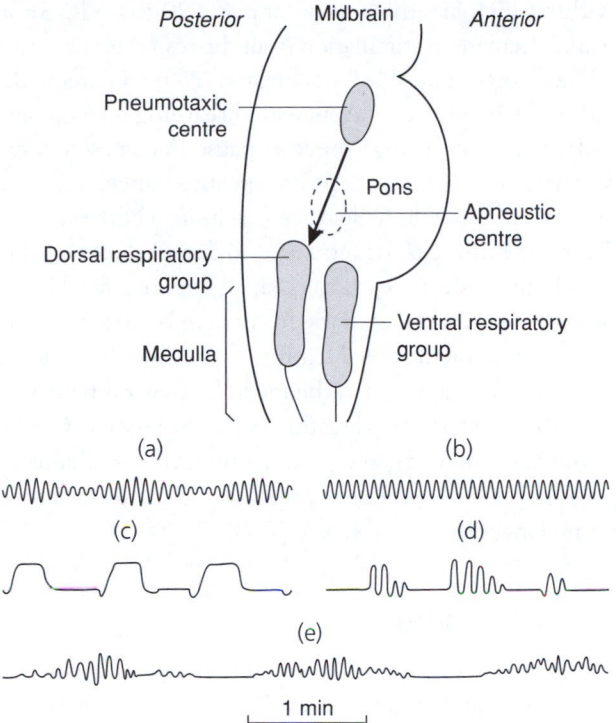

FIGURE 4.5 The respiratory centre of the brain stem and irregular forms of breathing. The dorsal respiratory group provides inspiratory signals at all times, and the ventral respiratory group helps to trigger inspiration during times of greater pulmonary need, e.g. exercise. The pneumotaxic centre of the pons influences the cut-off point for inspiration to prevent over-inflation of the lungs. This cut-off signal may be itself blocked by the apneustic centre under various conditions, thus allowing increased inspiration. Abnormal forms of breathing are shown. (a) Cheyne–Stokes; (b) central neurogenic hyperventilation; (c) apneustic breathing; (d) cluster breathing; (e) Biot's (ataxic) breathing (see text for explanation).

The medullary breathing centre has morphine receptors, i.e. cell surface proteins that bind drugs such as morphine. These are known as μ-receptors (pronounced 'mu'). Elsewhere in the medulla, morphine-like drugs binding to μ-receptors block pain. On the respiratory centre, however, morphine binding to these receptors causes respiratory depression, i.e. breathing will slow down and become shallow. Any patient receiving morphine for pain should be observed for shallow, slow breathing as a side effect of the drug. In these cases it may prove detrimental to the patient, especially elderly people or those with chronic respiratory disease, and the drug should be reduced or replaced.

Abnormalities of the breathing pattern (Figure 4.5) are sometimes due to disturbances affecting the respiratory centre, e.g. after **head injury** or due to **raised intracranial pressure (RICP)**. **Cheyne–Stokes respiration** is a rhythmic coming and going (waxing and waning) of the depth and rate of breathing interspersed by periods of apnoea. The cycle occurs over about 1 minute, within which breathing stops for about 20 seconds. An increase in carbon dioxide sensitivity and decrease in stimulation from the respiratory centre result in this pattern of breathing. The lesion responsible is not clear; it is often bilateral, deep in the cerebral hemispheres or within the basal nuclei. **Apneustic breathing** refers to a prolonged inspiration of 2 or 3 seconds followed by a long expiratory pause. A complete respiratory cycle takes about 50 seconds, during which the patient has breathed once. The lesion responsible is within the pons area, often caused by a blockage (occlusion) of the main arterial blood supply in the area. **Cluster breathing** is the term used to describe a series of rapid breaths (five or six together) which diminish in depth to complete apnoea for 20 seconds or so before starting again. The lesion responsible is in the lower pons or upper medulla. **Biot's (ataxic) breathing** shows a random unpredictable breathing pattern with shallow and deep inspirations and periods of pause. The lesion is in the medulla. **Central neurogenic hyperventilation** is a continuous pattern of fast, deep breaths, caused by lesions probably in the midbrain or pontine area of the brain stem. Such rapid breathing causes **alkalosis** (raised blood pH level, i.e. above pH 7.4), since CO_2 is lost to excess, and clearly indicates that CO_2 stimulation of breathing is no longer the case (Hickey 2008).

Observations of breathing

Assessment of the respiratory system is critical to our understanding of the patient's oxygen delivery system to the tissues and of carbon dioxide excretion: the patient's cellular metabolism depends on both (Owen 1998).

Respiratory rate and depth

Respiratory rate, the number of breathing cycles per minute, is the usual respiratory observation made by nurses. As adults, we breathe on average about 12–18 times per minute, but the rate can climb to 30 or more as a result of exercise, which provides additional oxygen, or as a result of some respiratory and cardiovascular disorders. A breathing cycle consists of an inspiration, an expiration and a brief pause. Modest increases in respiratory rate and tidal volume improve respiratory efficiency, as we have noted happens in exercise. But too fast a rate is inefficient, and so too is a very slow rate, e.g. below 12 breaths per minute, unless there is a greater *depth* of breathing (i.e. increased TV). Fast respiratory rates (**tachypnoea**), i.e. up to 30 per minute, can also be seen in infections involving fever, especially respiratory infections. Fever involves increased breathing rates, probably to supply additional oxygen for the raised tissue metabolism caused by activation of the body's defences. Faster breathing may also help to cool the body (see Chapter 1) as panting does in dogs. **Hyperventilation** is over-breathing, which may be due to physical or psychological causes. Pain and stress can both cause hyperventilation, and it is a feature of emotional reactions such as panic. Hyperventilation itself can severely reduce the carbon dioxide levels in the blood, which would normally slow breathing down by taking away the main respiratory drive. However, the higher centres of the brain, i.e. those involved in the stress reaction, override this chemical stimulus and drive respiration independently of carbon dioxide levels. The low carbon dioxide causes an alkaline state in the blood, i.e. raised pH called an **alkalosis**, and this in turn reduces the amount of freely available calcium in circulation. This free calcium reduction causes symptoms such as peripheral tingling and numbness, stiff contractions of the hands and fingers, and a feeling of unreality; all of which may add to the patient's stress.

Normally, oxygen and carbon dioxide in the blood create between them a gas pressure (the **blood gas tensions**) (Figure 4.6), similar to the pressure created by the gas in an unopened fizzy drink bottle. Each gas contributes part of this total pressure, and this is known as the **partial pressure of oxygen (PO_2)** or the **partial pressure of carbon dioxide (PCO_2)**. They are not equal since they depend on the volume of each gas carried by the blood. The PO_2 of *arterial* blood is 13.3 kPa (kilopascals) (100 mmHg), whereas the PCO_2 is 5.3 kPa (40 mmHg). The values for *venous* blood reflect the loss of oxygen from the blood to the tissues and the gain of carbon dioxide from the tissues to the blood (venous PO_2 = 5.3 kPa or 40 mmHg; PCO_2 = 6.1 kPa or 46 mmHg, where 1 kPa = 7.5 mmHg) (Figure 4.6). Respiratory rate increases would therefore result from increased PCO_2 or decreased PO_2 in arterial blood. Accurate measurement of these values requires an *arterial* blood sample for analysis, since this records the results of gas exchange events taking place in the lungs (i.e. one of several lung function tests). A venous blood sample analysis would only reflect gas exchange in the tissues, and this is not useful for the diagnosis of lung disease.

Dyspnoea means difficulty in breathing, and is recognised by the patient becoming very anxious and struggling to breathe (called **air hunger**) including attempts to sit upright and

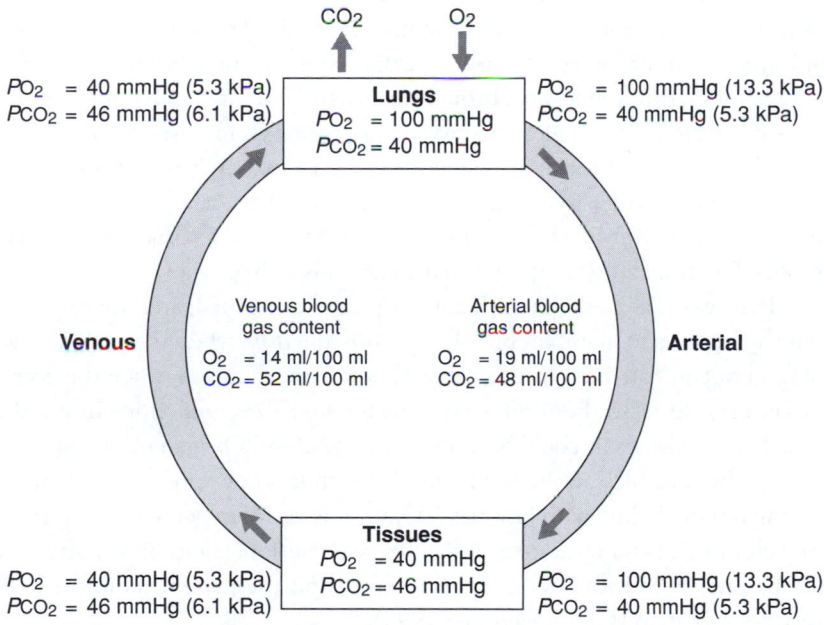

FIGURE 4.6 The blood gas tensions in arterial and venous blood compared with the gas tensions of the lungs and tissues. Notice that the arterial blood gas tensions adopt the same values as the lungs, and the venous blood gas tensions adopt the same values as the tissues (measured in mmHg and kPa). Blood gas contents are also shown for arterial and venous blood.

forward if possible (see p. 58), a rapid respiratory rate, cyanosis (see p. 69) and possibly various abnormal respiratory sounds (Grey 1995) (see p. 000). Fast intervention is needed to relieve both the lack of oxygen and the distress caused by dyspnoea, depending on the cause. Difficulty in breathing can occur in air containing less oxygen than required (called **rarefied air**), as noted at high altitudes in those not acclimatised to the situation. Not only is there less oxygen, but the altitude also involves lower air pressure, which exacerbates the problem. Deep-sea diving can also cause problems, because the increased water pressure on the body with depth allows more gas to be carried in the blood, additional gas that must be removed *slowly* (by decompression) as the diver comes to the surface. Failure to do this results in rapid release of the extra gas into the circulation, forming gas bubbles in the blood (called **gas emboli**, a condition known as **the bends**), which can cause the death of the diver.

Patients may often experience difficulty in breathing while lying flat (known as **orthopnoea**), which necessitates their sleeping in an upright position. The sitting-up position improves breathing because it allows for greater chest expansion (no restriction of chest wall movement caused by the bed) and improves the flattening of the diaphragm (gravity removes the pressure caused by the abdominal contents below). In addition, any fluids in the lungs drain by gravity towards the **base** while sitting up, freeing the **apical** (top) areas of the lungs, which then have a better air supply and are therefore more efficient for gas exchange. Sitting upright also allows for more efficient use of the secondary muscles of respiration (see p. 58).

In respiratory and heart diseases, the cause of an increased respiratory rate is a lack of oxygen (low PO_2), which the increased rate attempts to rectify. These diseases include **obstructive respiratory** (or **pulmonary**) **diseases**, include **asthma**, where bronchoconstriction and mucosal swelling narrow the airway; **bronchitis**, where chronic swollen mucous membrane with excessive secretions obstruct the airway; and **emphysema**, where breakdown of the alveolar wall reduces the surface available for gas exchange. **Chronic bronchitis** is a disease associated with a cold, wet climate and smoking. Over many years, the reduced gas exchange commonly identified in this disease causes persistently reduced oxygen (low PO_2) in the blood. The respiratory centre normally responds to **hypoxia** (low O_2) by stimulating breathing. In diseased and inefficient lungs, CO_2 can be retained, and the patient becomes reliant on the hypoxia to maintain breathing. Consequently, when the patient is admitted, nurses should not initiate oxygen therapy without medical advice, since the correction of the hypoxia may decrease the respiratory drive, worsen the lung efficiency and increase the retained CO_2. The result could be a respiratory acidosis. Oxygen may seem the obvious treatment for the breathless, cyanosed patient, but under these circumstances it may bring reality to the phrase 'killing with kindness'. Oxygen is useful in acute respiratory problems, but for the chronic sufferer it must be used with great caution. Caution will often mean that O_2 would be prescribed by a doctor in low dosage, and the patient monitored closely for respiratory deterioration (Forbes-Faulkner 1998).

Heart diseases can be a cause of increased respiratory rate, including **heart** (or **cardiac**) **failure**. **Left ventricular failure** (**LVF**) causes blood to accumulate in the pulmonary veins awaiting the opportunity to get into the left side of the heart. This 'traffic jam' of blood gets back to the lungs, where fluid from the plasma can leak into the alveolar spaces, causing **pulmonary oedema**. This prevents gas exchange across any alveolar space that is involved in collecting this fluid. This is sometimes referred to as the **backward problem** (see Chapter 2). **Right ventricular failure** (**RVF**, or **congestive cardiac failure**, **CCF**) can cause increased respiratory rates by reducing the amount of blood being pumped to the lungs, at the same time slowing down circulation in the tissues. The tissues become starved of O_2 and cannot pass their CO_2 quickly to the blood for excretion, and the resulting changes in the PO_2 and PCO_2 affect the respiratory centre. In acidosis, low blood pH (i.e. below the normal of pH 7.4) causes increased respiration in an attempt to remove CO_2 gas from the blood. Carbon dioxide is an acid gas since it combines with water to form carbonic acid, which liberates hydrogen ions (see p. 62).

Increased respiration also occurs as a result of lung collapse (called **atelectasis**), which can be due to chest trauma or can occur spontaneously. Atelectasis is the result of a loss of the negative pressure between the two layers of the pleura so they separate. A **tension pneumothorax** is where air is sucked in through a chest wound and builds up in the pleura, collapsing the lungs. A **pneumothorax** is air in the pleura from a burst **bulla**, or air blister, within the visceral layer of the pleura. A simple fractured rib can increase respiration rates because the patient cannot take deep breaths owing to the pain and compensates by faster but shallow breathing, which reduces respiratory efficiency. Respiratory changes due to the pain of fractured ribs may be inconvenient to the young but could be life-threatening to an elderly patient with other respiratory problems, such as chronic bronchitis.

Since blood tends to reach all the alveoli, the efficiency of gas exchange also depends on air reaching all the alveoli as well. This actually varies slightly, with more air than blood occurring in the **apex** (top) of the lung, and more blood than air occurring in the basal areas. The best 'blood–air' flow match occurs in the central regions, although fine tuning of the air flow to match the blood flow throughout the lungs means that small variations make little difference. However, big differences occur when serious 'air–blood' flow disturbances take place, as in **shunting**. In shunting, blood passes through large areas of unventilated alveoli, returning from the lungs without any gas exchange. This *high PCO_2/low PO_2* blood then mixes with blood that has exchanged gases, altering the blood gas tensions of arterial blood (a good example of how arterial blood gas measurements record lung function efficiency). If shunting is severe enough, it will affect oxygenation of the tissues, causing respiratory increases, cyanosis and dyspnoea. Shunting occurs in atelectasis, fluid accumulating in the alveoli, such as in **lobar pneumonia** or pulmonary oedema, or in tension pneumothorax. Lobar pneumonia is a lung infection characterised by **exudate** (leaked fluid accumulating in the tissues) collecting in the alveoli and preventing air from entering the gas exchange compartment. **Bronchial pneumonia** is similar, where the fluid collects in the bronchus, higher up the respiratory tract. A tidal volume that is too low (i.e. very shallow breathing) is also important as an estimate of respiratory efficiency. Low inhaled volumes will be mostly dead space with little alveolar air. A slow respiratory rate associated with deep breathing can be a feature of some periods of sleep. If slow rates are accompanied by shallow breaths, i.e. low tidal volume, which means low alveolar air volumes, this indicates poor respiratory efficiency. This kind of breathing pattern is very serious, and it is often seen when the patient is close to death. If it happens during sleep, as sometimes is the case, it is known as **sleep apnoea** (apnoea = cessation of breathing), a potential complication that should be investigated (Strohl 1996).

Peak flow

When asked, 'What does a **peak flow** meter measure?' a common answer is that it measures an air *volume* of some kind. This is not the case, however, as peak flow measures air *speed*, or more exactly, the maximum speed (peak) of air leaving the lungs (flow) during a *forced* expiration. Like a car speed, where a distance is compared with a time (miles or kilometres per hour), so peak flow compares an air volume with a time (litres per minute). The adult variation for peak flow is large, owing to differences in sex, age, build, smoking habits, and so on. The average adult peak flow is about 400 litres per minute, with men's values usually slightly higher than women's. Four hundred litres is a large volume, much bigger than any human lungs could contain. In addition, the expiration used to gain this result lasts only a second or two, with only a few litres leaving the lungs. Since the meter is not measuring *all* the 400 litres, the result is an *assumption* that 400 litres *would be* expelled from the lungs if the current maximum speed *had been* maintained for 60 seconds. The value is dependent on healthy **lung compliance**, the lungs' ability to stretch to accommodate incoming air, and on the patency of the air passages. Reduced lung compliance, which limits the lungs' air capacity, or partial airway obstruction (e.g. an asthma attack) will reduce the peak flow significantly. A narrow airway will significantly reduce the speed that air can achieve when leaving the lungs. Peak flow is achieved by blowing as hard and as fast as possible into a peak flow meter, after taking the greatest possible deep breath (inspiratory reserve volume). The full peak flow involves expelling as much of the vital capacity as quickly as possible. The accepted result is the best of three attempts. Severely breathless patients may not be able to perform this test, and it is therefore better used as a predictor of deteriorating respiratory performance before an acute attack.

Cough

Coughing and sneezing are respiratory phenomena with a purpose: that of clearing the airway of obstructions or irritants. The cough reflex centre is in the medulla, in association with the respiratory centre, and initiates coughing from stimuli received from the upper respiratory tract. Choking is an emergency that may occur after the failure of severe coughing to relieve an acute upper respiratory obstruction, such as food. But coughing can also be chronic and persistent, and the nurse should look for a pattern that will shed light on the cause of the cough. Some information needs to be known:

- Is the cough dry (nothing coughed up) or productive (coughing produces something from the lungs)?
- Is the cough accompanied by a sore throat or hoarse voice?

A dry cough suggests that a throat irritation is the cause, possibly an **upper respiratory tract infection (URTI)** such as the common cold. A sore throat and a hoarse (or lost) voice would further confirm this scenario. A productive cough recovers some substance, usually mucus, from the lungs, suggesting the problem is probably lower in the respiratory system.

Mucus could be substantial, as is often the case with chronic bronchitis, being coughed up every few minutes throughout the day. It may be infected, being mixed with pus, and may appear green. Blood coughed from the lungs (**haemoptysis**) is potentially very serious on two counts: (1) it is blood lost from circulation, potentially causing shock; and (2) it fills the airway, preventing inhalation and gas exchange. The result can be death if there is much bleeding and it is not treated quickly. Haemoptysis has various causes: **lung cancer** that has eroded through a main blood vessel; left ventricular failure, where a backflow of blood creates pulmonary congestion; or erosion and enlargement of alveolar lung tissue (cavitations of the lung called **emphysema**) caused by the persistent long-term cough of chronic bronchitis. Emphysema is a permanent complication of smoking that causes chronic dyspnoea. Since smoking is a lung irritant, it is a major cause of several lung and heart disorders, such as cancer, chronic bronchitis, emphysema and coronary thrombosis. Knowledge of a patient's history of smoking is important in any lung assessment as smoking could be the reason for many chronic coughs with mucus production.

Respiratory sounds

Respiration is essentially silent, so nurses observing any sounds that occur during breathing should report their findings, with the understanding of what they could represent. **Rales** are crackles or bubbling noises heard mostly on inspiration when air enters parts of the airway that has abnormal fluid present, as in pulmonary oedema due to heart failure or pneumonia. They are unaffected by coughing. **Rhonchi** are wheezes heard mostly on expiration and often clear after coughing. High-pitched rhonchi (**sibilant rhonchi**) come from the small branches of the respiratory passages and are heard, for example, in patients suffering from asthma. Lower-pitched rhonchi (**sonorous rhonchi**) are from the larger bronchi and occur in **bronchitis**. These sounds can be identified using auscultation, i.e. listening to the chest through a stethoscope, but severe forms of the sound may be heard while in close proximity to the patient without any listening aids. Such observations should be reported urgently to the doctor since intervention may be necessary to improve the patient's breathing. **Stridor** is one such urgent problem; it is a loud, harsh, high-pitched and vibrating sound, sometimes called 'crowing', during mostly inspiration, and caused by partial obstruction of the larynx (**laryngeal stridor**) or trachea. Sometimes this can happen in newborn babies and is known as **congenital laryngeal stridor**. The cause in the newborn is a congenital defect of the upper opening of the larynx, but the sound usually disappears by around one year of age. Stridor can be heard in **croup**, an acute upper-respiratory (larynx and trachea) infection, which is often viral in origin, and affects mostly children. It is accompanied by dyspnoea and distress, and sometimes sternal and ribcage retraction, when the chest wall is pulled back during inspiration. If inadequate air reaches the lungs, cyanosis may occur.

Cyanosis

Cyanosis is generally regarded as a grey, blue or mauve discoloration of the skin, depending on the degree of severity. It is caused by a lack of oxygen in the tissues (**tissue hypoxia**), but the skin colour change is due to an accumulation of **reduced haemoglobin** in the tissues. Reduced haemoglobin is haemoglobin without oxygen that takes on a hydrogen ion (H^+) in order to buffer these ions and prevent pH changes in the circulation (see blood gas transport,

p. 65, and Chapter 1). Excess reduced haemoglobin occurs as a result of inadequate oxygenation, when there is an excess of vacant haemoglobin capable of binding hydrogen ions. In general, if the colour change is observed in the periphery (i.e. the hands and feet), this is due to normal adequate arterial blood oxygenation, but the tissues are extracting excess oxygen from this blood, leaving larger than normal quantities of reduced haemoglobin in the very small veins (called **venules**). These tiny veins contribute to the visible colour of the skin. Restriction of blood supply to a part or whole of a limb may cause a degree of peripheral cyanosis in that affected limb. If the cyanosis is observed more centrally (i.e. the trunk or face), it is due to the lack of oxygenation of arterial blood by the lungs. The greater the volume of reduced haemoglobin, the more severe is the colour change from grey to deep purple. Central cyanosis can be treated with oxygen, which will occupy larger quantities of haemoglobin and therefore lower the level of reduced haemoglobin in the tissues.

Oxygen blood saturation (pulse oximetry)

Each haemoglobin molecule in the blood can bind and carry four oxygen molecules to the tissues, and, as such, haemoglobin would be 100% saturated. A haemoglobin molecule with only three oxygen molecules is 75% saturated, with two oxygen molecules, it is 50% saturated, and so on. A mixture of millions of haemoglobin molecules, some at 100%, some at 75%, some at 50%, and so on, results in a saturation value for *whole* blood at figures between those stated, e.g. 95% saturated. The amount of oxygen carried on haemoglobin should normally be very close to 100% (i.e. fully saturated). This can be monitored easily by attaching the patient's finger to a clip-on sensor that gives an instant readout of both the pulse and oxygen saturation level: the pulse oximeter. Low levels of oxygen saturation, e.g. less than 97%, indicate a problem in the lungs that is preventing full oxygenation of the blood. Such problems include many of the lung conditions discussed here, such as chronic bronchitis and pneumonia. The importance of this on-the-spot method of noting the oxygen saturation when compared with repeated arterial blood sampling and the delay while awaiting the results becomes obvious. Rapid changes in oxygen saturation can be detected quickly and corrective treatment can be carried out at once. Oxygen saturation of blood is affected by the blood gas tension of oxygen (PO_2), and a correlation of oxygen saturations over a range of PO_2 is shown by the oxygen saturation curve (Figure 4.7).

The difference between the two is that saturation involves the *volume* of oxygen carried, whereas the gas tension is the *pressure* it exerts. Naturally, the greater the volume carried, the greater is the pressure exerted. The curve shows a high saturation (98.5%) in the lungs giving a PO_2 of 100 mmHg, and a lower saturation (75%) in the tissues giving a lower PO_2 of 40 mmHg (see blood gas tensions, p. 65). This represents an off-loading of oxygen in the tissues that de-saturates haemoglobin by about 23%, and a corresponding on-loading of oxygen in the lungs. Under exercise conditions, oxygen is used faster than usual, which lowers the PO_2 in the tissues below 40 mmHg. Because of the shape of the left half of the curve (i.e. the steep section), a drop in the PO_2 in the tissues below 40 mmHg causes a steep drop in the oxygen saturation. For example, if the PO_2 in the tissues drops to 30 mmHg (i.e. a 10 mmHg drop) during exercise, this causes a de-saturation of haemoglobin from 74% down to 43%. This de-saturation off-loads a lot of oxygen to tissues to accommodate for the exercise.

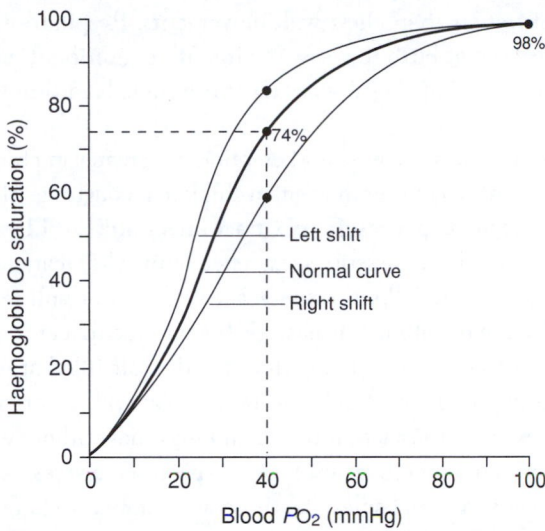

FIGURE 4.7 The oxygen saturation curve. The percentage of oxygen saturation of haemoglobin is plotted against the oxygen blood gas tension (PO_2). The normal curve (centre) shows an off-loading of oxygen to the tissues from 98% to 74% saturated (PO_2 of tissues being approximately 40 mmHg) and a loading of oxygen to the haemoglobin from 74% to 98% saturation in the lungs (PO_2 of the lungs being approximately 100 mmHg). Shifts of the curve to the left or right can happen (see text).

Compare this with the same (10 mmHg) drop in PO_2 in the tissues in the upper (flatter) part of the curve, i.e. from 100 mmHg down to 90 mmHg, with only a corresponding drop in saturation from 98% to 96%.

Shifts in this curve (Figure 4.7), either to the right or left, occur as a result of various changes in certain physical parameters. Shifts to the *right* can be caused by an increase in the PCO_2 (i.e. more haemoglobin will be carrying CO_2, less O_2). This is the **Bohr effect.** Similarly, low PCO_2 causes the curve to shift to the *left*, the **Haldane effect**, allowing more haemoglobin for carrying O_2. Blood pH also affects the curve. Increasing acidity (lower pH) shifts the curve to the *right*, while alkalinity (higher pH) shifts the curve to the *left*. Higher blood temperatures shift the curve to the *right*, and lower blood temperatures shift the curve to the *left*. An end product of red blood cell metabolism is **DPG (2,3-diphosphoglycerate)**. If DPG increases, the curve shifts to the *right*, but it shifts to the *left* if DPG levels drop (as can be the case with stored blood in the blood bank).

Childhood breathing

Normal respiration rates vary in childhood according to age. At birth, the rate is from 30 to 80, in early childhood it is from 20 to 40 and in late childhood from 15 to 25. All the infant lung volumes are much smaller than the adult, the tidal volume being about 15 ml, with a corresponding smaller dead space. Diaphragmatic breathing is dominant over chest wall movements during the early years of life, and as a result the nurse may find it easier to count abdominal movements rather than chest wall movements. Respiratory effort forms part of the **Apgar score** carried out at birth to assess the infant's condition, (i.e. 0 = absent breathing, 1 = gasping or irregular breathing, 2 = crying or rhythmic breathing) (Figure 4.8) (Letko 1996).

Breathing responses to illness, exercise and emotion are greater in children than in adults. Probably the most common respiratory symptom in children is coughing, which is usually caused by a throat irritation or a mild **upper respiratory tract infection (URTI)**, such as the common cold. Just occasionally it may be more serious, e.g. pneumonia (Kambarami *et al.* 1996).

The child who is born before full term is *premature*, and as a result may suffer severe respiratory problems. **Hyaline membrane disease (HMD)** is due to a lack of **surfactant** on the alveolar wall. Lungs must switch from being fluid-filled to air-filled at birth, and surfactant produced in the lungs lowers the resistance of the alveolar wall to stretching (i.e. it lowers the **surface tension**). A lack of surfactant results in lungs that will not expand properly and therefore will not admit enough air. It results in **respiratory distress syndrome (RDS)**, a complication seen in very preterm babies, i.e. those with immature lungs, but the condition is rare after 37 weeks' gestation. RDS involves respiratory rates over 100 breaths per minute, expiratory **grunting** sounds (due to expiration against a partially closed **glottis**, the narrowest part of the airway inside the larynx) and chest wall retraction. In severe cases the baby is cyanosed, with gasping respirations and even apnoea, and will need resuscitation, oxygen and assisted breathing, possibly ventilation. Hypoxia must be prevented because it can cause brain damage and less surfactant production; a high oxygen level is also dangerous since it can cause blindness by damaging the retina. Oxygen supplementation should be medically prescribed and strictly monitored.

Young children are more prone than adults to lung infections, mostly because they have an immature immune system which is exposed to a world of infectious agents (**antigens**)

Assessment	Score		
	0	1	2
Heart rate	Absent	Slow (<100/min)	Over 100/min
Respiratory effort	Absent	Slow or irregular	Good crying
Muscle tone	Limp	Some flexion of extremities	Action motion
Response to stimulation	None	Poor, with grimace	Good crying
Colour	Blue or pale	Body pink extremities blue	Completely pink

Score 0–3 = severe distress of infant
Score 4–7 = moderate distress of infant
Score 8–10 = no difficulty of infant to adjust to extrauterine life

FIGURE 4.8 The Apgar score.

that are new to them. Some conditions, such as **cystic fibrosis**, make this problem worse. Cystic fibrosis is a genetic congenital disorder of exocrine gland secretion that affects mostly the mucus of the lungs and digestive system. Mucus becomes thick and sticky, with repeated infections, not only causing malabsorption and malnutrition but also chronic respiratory obstruction with breathing difficulty. Children born with the condition in the past had a limited life expectancy, but now they are surviving into adulthood as a result of the advances that have been made in care and treatment.

Drugs affecting the respiratory system

Drugs active on the respiratory system include:

- **Bronchodilators**, which cause widening of the airway to improve air flow into and out of the lungs. They are used to treat conditions such as asthma, where the airway passages are severely narrowed. There are several groups of bronchodilators, which work differently. The **β_2-selective agonists** (i.e. drugs that stimulate the β_2 receptors) cause smooth muscle cells to relax in the airway wall, thus dilating the airway (Figure 4.9).

  These β_2 receptors are one of three classes of receptors (α, β_1, β_2) which are acted on by the **sympathetic nervous system** on muscle tissue. Examples of these drugs are **salbutamol, terbutaline** and **salmeterol**. The **antimuscarinic** bronchodilators cause dilation of the airway by blocking the muscarinic receptors, i.e. receptors which normally bind acetylcholine. These receptors are part of the **parasympathetic nervous system**,

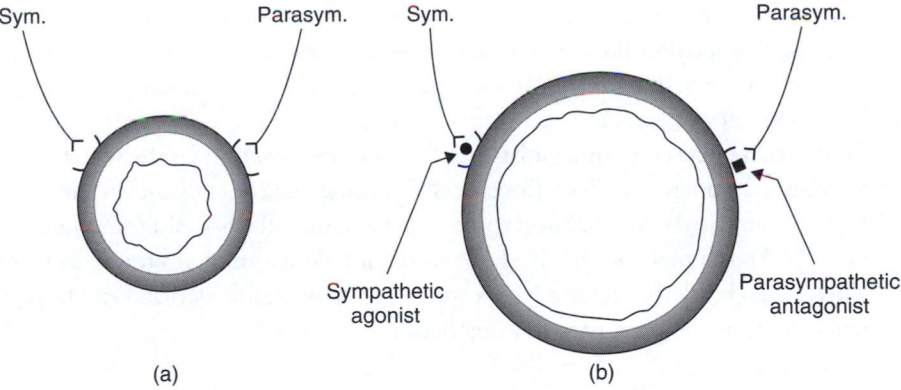

(a) (b)

FIGURE 4.9 The bronchodilator drugs. Cross-sections of the bronchioles showing the darker outer layer (smooth muscle) with the white inner lining (mucous membrane). (a) bronchoconstriction, where the lumen is narrowed, often due to an imbalance between the sympathetic nervous system (sym.) and the parasympathetic nervous system (parasym.); (b) sympathetic agonists can be used to increase (+) sympathetic activity, which then dilates the bronchus; or parasympathetic antagonists can be used to block (–) parasympathetic activity, which then does not oppose sympathetic bronchodilation.

which normally acts on smooth muscle in the airway to cause constriction. Thus, by blocking these receptors, the airway dilates. **Ipratropium** is the best example of this class of drugs. The **methylxanthine** bronchodilators act, it is thought, by raising cAMP levels inside respiratory muscle cells, and this higher cAMP level promotes muscle relaxation and thus bronchodilation. However, the uncertainty is due to the fact that at least two other mechanisms of action have been proposed, so it may be a combination of mechanisms that is responsible for the final bronchodilation effect. The best-known drugs in this group are **theophylline** and **aminophylline** (which is a complex of theophylline with ethylenediamine). Bronchodilators are required to treat acute respiratory distress due to bronchoconstriction, as in acute asthma attacks, and as such are better administered directly into the lungs by inhalation. This not only promotes rapid relief of symptoms but reduces side effects because the drug is not as well absorbed into circulation from the lungs as it would be from the digestive system. However, methylxanthine aminophylline, not normally a first choice drug, is usually given by slow intravenous injection.

- **Mast cell stabilisers**, or **cromones**, are drugs that reduce the risk of histamine release from mast cells. Mast cells store histamine and this is released in an immune reaction to an antigen. Histamine release triggers a number of different effects leading to an inflammatory response, including bronchoconstriction if the mast cells releasing histamine are in the respiratory tract. This would happen particularly if the antigen was inhaled, such as pollen or pollutants in the air. Drugs in this group include **cromoglycate**.

- **Corticosteroids** are anti-inflammatory drugs, and those used in respiratory disorders include **beclometasone** and **budesinide**. These are normally used as a daily preventative measure by inhalation as they reduce or prevent inflammation of the respiratory mucosa, thus reducing airway obstruction caused by swollen mucus. Some of these drugs, such as **prednisolone** and **hydrocortisone** (**cortisol**), can be given by the intravenous or oral route in acute asthmatic attacks, as an additional treatment along with the bronchodilators, to reduce acute inflammation.

- **Leukotriene receptor antagonists**, such as **montelukast** and **zafirlukast**, are orally administered drugs that block the effects of specific leukotrienes within the respiratory tract. Leukotrienes are chemicals produced by mast cells, basophils and macrophages (see p. 23) and they are involved in causing inflammation and bronchoconstriction. These drugs block the leukotriene receptors (i.e. they are antagonists) and thus prevent leukotriene activity and bronchoconstriction.

Key points

- We need oxygen (O_2) from the air, but the primary driving force of breathing is carbon dioxide (CO_2).
- In acidosis, blood below pH 7.4 causes increased respiration in an attempt to remove carbon dioxide, an acid gas, from the circulation.
- Movement of gases across the alveoli uses gas concentration gradients.

- The lungs are held tightly against the chest wall by a negative pressure, or vacuum, existing between the visceral and parietal layers of the pleura.
- The volume of air taken in with each breath is the tidal volume, about 500 ml in adults, subdivided into the alveolar air, which will exchange gas, about 350ml, and the dead space, which will not exchange gas, about 150 ml.
- Respiration depends on the respiratory centre, which is shared between the medulla and the pons, in the brain stem.
- The average respiratory rate in an adult is about 15–18 times per minute, but the rate can rise to > 30 times per minute during exercise or when there is a respiratory or a cardiac disorder.
- Breathing consists of an inspiration, an expiration and a brief pause.
- Oxygen and carbon dioxide in the blood create a gas pressure, the blood gas tensions. The PO_2 of arterial blood is 13.3 kPa, or 100 mmHg; the PCO_2 is 5.3 kPa, or 40 mmHg. Venous blood PO_2 = 5.3 kPa or 40 mmHg; PCO_2 = 6.1 kPa or 46 mmHg.
- Pneumothorax is air in the pleural space.
- Left ventricular failure (LVF) causes blood to back up into the pulmonary veins, and fluid from the plasma leaks into the alveoli, causing pulmonary oedema and dyspnoea.
- Shunting involves blood passing through areas of unventilated alveoli, returning from the lungs without any gas exchange.
- Cyanosis is a grey to mauve discoloration of the skin caused by a lack of oxygen resulting in an accumulation in the tissues of reduced haemoglobin (i.e. haemoglobin that has a hydrogen ion attached).
- Stridor is a loud, harsh high-pitched sound during inspiration caused by partial obstruction of the larynx (laryngeal stridor) or trachea.
- Peak flow measures the maximum speed of air leaving the lungs during a forced expiration.
- Respiration is silent. Nurses observing abnormal breath sounds should report their findings, with the understanding of what they represent.
- Respiratory distress syndrome (RDS) is sometimes seen in very preterm babies. It involves respiratory rates over 100 per minute, expiratory grunting and chest wall retraction. In severe cases, cyanosis with gasping respirations and even apnoea occur.
- Smoking is a lung irritant and a major cause of lung cancer, chronic bronchitis, emphysema and heart diseases. Knowledge of a patient's smoking history is important in any lung assessment.
- The main drugs used in bronchoconstriction disorders (such as asthma) are the bronchodilators (as a treatment of acute attacks) and corticosteroids (as both a preventative measure and as a additional treatment of acute attacks).

References

Forbes-Faulkner L. (1998) Oxygen therapy: challenges for nurses. *Kai-Tiaki: Nursing New Zealand*, **4**(3): 17–19.

Grey A. (1995) Breathless . . . dyspnoea. *Nursing Times*, **91**(27): 46–47.

Hickey J.V. (2008) *The Clinical Practice of Neurological and Neurosurgical Nursing*, 6th edition. Lippincott Williams & Wilkins, Philadelphia, PA.

Kambarami R. A., Rusakaniko S. and Mahomva L. A. (1996) Ability of caregivers to recognise signs of pneumonia in coughing children aged below five years. *Central African Journal of Medicine*, **42**(10): 291–294.

Letko M.D. (1996) Understanding the Apgar score. *Journal of Obstetric, Gynecologic and Neonatal Nursing*, **25**(4): 299–303.

Owen A. (1998) Respiratory assessment revisited. *Nursing*, **28**(4): 48–49.

Strohl K. P. (1996) The biology of sleep apnea. *Science and Medicine*, **Sept/Oct**: 32–41.

Chapter 5 **Fluid balance**

Introduction

Water is fundamental to life on Earth, and therefore life, especially human life, only exists where water is readily available. This limits where humans can live and travel, unless special arrangements are made for water to be available. The water molecule (H_2O) (Figure 5.1) is made from two hydrogen atoms covalently bonded to an oxygen atom. This creates a dipole, i.e. 'two poles', in this case, a molecule with a *positive* pole at one end (the hydrogen end), and a *negative* pole at the other end (the oxygen end) (Figure 5.1).

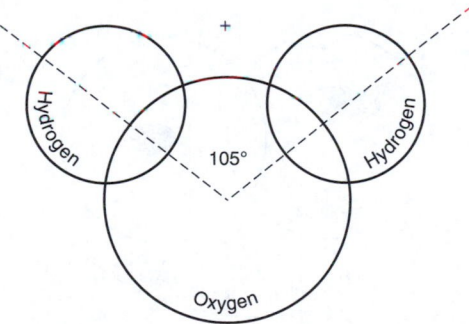

FIGURE 5.1 The water molecule. Two hydrogen atoms bonded to one oxygen atom at an angle of 105° to make one water molecule. The hydrogen end is positively (+) changed, and the oxygen is negatively (−) changed, so the whole molecule becomes a dipole (i.e. two poles).

This arrangement allows water to have some interesting and biologically valuable properties, such as, it is an excellent solvent for many other molecules and it has a high **heat capacity**. This means that it absorbs and loses large amounts of heat with little change in temperature, important as part of stabilising body temperature.

Water in the body

The human body contains any amount of water from 55% to 78% depending on body size, and this water is recycled and renewed multiple times a day. A typical 70 kg person is carrying about 45 litres of water (about 70% of the body weight). Water is critical in the body because:

- Cellular metabolism depends on water; many chemical reactions involve waters and other reactions that do not use water directly work through the medium of water (i.e. they would not happen if the components were dry).
- Water is vital for movement of substances around the body, notably by the blood and the lymphatic systems, which are both important water-based transport systems. This is because water is an excellent **solvent**, and many compounds are dissolved in water in the human body. At a cellular level, water is instrumental in the movement of dissolved substances across membranes.
- Water is vital also for elimination purposes, not just through urine, but also through the other water-based excretory systems: faeces and sweat. Many waste substances for excretion are dissolved in water (e.g. urea).
- Water helps to keep cells in their correct shape through internal pressures, and water shortage in the cells causes shrinkage with a corresponding reduction in function.

The body requires between 1 and 7 litres of water intake per day to avoid dehydration. The exact amount is dependent on levels of activity, the body and ambient temperatures, the atmospheric humidity and other factors, but averages about 2–2.5 litres per day for most people.

Water occupies three body compartments (Figure 5.2):

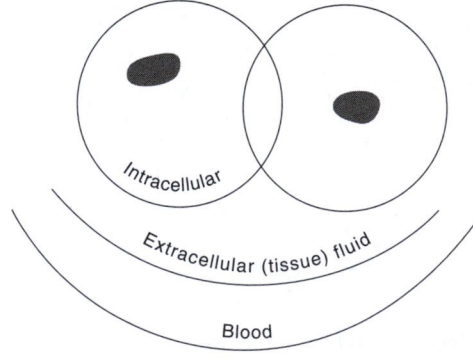

FIGURE 5.2 The three body water compartments. Water occupies the intracellular (inside the cells), extracellular (outside the cells, also called tissue fluid) and blood compartments.

1   **intracellular**, i.e. inside the cells, the largest fluid compartment, with an average of about 30 litres of water;
2   **extracellular**, i.e. outside (or between) the cells, also called **tissue fluid**, with an average of about 12 litres of water;
3   **blood**, both inside the blood cells and as the main constituent of plasma, with an average of about 3 litres of water.

The total for all three compartments is about 45 litres. However, water is never static in these compartments but moves across **semi-permeable membranes (SPMs)** from one compartment to another, and is also replaced all the time by new water. The movement and replacement sequence for water are as follows: new water entering the digestive system from drinking is absorbed into the blood, then passes into extracellular fluid, then intracellular fluid, back to extracellular fluid, then blood again, either directly or via the lymphatic system, and is finally excreted (Figure 5.3).

Water moves down its own concentration gradient, i.e. it flows from areas of high concentration to areas of low concentration, a process called **osmosis** (Figure 5.4).

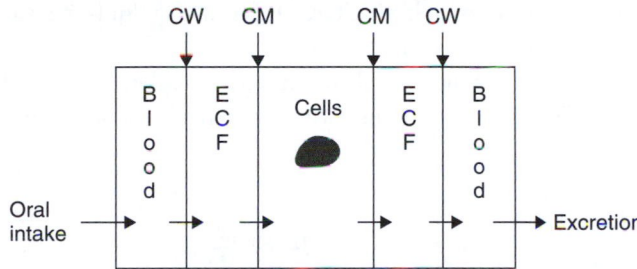

FIGURE 5.3   Water passes from input (oral) to output (excretion) through the three body compartments: blood, ECF (extracellular fluid) and cells. CW, capillary wall; CM, cell membrane.

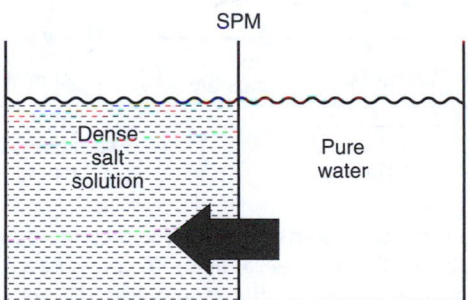

FIGURE 5.4   Osmosis. In this example, pure water can be considered as a high concentration when compared with the same volume of a dense salt solution. Water will pass through a semi-permeable membrane (SPM) until the concentration of water is equal on both sides. This would *increase* the volume on the salt side and *decrease* the volume on the pure water side. This process, called osmosis, is in action in the body, and is one means by which water moves from one compartment to another.

In addition, water will also move down pressure gradients. This process allows the formation of tissue fluid, derived from the *net outflow* of fluid from plasma at the highest pressure (arterial) end of the capillary. Meanwhile, fluid is returning to the plasma, caused by the *net inflow* of fluid at the lowest pressure (venous) end of the capillary (Figure 5.5).

Water gain versus water loss

The fluid balance chart

Humans gain and lose water constantly throughout the day. Some of these gains and losses are known to us, and to some extent they are under our control. However, other gains and losses are invisible to us (known as **insensible** gains or losses), and they function without any conscious control by us.

Humans gain water mainly through drinking (oral intake, about 2500 ml per day) at regular intervals throughout the day (Figure 5.6). This may be as plain water or flavoured as in tea, coffee or soft drinks. Even alcoholic drinks contain a large proportion of water, notably beer. Drinking water is not only driven by thirst but we take in fluids for pleasure and comfort. Thirst is the *bottom line* as a driving force for drinking fluids, i.e. we should never wait for thirst to occur before taking fluids by mouth.

Apart from oral intake of fluids, we also gain much smaller quantities (about 300–500 ml per day) from tissue metabolism. This quantity is too small to sustain life, so oral intake daily becomes essential.

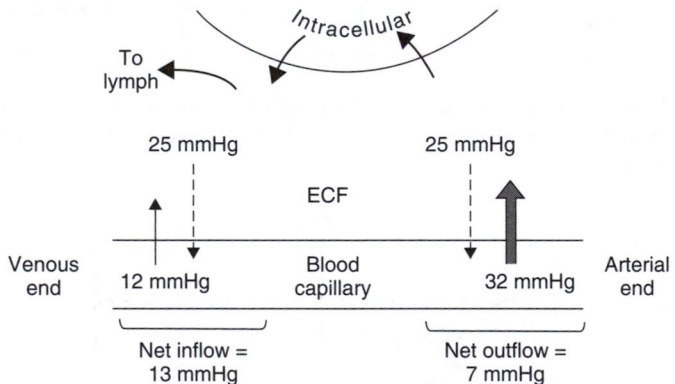

FIGURE 5.5   The formation and return of tissue fluid. Blood pressure in the capillary forces water out of plasma into the ECF (extracellular fluid). The pressure at the arterial end (32 mmHg) is higher than the pressure at the venous end (12 mmHg) as blood pressure falls throughout the capillary bed. The plasma proteins pull water back into the capillary with an attractive force (measured as a pressure of 25 mmHg) across the capillary bed. Therefore, at the arterial end there is a net *outflow* from the capillary (i.e. 32−25 = 7 mmHg), which constantly creates new tissue fluid from blood plasma, and at the venous end there is a net *inflow* into the capillary (i.e. 25−12 = 13 mmHg), which constantly returns water back to the blood plasma. The cells interchange water with the ECF, and some extra water escapes the ECF to become lymphatic fluid.

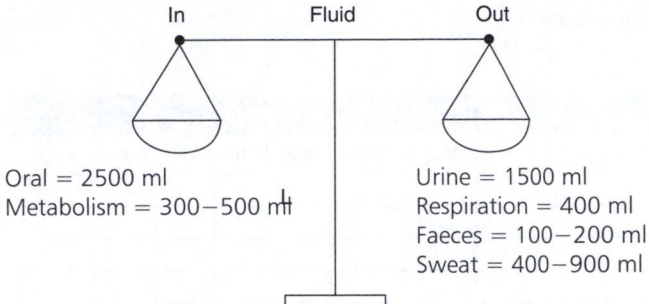

In   Fluid   Out

Oral = 2500 ml   Urine = 1500 ml
Metabolism = 300–500 ml   Respiration = 400 ml
                                  Faeces = 100–200 ml
                                  Sweat = 400–900 ml

FIGURE 5.6   Fluid balance. To balance on both sides, input (oral and metabolism) must equal output (urine, faeces, respiration and sweat).

Humans lose much of their daily fluids through urine output (about 1500 ml per day, see Chapter 7 and Figure 5.6), but an important loss is also through the skin by evaporation of sweat (400–900 ml per day, see Chapters 1 and 9). This skin loss is part of our **insensible loss** since it cannot be directly measured and has to be estimated. Other forms of insensible loss are water vapour exhaled through the lungs (about 400 ml per day) and water lost in faeces (about 100–200 ml per day). These insensible losses must be part of the estimation.

Fluid balance records the amount of intake versus output to see if there is net gain or loss of fluid over a 24-hour period. Everything the patient drinks and passes as urine for 24 hours is measured (in millilitres, ml) and recorded on a fluid balance chart (Figure 5.7).

The insensible losses and gains are estimated and recorded, and a net total is achieved. The object is to try and maintain a *neutral* fluid balance over 24 hours, i.e. no excess of intake (*positive* balance) or excess of output (*negative* balance). Excess water intake or output over one or two periods of 24 hours is not normally a problem in health as the body makes adjustments (usually to urine output) to correct any deficits.

Producing a lower urine output will conserve water if intake is low. Similarly, a higher urine output will correct the balance if oral intake is high (e.g. the person drinking lots of beer who then needs to go to the toilet frequently!) (the physiology of these changes can be found in Chapter 7).

If fluid balance recordings show a persistent excessive loss or gain of fluid over several days or weeks, this will indicate that there is a problem that needs investigation and attention. Special considerations must be made in relation to fluid balance under certain circumstances, as follows:

- Patients on **intravenous** (IV) infusions and **blood transfusions** must have the volumes of administered fluid measured and included in the fluid balance record. Giving fluids by the intravenous route is an effective way of rehydrating patients who cannot drink enough, but it raises the risk of rapid fluid overload if renal output is poor.
- Patients who are designated as **nil by mouth (NBM)**, i.e. eating or drinking nothing for longer than a few hours, require careful fluid monitoring to identify any risk of dehydration. Patients who cannot eat or drink long term will need alternative fluid

Fluid Balance Chart

Date _____

Oral/Enternal intake					Output				
Time	Description	Oral	Enternal	Total	Time	Urine	Stool	Other	Total
	Total				Total				
		Oral/IV intake 24-hour total					Output 24-hour total		

FIGURE 5.7 The 24-hour fluid balance chart. The patient's input and output are measured and entered on the chart along with the time. Totals for the 24 hours are calculated, taking into account the insensible losses. IV, intravenous.

replacement, either by the IV route or by feeding tube. These include coma patients and some of those in critical care.

- Patients who are vomiting or have no appetite for food and drink. A single bout of vomiting is not a major problem, but if this persists for more than a few hours then fluid balance may need to be monitored and an alternative fluid input considered. Because of their smaller size, children may be particularly prone to dehydration due to persistent vomiting.

Central venous pressure (CVP) is a measure of the pressure of the *venous blood* return to the heart, i.e. the blood pressure in the major *veins* close to the right atrium (see Chapter 3). Normal CVP is 3–10 mmHg (or 5–12 cmH$_2$O). CVP will be altered (higher or lower) when blood volume changes occur, and severe under-hydration or over-hydration will affect blood volumes, as will, of course, significant blood loss. Therefore, CVP measurements may be important when rehydrating patients rapidly.

Problems of water imbalance

Oedema

Oedema is excessive fluid in the tissues causing the tissues to swell. This excess of water is mostly in the extracellular (tissue fluid) compartment, with very little in the intracellular compartment, as the cells would rupture if they took on too much water. Some extra fluid can be housed in the blood compartment, but this is limited because excess water in circulation boosts blood volume, and thus raises blood pressure. High blood pressure (**hypertension**) can be treated using drugs that promote water loss from the blood compartment through the kidneys (drugs called **diuretics**, see Chapters 3 and 7).

Oedema results either from the intake of water persistently exceeding the output, i.e. a *positive* fluid balance, over several days or weeks, or due to the body's failure to handle water properly (i.e. heart failure or kidney failure). A poor outcome in acute renal failure has been linked to positive fluid balance (Payen *et al.* 2008). In normal health, it is difficult to achieve a persistent positive balance because the kidneys remove the excess water and therefore improve the output, thus restoring the balance (i.e. the more you drink, the more you pass urine). There are also *local* causes of oedema, i.e. specific causes of oedema occurring in a particular part of the body. Oedema is therefore a pathological state, i.e. a symptom of some underlying pathology. The problem of tissue oedema can be narrowed down to five causes:

1 *Obstructed venous return* of blood, as seen in **heart failure**. *Right* ventricular failure causes a backlog of blood waiting to get into the right side of the heart and this backlog can increase venous pressure sufficiently that the veins can no longer accept blood from the capillaries, which then engorge and leak fluid into the tissues (called **systemic oedema**). *Left* ventricular failure causes a backlog of blood from the lungs waiting to enter the left ventricle, and this increases the venous blood pressure coming from the lungs, which then causes fluid to spill out of the capillaries in the lungs. Fluid then collects in the

alveoli (called **pulmonary oedema**). At a more local level, congestion of venous return can occur if there any tight restrictions to a limb preventing venous return, for example an inflated blood pressure cuff left on for too long.

2   *Excess sodium* in circulation and the tissues. The kidneys remove excess sodium from the body by excreting it in the urine. Kidney problems can cause a failure to remove sodium, which then accumulates in the blood (called **hypernatraemia**) and in the tissues. One property of sodium is that it attracts water. If sodium is retained in the body, so will water, causing an oedematous state. Excessive sodium intake will also contribute to oedema, especially again if the kidneys are unable to excrete it all. The hormone **aldosterone** (from the adrenal cortex) conserves sodium in the body, and excess of this hormone may also contribute to a hypernatraemia, and thus oedema.

3   *Inadequate plasma protein* concentration. One of the vital functions of proteins in plasma is to attract fluid back to the blood from the extracellular compartment. This attracting force draws water back at a pressure of 25 mmHg along the capillary length (Figure 5.5). Capillaries have semi-permeable walls to allow this water to pass through. In the event of low plasma proteins, this attractive force is reduced (i.e. the 25 mmHg pressure drops), and water is then added to the tissues faster than it is withdrawn, and thus it accumulates in the tissues. Low plasma proteins can occur in starvation (especially very low dietary protein intake), and in liver disease since the liver produces **albumen**, the most abundant of the plasma proteins.

4   *Obstructed lymphatic drainage* of the tissues. Normally, the lymphatic system drains away any excess fluid from the extracellular tissue space, thus preventing any fluid build-up (Figure 5.5). Anything that obstructs this drainage will cause oedema. Examples of this are new growths or inflammation of the lymphatic glands (or nodes) and any external pressures on the lymphatic vessels.

5   *Increased capillary wall permeability*. This occurs as a process of **inflammation**. The normally permeable capillary wall becomes even more permeable (i.e. 'leaky') as a result of the inflammatory process. This causes more water to escape into the tissues. Proteins in the plasma are normally too big to pass through the capillary wall, but in inflammation capillaries can become leaky enough to allow proteins to escape the plasma into the tissue fluid. The protein-rich environment around the capillaries attracts even more water out of the capillaries and causes local swelling (localised oedema) of the tissues. Swelling is one of the cardinal signs of inflammation, along with redness, pain and heat.

Pulmonary oedema is a very serious problem that is recognised by acute dyspnoea (breathlessness), severe cyanosis (due to **shunting**, see Chapter 4) and cough. The surprise is the fact that symptoms of pulmonary oedema occur so quickly after left ventricular failure has occurred. This is because the distance between the left heart and the lungs is very short, and any backlog of blood flow reaches the lungs rapidly. **Loop diuretics** (see Chapter 7) are drugs used to treat pulmonary oedema caused by left ventricular failure. They work by promoting fluid loss from the kidneys, which in turn withdraws fluid from the lungs.

Systemic fluid overload can be identified by the following observations: weight gain, raised blood pressure, fast pulse and breathing rates, raised urine output if the kidneys are functioning normally, or lower urine output if the heart is in failure, and oedematous swelling of tissues (Mooney 2007). The swelling of the tissues is mostly in the limbs (i.e. tissues furthest from the heart), especially the legs and ankles as fluid drains downwards to the lowest points due to gravity. This gravity-driven oedema is known as **dependent** oedema. Dependent oedema also occurs in the back and sacral areas in patients lying on their backs while confined to bed, and may contribute to pressure sore formation. Dependent oedema can also be recognised by applying gentle pressure from a finger on the skin to create a shallow dent. If this dent remains when the finger is withdrawn, it is systemic oedema. Reduction of this oedema can be assisted by seating the patient with legs elevated, thus employing gravity to gradually drain the tissues of fluid back into circulation. Also, it can be prevented by the application of bandages or pressure stockings, which stop fluid leakage into the tissues.

Cerebral oedema is swelling of the brain, due to inflammation of the brain or its coverings, or sometimes due to head injury (i.e. **concussion**, which is 'brain shaking'). Because the brain is encased in the skull, the problem with swelling is the risk of increasing intracranial pressure (**raised intracranial pressure, RICP**), which will put the brain under pressure.

Dehydration

Insufficient fluid in any or all of the three tissue compartments is called **dehydration**. This is due to the following three conditions:

1 A *persistent negative fluid balance*, where output exceeds input for more than a few days. The exact time it takes to establish dehydration depends on how poor the fluid intake is, or how large the fluid loss is. A total lack of all fluid intake will start to cause minor dehydration within hours. Thirst is the normal body response to early dehydration, i.e. before tissue harm is caused, in an attempt to correct the fluid balance by increasing oral intake. The causes of negative fluid loss includes persistent vomiting, diarrhoea, both diabetes mellitus and diabetes insipidus, polyurea (a large urine output), excessive use of diuretic drugs, and fever (see Chapter 1).

2 *Extensive blood loss* causing **hypovolaemia** (low blood volume), usually rapidly, i.e. before the volume loss can be corrected. Blood volume losses can be from internal or external haemorrhage, or plasma loss from extensive burns.

3 *Maldistribution of fluid*, i.e. fluid is unevenly distributed around the body, with accumulation in some areas while other areas suffer dehydration (Kreimeier 2000).

Severe dehydration causes weight loss, reduced pulse pressure (see Chapter 3), rapid shallow breathing, fast weak pulse, low volumes of highly concentrated urine, dry wrinkled skin, poor production of thick saliva from a dry mouth (see below), thirst, and shrunken tissues (Mooney 2007). Folds of skin formed by gentle external digital pressure remain as folds when the finger pressure is removed. Tissues around the eyes shrink and the eyes appear sunken in their sockets in severe depletion of fluids. The mouth in particular becomes very dry with little or no saliva. This causes the mouth to become very dirty and at risk of oral infections. This is partly because oral fluid intake is an important cleansing mechanism for the mouth, and absence predisposes the mouth to poor hygiene. The dehydrated dirty mouth becomes very hard to clean properly. An oral infection leads to throat, chest, middle ear and even brain infections if left untreated. Management of dehydration is, of course, rehydration, preferably by mouth. However, some patients require an alternative route for fluid replacement, which is normally the intravenous (IV) route. These patients include:

- those who are severely dehydrated and need urgent rehydration, and oral intake is not adequate enough to rehydrate the patient quickly;
- those unable to drink and swallow properly, e.g. unconscious, nil by mouth and post-operative patients.

Electrolyte balance

Water balance in the body is linked to the balance of electrolytes within the three compartments (cells, tissue fluid and blood, Figure 5.8).

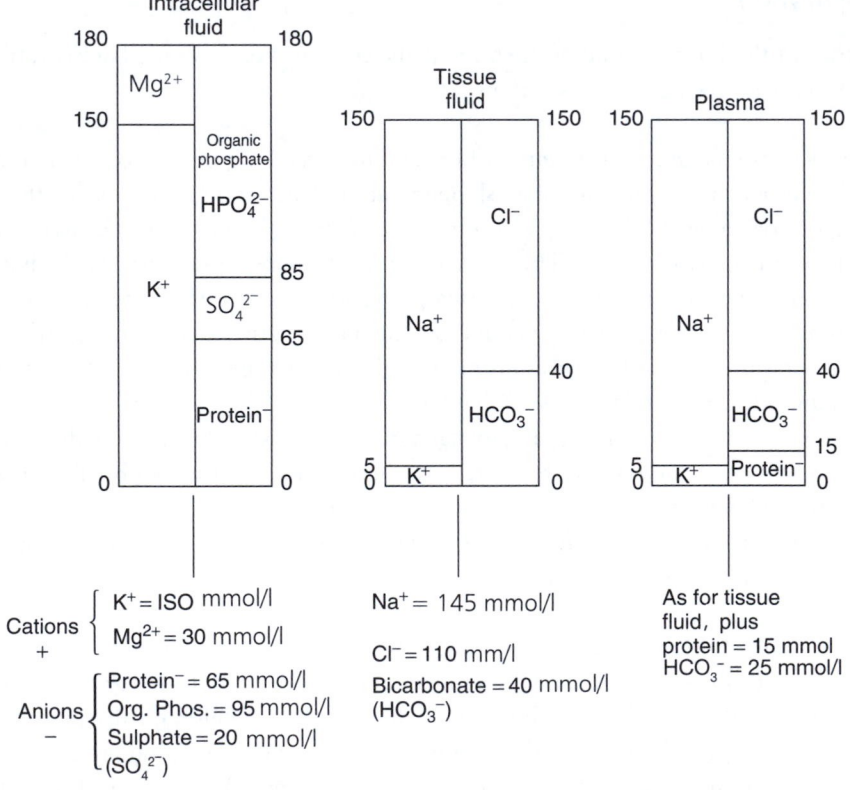

FIGURE 5.8   The relative concentrations and amounts of the major electrolytes are shown in the three body compartments. Values (mmol/l) are in millimoles per litre.

Electrolytes refer to ionised particles in solution. They are usually minerals derived from the diet, such as sodium, potassium and calcium. Ionised means they have either *lost an electron* and as a result taken on a *positive* electrical charge (e.g. **sodium = Na$^+$**), called **cations**, or they have *gained an electron* and as a result gained a *negative* electrical charge (e.g. **chloride = Cl$^-$**), called **anions**. The electrolyte contents and amounts that are found in body fluids are shown in Figure 5.8. From these values, it becomes obvious that the bulk of the potassium is inside the cells (intracellular), while the bulk of the sodium is outside the cells (tissue fluid and blood plasma). Blood plasma also has proteins that carry negative charges and are thus considered to be anions, while intracellular fluid has **organic phosphates (HPO$_4$$^{2-}$)**, which are also negatively charged. Blood and tissue fluid have **bicarbonate (HCO$_3$$^-$)**, which is an electrolyte important in buffering acids (by binding **hydrogen ions, H$^+$**) to prevent excessive acidity.

Some important electrolyte functions include:

- Sodium (Na$^+$) is essential for nerve conduction and water balance (see p. 84).
- Potassium (K$^+$) is also essential for nerve conduction, and is important in muscle contraction (including the heart muscle) and regulation of blood pressure.
- Chloride (Cl$^-$) works in chemical combination with sodium (as **sodium chloride, NaCl**) and with potassium (as **potassium chloride, KCl**). As sodium chloride it is essential for maintenance of fluid balance in blood and extracellular fluids.
- Calcium (Ca^{2+}) is essential for nerve conduction, muscle contraction and blood clotting and as part of the mineralisation of bones and teeth.
- Magnesium (Mg^{2+}) is essential for more than 300 metabolic reactions, including energy production and muscle relaxation between contractions.

Because electrolytes have a wide range of vital functions in the body, electrolyte imbalance causes serious upsets in fluid balance, cardiac and neurological function, acid–base balance, and other cellular functions. Imbalance is caused by many disorders, such as eating problems (malnutrition and starvation, see Chapter 6), dehydration and acidosis, but most important is **renal failure** because it is the kidney's role to regulate the electrolyte levels by eliminating any surplus. Electrolyte imbalance, such as hypernatraemia or hyperchloraemia, can also be the consequence of prolonged or excessive intravenous infusion of sodium chloride. Medical staff must be careful about balancing electrolyte input for those patients on long-term intravenous infusions. Hyperchloraemia may cause an acidosis (excessive acid conditions in the blood and tissue fluids), but this may have some beneficial effect by causing extra download of oxygen from the blood into the cells (see Bohr effect, Chapter 4) (Handy and Soni 2008).

Table 5.1 shows the terms used to describe the various abnormal levels of the major electrolytes and the symptoms that they produce.

TABLE 5.1 Four major electrolytes present in body fluids, the terms used to denote excess and insufficiency, and the symptoms

Electrolyte	Excess	Symptoms of excess	Insufficient	Symptoms of insufficiency
Sodium (Na⁺)	Hypernatraemia	Weakness, irritability, oedema, fits, coma	Hyponatraemia	Headache, confusion, fits, muscle cramps, tiredness, nausea, vomiting, restlessness
Potassium (K⁺)	Hyperkalaemia	Nausea, fatigue, muscle weakness, bradycardia, cardiac arrest	Hypokalaemia	Muscle weakness, aches and cramps, palpitations, cardiac arrhythmias
Chloride (Cl⁻)	Hyperchloraemia	Vomiting, dehydration, diarrhoea, Kussmaul breathing (see Chapter 4), weakness, thirst, possibly acidosis	Hypochloraemia	Vomiting, dehydration, diarrhoea
Magnesium (Mg²⁺)	Hypermagnesaemia	Loss of deep tendon reflexes, flaccid paralysis, apnoea. urinary retention, bradycardia, hypotension	Hypomagnesaemia	Hypokalaemia, hypocalcaemia, tetany, fits, cardiac arrhythmias

Key points

- The body consists of 55–78% water.
- A 70 kg person is carrying about 45 litres of water, about 70% of the body weight.
- Water occupies three body compartments: intracellular, extracellular (tissue fluid) and the blood.
- Water moves down its own concentration gradient, from high concentration to low concentration, a process called osmosis.
- Humans gain water through drinking about 2500 ml per day, with some additional gain from metabolism.
- Humans lose fluids through urine output (about 1500 ml per day), but with additional losses through the skin (400–900 ml per day), respiration (about 400 ml per day) and in faeces (about 100–200 ml per day).

- Fluid balance records the amount of intake and output to see if there is net gain or loss of fluid over a 24-hour period.
- Central venous pressure (CVP) is a measure of the pressure of the venous blood returning to the heart.
- Oedema is excessive fluid in the tissues, causing the tissues to swell.
- There are five causes of oedema: poor venous return, low plasma proteins, excess sodium in the tissues, obstructed lymphatic drainage and increased capillary wall permeability.
- Dehydration is insufficient water in the tissues.
- Dehydration is caused by persistent low oral fluid intake, severe blood loss or uneven water distribution in the tissues.
- Dehydration causes tissues to shrink and the mouth to become dry.
- Dry mouths can get infected, leading to throat, chest, middle ear and even brain infections.
- A dehydrated patient needs regular mouth hygiene to promote oral moisture and to prevent infection.
- Rehydration is required urgently, preferably by mouth, but supplemented by intravenous intake if oral fluids are insufficient or the patient cannot swallow.
- Water balance is linked to electrolyte balance in the three compartments: the cells, tissue fluid and blood.
- Electrolytes are ionised (charged) particles in solution.

References

Handy J. M. and Soni N. (2008) Physiological effects of hyperchloraemia and acidosis. *British Journal of Anaesthesia*, **101** (2): 141–150.

Kreimeier U. (2000) Pathophysiology of fluid imbalance. *Critical Care*, **4** (supplement 2): S3–S7.

Mooney G. P. (2007) Fluid balance. Available at: http://www.nursingtimes.net/199391.article.

Payen D., Cornélie de Pont A., Sakr Y., Spies C., Reinhart K. and Vincent J. L. (2008) A positive fluid balance is associated with a worse outcome in patients with acute renal failure. *Critical Care*, **12**: R74.

Chapter 6 **Nutrition**

- Introduction
- Proteins
- Fats
- Carbohydrates
- Vitamins
- Minerals
- Fibre
- Nutrition in the young and the elderly
- Disorders of nutrition
- Observations of the nutritional state
- Key points
- References

Introduction

Observing the nutritional status of patients involves a number of specific assessments that together will give insight into the dietary needs of the patient. Nutritional assessment often starts with the *diet*, i.e. not just the current diet but the *dietary history*, which is especially important on admission. Information on nutritional status should be ascertained from what the patient and relatives say about the patient's eating habits at home, and whether or not they have been eating a **balanced diet**. This phrase means a diet containing all the necessary daily portions of protein, carbohydrate, fats, fluids and fibre. Vitamin and mineral intake is harder to judge, and if deficiency is suspected, this would require investigation. The patient is weighed and any previous weight loss identified is noted.

Energy is, in a popular sense, thought of as the power and sustainability of muscle action, but energy is much more than this. Every cell needs energy to function, and therefore must produce it. This requires energy-giving foods as a requirement of our daily diet. The process of energy production within cells is discussed in Chapter 1 (see Figure 1.1).

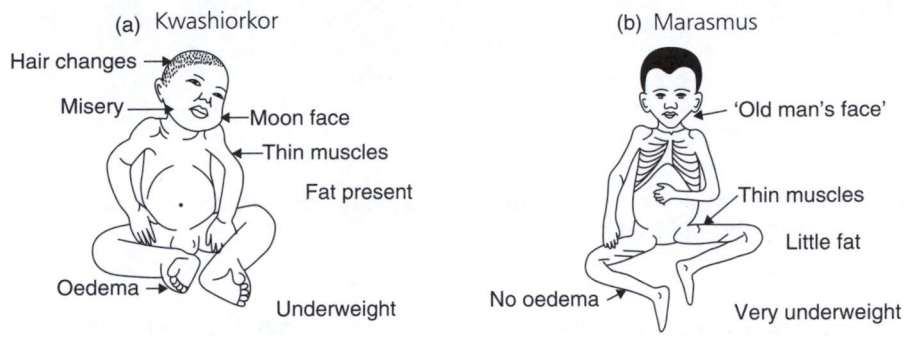

FIGURE 6.1   (a) Kwashiorkor (protein deficiency) and (b) marasmus (energy deficiency) in children.

The energy value of specific foods is measured in **kJ (kilojoules)** or **kcal (kilocalories)**, where 1 kcal = 4.184 kJ. **Energy balance** refers to the person's energy intake compared with their energy use. If the balance is *neutral*, then their energy intake matches their energy use. They neither gain nor lose energy. In *positive* balance the energy intake exceeds the amount used and surplus energy must be stored in the body. This is not a problem in the short term, but persistent and long-term positive balance leads to obesity. In *negative* balance the intake is less than the energy used. Again, in the short term, this is not a problem and the shortfall can be made up. However, in the long term, chronic negative balance leads to severe weight loss and can result in death. The body uses glucose (a simple carbohydrate) as the *first-line energy* source, but if this is not available (e.g. due to a poor diet of low-energy foods) the body turns to fats as a *secondary* source of energy. Ultimately, and as a last resort, protein from skeletal muscle can be used as an energy source. This only happens in critical situations, for example, in severe ill health when the patient is deteriorating towards the end of life. **Marasmus** (Figure 6.1b) is a disorder of negative energy balance, where there is a lack of energy (low calorie) intake, seen mostly in very young children. It causes depletion of glucose and fat stores in the body, and this leads to muscle wasting. There is severe weight loss and failure of growth. This is a long-term chronic disorder because it takes time to convert, first, fat, then muscle to energy. Equally, it takes time to replenish the energy stores, therefore treatment improves the condition gradually.

Proteins

Proteins are the body's source of **nitrogen** (see protein energy source, Chapter 1). Since the body is largely made from protein (proteins are a component of just about every body tissue, including blood), it makes sense that we need a regular daily intake of protein to satisfy demands made by cells during metabolism, cell replacement, tissue growth and repair. Proteins are made from **amino acids**, which contain an **amino group** (NH_2), a **carboxyl group** (**COOH**) and a **radical group** that differs from one amino acid type to another (Figure 6.2).

Proteins, as part of our diet, are reduced by digestive enzymes to 23 different types of amino acids (see Table 6.1) and these are absorbed into the blood. The liver uses a large number of amino acids to produce blood proteins (largely **albumin**) and also stores many more amino

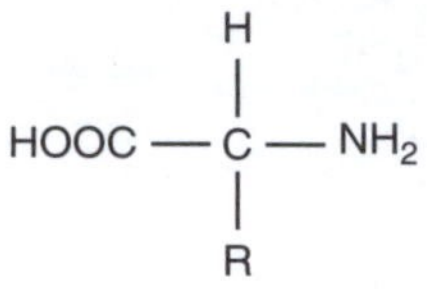

$$HOOC - \underset{\underset{R}{|}}{\overset{\overset{H}{|}}{C}} - NH_2$$

FIGURE 6.2 The amino acid molecule with an amino group (NH$_2$), a carboxyl group (COOH) and a variable radical (R).

TABLE 6.1 Essential and non-essential amino acids. Essential means they must be present in the diet because the liver cannot synthesise them. Non-essential amino acids can be synthesised by the liver if they are lacking in the diet

Essential	Non-essential	
Isoleucine	Alanine	Selenocysteine
Leucine	Asparagine	Serine
Lysine	Aspartic acid	Tyrosine
Methionine	Cysteine	Arginine
Phenylalanine	Glutamic acid	Histidine
Threonine	Glutamine	Ornithine
Tryptophan	Glycine	Taurine
Valine	Proline	

acids (known as the liver's **amino acid pool**). The liver has some ability to convert one amino acid type to another type as the body requires. Human proteins are assembled inside the body's cells by the process called **protein synthesis**, using the **deoxyribonucleic acid (DNA)** code provided by the genetics of the cell. Each individual **gene** codes for one type of protein, which will be any of the wide range of possible proteins:

- **hormones**, which regulate tissue function;
- **antibodies**, which fight infections;
- **enzymes**, which drive cellular metabolism;
- **plasma proteins**, which have multiple functions in the blood;
- **structural proteins**, which build and support the body, and many other protein types.

It is evident from this that a shortage of protein in the diet results in a severe lack of amino acids and therefore an inability for the cells to sustain protein synthesis. This causes disturbed metabolism, poor hormonal function, high risk of infections, potential structural weaknesses and multiple other problems. On a chronic (i.e. long-term) basis this causes a condition known as **kwashiorkor** (Figures 6.1a and 6.3). In this disorder, the deficiency is mainly protein, but vitamin deficiency may also be present. A significant stress level is also involved in the cause of this disorder. The symptoms include moon-shaped face, oedema

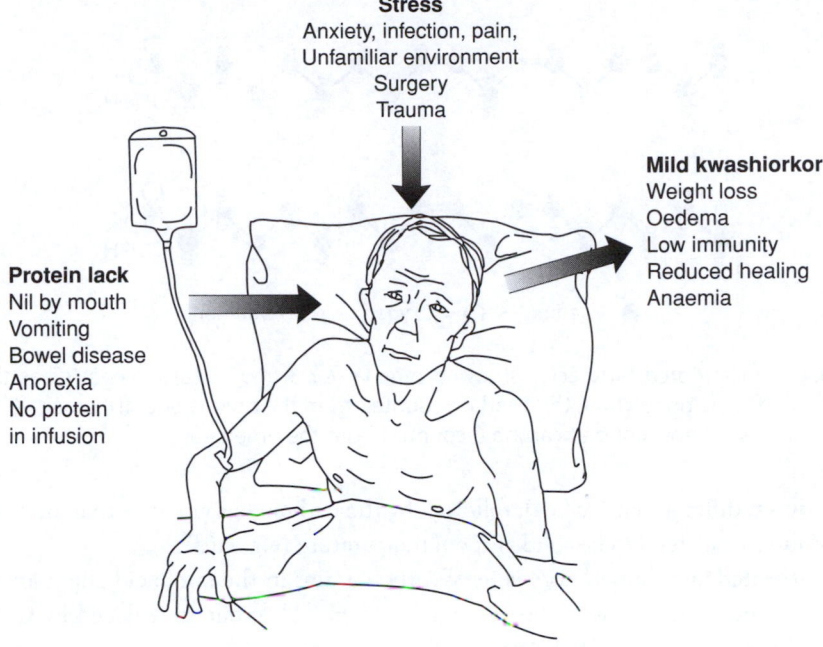

Stress
Anxiety, infection, pain,
Unfamiliar environment
Surgery
Trauma

Mild kwashiorkor
Weight loss
Oedema
Low immunity
Reduced healing
Anaemia

Protein lack
Nil by mouth
Vomiting
Bowel disease
Anorexia
No protein
in infusion

FIGURE 6.3   Mild kwashiorkor in hospital patients, due to protein lack and stress.

due to low blood proteins (see Chapter 5), growth and mental development are retarded, muscle wasting with retained fat, poor immunity which increases the risk of infections, delayed wound healing, anaemia, hair loss, mild weight loss and liver degeneration.

A mild form of kwashiorkor could be happening in some patients in hospital. Contributing to this are the fact that hospital patients may have insufficient dietary intake, especially protein, due to nausea and vomiting, prolonged periods of nil by mouth or anorexia. Added to this is the presence of stress, mostly from pain, surgery, abrupt change of environment on admission, infection and injury. Protein deficiency in hospitalised patients will delay healing, especially wounds and fractures, and allow increased risk of infections. Assessment of the nutritional status of the hospitalised patient should consider the possibility that they may be lacking protein.

Fats

Fats are our *second-line energy* source (see Chapter 1) and are made from carbon, hydrogen and oxygen. Fats are **triglycerides**, that is, molecules composed of a glycerol backbone to which is attached three **fatty acids** (Figure 6.4). Fatty acids are long chains of carbon atoms ending in a carboxyl group, COOH (which can liberate hydrogen and hence is acidic).

Saturated fatty acids have the general formula $CH_3(CH_2)_nCOOH$, indicating that a carbon atom with three attached hydrogen atoms occupies one end of the molecule and is followed by a chain of n carbons each with two attached hydrogens (where the number n

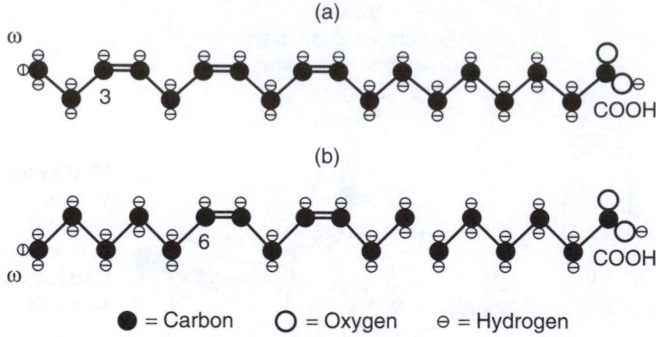

FIGURE **6.4**   Unsaturated fatty acids showing omega (ω) 3 and 6. (a) Omega 3 has the first double bond at the third carbon counted from the omega end; (b) omega 6 has the first double bond at carbon 6 counted from the omega end.

varies between different fatty acids), followed by the carboxyl group. Fats that are based on saturated fatty acids tend to be solid at room temperature (e.g. lard).

In **unsaturated** fats, one or more pairs of carbon atoms in the fatty acid chain are linked by a double rather than a single bond (that is, a CH_2CH_2 group is replaced by CH=CH, with two fewer hydrogens). Thus, 'saturated' means that all the carbons are saturated with hydrogen, while 'unsaturated means that some carbons are missing hydrogen. In a **mono-unsaturated** fatty acid, only one carbon–carbon single bond is replaced by a double bond; in a **poly-unsaturated** fatty acid, this occurs at more than one place in the carbon chain. Poly-unsaturated fats tend to be liquid at room temperature (e.g. oils, such as cooking oil).

In an unsaturated fatty acid, the **omega** (ω) count indicates the position of the first double bond in the chain, counted from the end furthest from the carboxyl group (the omega end), which is the end that is most stable during physiological reactions (Figure 6.4). In a triglyceride molecule, the omega end is furthest from the glycerol backbone (Figure 6.5). Table 6.2 shows two typical examples.

Fats are essential in the diet because from them are derived the steroid hormones (e.g. cortisol, the oestrogens, the testosterones and others), structural fats (e.g. cell membranes

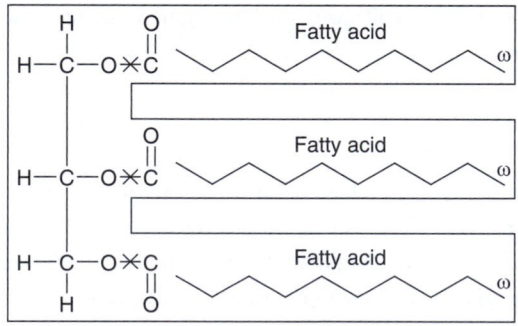

FIGURE **6.5**   The triglyceride molecule consists of three fatty acids attached to a glycerol backbone. The free ends of the fatty acids are the omega (ω) ends.

TABLE **6.2** Eicosapentaenoic acid (EPA) and linoleic acid, showing omega numbers

Fatty acid	Molecule	Omega
Eicosapentaenoic acid (EPA)		Omega 3
Linoleic acid		Omega 6

and adipose tissue) and cytokines (cell signalling molecules), and because they allow the intake of fat-soluble vitamins (i.e. vitamins A, D, E and K). Generally, the healthier option is to reduce the intake of saturated fats and make up the difference with unsaturated fats. This is because saturated fats have been linked to obesity and to coronary arterial disease, which causes potentially fatal heart disorders.

Carbohydrates

Similar to fats, carbohydrates are made from carbon, hydrogen and oxygen. The difference is that the hydrogen and oxygen have the same ratio as water, i.e. two hydrogen for every oxygen (2H:O). Carbohydrates, therefore, could be viewed as *hydrated carbon* (hence the name). They exist at three levels of complexity:

1   **Monosaccharides** are simple sugars made from three to seven carbons bonded to hydrogen and oxygen. They may exist in straight line or ring structures. **Glucose** is the best-known monosaccharide in human physiology as it is the *first-line energy* source used in cellular metabolism (see Chapter 1).

2   **Oligosaccharides** are more complex molecules made from various numbers of monosaccharide sub-units bonded together. The simplest oligosaccharides are the **disaccharides**, sugars that are built from two monosaccharides (di = two), e.g. **maltose**, made from two glucose molecules, and **sucrose**, made from one glucose and one **fructose**. Sucrose (disaccharide) is table sugar, maltose (disaccharide) is a constituent of malt (see Figure 6.6) and fructose (monosaccharide) is fruit sugar. More complex oligosaccharides consist of three or more monosaccharide molecules, and these are found commonly in plants. As such, they occur regularly in the human diet. Some of these can be digested by humans, other cannot. The undigested molecules become dietary fibre (see the section on fibre).

3   **Polysaccharides** (also known as **glycans**) are the most complex and the most common carbohydrate structures found in nature. They are built from multiple monosaccharide sub-units, of which glucose is the most common. Polysaccharides are important in humans as energy storage as well as structural and protective components. **Starch** is a well-known form of polysaccharide that comes in two forms: **amylose** and **amylopectin**. Plants

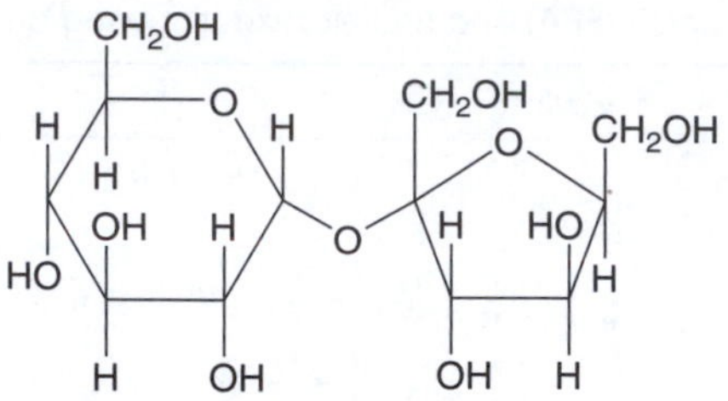

FIGURE 6.6 Disaccharides. (a) sucrose; (b) maltose. Sucrose is made from a combination of a glucose (shown here on the left) and a fructose molecule (on the right). Maltose is made from a combination of two glucose molecules.

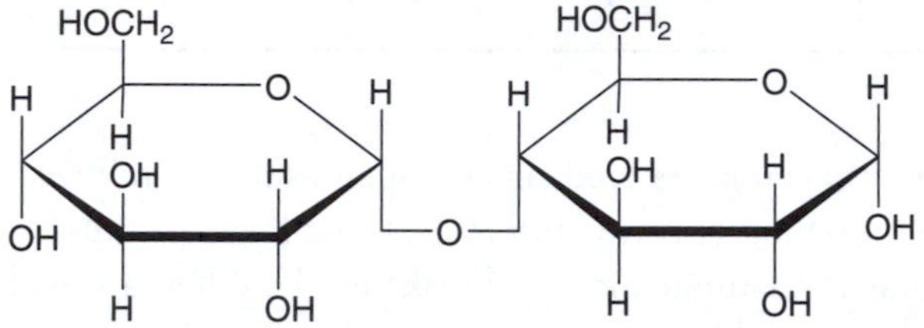

store starch and therefore it is eaten regularly in the human diet. Digestive enzymes break down starch, starting in the mouth with the enzyme **salivary amylase**, a component of saliva. **Glycogen** is the main energy storage in humans. It is a polysaccharide made from vast numbers of **glucose** molecules linked together. It is found in the liver and skeletal muscles, the two structures that need high energy levels, and it can be broken down by enzymes to release glucose, which is used to provide cellular energy and to stabilise blood sugar levels. **Cellulose** is one of nature's most common structural polysaccharides, being a major component of plants. Because it is found in plant cell walls, it becomes another component of our diet. However, cellulose cannot be digested in humans by our enzymic action, and it therefore becomes a major part of our fibre intake (see the section on fibre). Normal bacteria in the digestive system of some animals (i.e. the ruminants such as cattle) can digest cellulose, releasing glucose that the animal can then absorb. Many human structural polysaccharides are bonded to protein or lipid molecules.

Vitamins

The word **vitamin** comes from the two words 'vital amine'. Two aspects make vitamins a cohesive group of nutrients:

1   Vitamins are organic nutrients required in small quantities, unlike proteins and carbohydrates, which are required in much larger daily amounts.
2   Vitamins are necessary in the diet since the body cannot synthesise them for itself.

Having said that, there are 13 different organic compounds that carry out a wide range of diverse functions in the body. They all have a name but are given a letter of the alphabet for convenience (e.g. ascorbic acid is vitamin C), but several of these vitamins include a number of closely related compounds, of which one is usually the active form and the others can be converted to this active form (e.g. vitamins A and D). Some vitamins are water-soluble (e.g. the eight vitamins of the B group and C), and others are fat-soluble (e.g. vitamins A, D, E and K). Table 6.3 shows details of the main vitamins in the human diet, including the important vitamin deficiency disorders.

Minerals

Minerals are inorganic chemical elements required in the diet in varying amounts, some in quite small daily amounts (called **trace elements**). They are essential because the body cannot produce them for itself. Table 6.4 gives details of the main minerals elements required by the body, including the important disorders and symptoms linked to excess or deficiency of these minerals.

Minerals are usually consumed in compound form, i.e. two or more mineral elements bound together chemically, e.g. NaCl (sodium chloride). In this form they are usually electrically neutral, i.e. they have no charge. In the body, these compounds are often dissolved in water (e.g. in blood and tissue fluid), where they normally disassociate (i.e. break up) into their component elements. In this process, each of the two elements takes on a charge, for example, in the dissociation of sodium chloride, $NaCl \rightarrow Na^+ + Cl^-$, where sodium loses an electron and becomes a positively charged **ion** (a **cation**) Na^+, while chlorine gains an electron and becomes a negatively charged ion (an **anion**) Cl^-. These are now **electrolytes**, that is, charged particles in solution. In the body, the vast majority of electrolytes are minerals (with some exceptions), e.g. sodium, potassium (K^+), chlorine, magnesium (Mg^{2+}) and calcium (Ca^{2+}). Notice that magnesium and calcium have a double-positive charge because they each lose two electrons when their compounds dissociate (rather than a single electron in the case of sodium and potassium). **Electrolyte balance** is the term used in stabilising electrolytes levels within normal limits in the body. Ill health can be caused by disturbance of electrolyte levels in the blood and tissue fluids: either excess or deficiency of one or more electrolytes. The symptoms of this **electrolyte imbalance** depend on several factors, e.g. which element is involved and if the problem is too much or not enough of that element. Table 6.4 shows the main electrolyte imbalances and their symptoms. Electrolyte imbalance can be caused by:

- body fluid loss as a result of prolonged vomiting, diarrhoea, excessive sweating or high fever;
- poor diet including inadequate minerals, vitamin and fluid intake;
- poor absorption of these nutrients;
- endocrine (hormone) disorders;
- renal disease, because the kidney normally regulates electrolyte levels by excreting the excess, or conserving electrolytes if they are low, and this function may be lost in kidneys disorders;
- some drugs, e.g. diuretics (which promote electrolyte loss) and hydrocortisone.

TABLE 6.3 The major vitamins, food sources, need and deficiency

Vitamin	Full name	Food source	Vitamin needed for	Effects from lack of vitamin
A	Retinol	Liver, fish liver oils, butter, cream, cheese, whole milk, egg yolk	Growth, vision, healthy tissues, immunity	Night blindness, dry and itching skin, reduced taste, bone growth failure
B_1	Thiamine	Yeast, cereals, legumes	Heart and circulation, growth, nervous system, energy	**Beriberi** (fatigue, low appetite, weight loss, muscle wasting, diarrhoea, heart failure, oedema, paralysis), plus parasthesia, **depression**
B_2	Riboflavin	Cereals, yeast, milk, eggs, green vegetable leaves, lean meat	Healthy skin, tissue healing, immunity, red blood cells	**Cheilosis** (oral cracks and fissures, scaling of lips), sore tongue (**glossitis**), sensitivity to light (**photophobia**), and **dermatitis**
B_3	Niacin or nicotinic acid	Yeast, liver, kidney, meat, cereals, green vegetables and bran	Energy, skin, nervous system, cell metabolism	Weakness, skin rash, memory loss irritability, insomnia, **Pellagra**: (dermatitis, glossitis, diarrhoea, mental disturbance e.g. depression, confusion, hallucinations, delirium, leading to death)
B_5	Pantothenic acid	All plant and animal food; especially eggs, kidney, liver, salmon, yeast	Energy production, immunity, hormones	Weakness, depression, low infection resistance
B_6	Pyridoxine	Pork, organ meats, fish, corn, legumes, seeds, grains, wheat, leafy vegetables, green beans, bananas	Protein metabolism, haemoglobin, nervous system	Fatigue, nervous dysfunction, anaemia, irritability, skin lesions
B_9	Folic acid	Green leafy vegetables, liver, beef, fish, lentils, asparagus, broccoli	RBC maturation, growth, healthy tissues	Anaemia, neural tube defects during very early pregnancy

B$_{12}$	Cyanocobalamin	Only from animal foods, liver, meat, milk, eggs, oysters	RBC (haemoglobin), growth, nervous system	**Pernicious anaemia** (fatigue, glossitis, nerve degeneration)
B$_{15}$	Pangamic acid	Sesame seeds, pumpkin seeds, whole brown rice, liver, organ meats	Unknown function	No deficiency symptoms known
B-factor	Choline	Yeast, milk, eggs, wheat germ, soya, organ meats	Nerve transmission, liver, cell membranes	Growth problems, reduced liver and nerve function
B-factor	Inositol	Milk, yeast, meat, fruit, nuts	Nerve transmission, fat metabolism	Eye problems, constipation, hair loss
C	Ascorbic acid	Citrus fruits, strawberries, tomatoes, cabbage, potatoes, parsley, broccoli, sweet peppers	Collagen maturity, wound healing, maintains healthy gums, skin, immunity and blood	Bruising, slow wound healing, anaemia, gingivitis, **Scurvy** (fatigue and bleeding, later gum disorder)
D	Calciferol	Milk, fish oil, liver, butter, egg yolk, and ultraviolet light (UVL) in sunlight acting on skin	Absorption of calcium from the diet, good bones and teeth	**Rickets** (children: soft bent and fragile bones, deformity), **Osteomalacia** (adults: soft and painful bones, fractures)
E	Tocopherol	Vegetable oil, whole grains, wheat germ, egg yolk	Antioxidant, maintenance of circulation and cell protection	Poor muscle performance and circulation, RBC haemolysis
F	Unsaturated fatty acids	All sources of unsaturated fatty acids	Skin, blood and glandular products	**Acne**, allergies, dry skin, brittle hair, **eczema**, brittle nails
H	Biotin	Liver, meat, eggs, nuts, milk, most vegetables, tomatoes, grapefruit, water melon and strawberries	Skin, blood circulation, metabolism	**Depression**, anorexia and non-specific skin rashes
K	Menadione	Lettuce, spinach, cauliflower, cabbage, egg yolk, soya bean oil, liver	Blood clotting mechanism	Bleeding and diarrhoea
P	Bioflavonoids	Fruit, especially citrus	Healthy blood vessel walls	Bleeding and bruising, colds, **eczema**

TABLE 6.4 The major minerals

Mineral (chemical symbol)	Mineral function	Food source	Effects from lack of mineral
Calcium (Ca)	Bones, teeth, muscle and nerve function, blood clotting mechanism	Milk and other milk products	Weak bones and teeth, weak muscles, bleeding, poor nerve function Severe loss of blood calcium levels causes **tetany** (a state of continuous muscle contraction)
Chromium (Cr)	Glucose metabolism, amino acid transportation, blood lipid and glucose levels	Full cream milk, seafood (e.g. oysters), wholegrain, cheese, fresh fruit, nuts, vegetables, brewer's yeast and variable amounts in water	Glucose imbalance, impaired growth, obesity, tiredness, increased cancer risk, heart disease and diabetes
Copper (Cu)	Haemoglobin in blood, collagen, heart function, energy production, iron absorption	Grains, nuts, liver, oysters and legumes	Anaemia, muscle weakness, abnormal collagen synthesis, neurological defects
Iodine (I)	Thyroid hormones	Seafood	Low thyroid hormone levels, goitre, cretinism, **myxoedema**
Iron (Fe)	Haemoglobin in blood, immunity, brain function	Liver, shellfish, oysters, lean meat, poultry, kidney, fish, beans and vegetables	**Anaemia**, attention and learning difficulties, increased risk of infections
Magnesium (Mg)	Nerve and muscle function, bone formation	Leafy green vegetables, nuts, wholegrain, peas, beans, dairy products, fish, cereals, legumes, meats	Weakness, dizziness, abdominal distension, convulsions
Manganese (Mn)	Involved in calcium and phosphorus metabolism and bone formation	Legumes, nuts, wholegrain cereal, tea, green leafy vegetables	No specific deficiency syndrome identified
Phosphorus (P)	Bones and teeth, energy production, DNA formation, metabolism	Meat, poultry, fish, eggs, peanuts	Serious problems with the nerve supply to muscles; skeletal, blood and kidney problems

Mineral	Function	Food sources	Deficiency/excess
Potassium (K)	Intracellular electrolyte, factor in nerve conduction	Bananas, oranges, grapefruit juice, melons, nectarines, prunes, pears, avocados, cucumbers, potatoes, peas, beans, tomatoes, nuts, legumes, seeds, milk products, meats of all kinds	Fatigue, depression, weakness, heart irregularities, dry skin, low blood pressure, oedema, muscle cramps
Selenium (Se)	Antioxidant, heart muscle, fat metabolism, tissue elasticity	Cereals, Brazil nuts, wholegrains, seafood, meat, poultry, fish, dairy products	Increased risk of cancer, myalgia (muscle pain) and muscle tenderness, heart disease (e.g. **Keshan disease** in China) and premature ageing
Sodium (Na)	Extracellular electrolyte, factor in fluid balance, blood pressure, muscle contraction, nerve conduction	Found widely in the diet, especially table salt, animal foods, processed foods	Deficiency very rare
Zinc (Zn)	Gene expression in tissue growth/repair, cell reproduction, child growth, sperm and testosterone	Meat, poultry, fish, oysters, eggs, legumes, nuts, milk, yoghurt, wholegrain cereals	Rare **acrodermatitis enteropathica** (rash over face, anus and distal parts), growth retardation in children, anorexia with diarrhoea, poor wound healing, depression, reduced reproductive ability

Fibre

Dietary fibre (sometimes called **roughage**) is a mix of large molecules in the diet which remain largely unchanged throughout the digestive system, and therefore are not absorbed, and so provide no direct nutritional value. By remaining in the digestive system, they become a major component of faeces (see Chapter 8). The term *fibre* includes some **oligosaccharides** and many of the **polysaccharides** (e.g. **cellulose**, **hemicellulose** and **pectin**) and also **lignin** (the tough component of wood but also found in plant stalks, etc.), and **gums**, which are also mostly derived from plant foods. Bacteria, normally present in the digestive tract (known as the **intestinal flora**), are *commensals* of the colon and caecum (commensals are harmless, even useful, organisms active in specific body sites). They are able to break down some of the fibre. These bacteria synthesise some nutrients, notably **niacin (nicotinic acid)**, **thiamine (vitamin B$_1$)** and **vitamin K**, which we can then absorb and use (fibre is covered in more detail in Chapter 8).

Nutrition in the young and the elderly

Nutrition in the young

The pre-school child from birth up to about 6 months old should be fed with breast milk preferably, or given formula (bottle) food if breast feeding is not an option. Children this young cannot cope well with fibre in their diet, and fibre increases the risk of malabsorption of nutrients. Therefore fibre in the diet should be avoided. Generally children aged from 6 months can be weaned onto more solid foods, although the actual age may vary between different children. Children should avoid certain foods at certain ages (see Table 6.5). Adequate nutrients to sustain growth is essential throughout childhood, especially during growth spurts when an increased rate of cell division and energy use puts greater demands on the diet.

In schoolchildren aged 5 years to teenage, growth rates slow down a little until the teenage growth spurt starts somewhere between 11 and 13 years old. Energy requirements reflect these changes in growth rate, for example:

- A boy aged 1 year requires about 234.3 kJ/kg/day (56 kcal/kg/day).
- A boy aged 10 years requires about 159 kJ/kg/day (38 kcal/kg/day).

These figures are given in kJ/kg/day = kilojoules per kilogramme per day; and kcal/kg/day = kilocalories per kilogramme per day. They reflect growth requirements, and variations in activity levels would add to these figures. Iron deficiency appears to be the most common dietary problem in adolescence, aggravated in girls by the onset of menstruation. Iron from animal sources is better absorbed than iron from plant sources, a point to consider in vegetarian diets. The addition of vitamin C and extra protein helps in iron absorption. During

TABLE 6.5 Foods young children should avoid

Food that should be avoided	Reason
High fibre	High fibre in a child's diet increases the risk of malabsorption of nutrients and may possibly lead to constipation or obstruction. Small children's bowels cannot cope with much fibre, and very young babies should have very low fibre content.
Honey	Honey may have spores of dangerous organisms.
Refined carbohydrates	Refined sugars (table sugar, sweets, etc.) release energy rapidly, which then triggers insulin release and the blood sugar then falls quickly. This destabilises blood sugar levels. Unrefined carbohydrates (e.g. potatoes, bread, pasta and rice) release energy gradually, which does not trigger a large insulin release and the blood sugar is better controlled.
Peanut butter	Any thick, sticky and oily food such as peanut butter may be hard for children to eat and swallow.
Cow's milk	Under 12 months of age, cow's milk is inappropriate and children should be preferably breast fed or given a baby formula food. The reason is that cow's milk contains proteins that small babies cannot digest and has mineral levels too high for immature kidneys to cope with. Over 12 months, children need the fat and calories found in whole milk for growth, so low-fat milk is inappropriate.

the adolescent growth spurt, the skeleton requires a great deal of calcium. This is because the skeleton stores 99% of the body's calcium, and 45% of the adult bone mass is added during the teenage years. The biggest gains in bone mass occur between 10 to 14 years in girls, and between 12 to 15 years in boys. About 30% of the dietary calcium is absorbed, and retention of calcium in the body is about 200 mg/day in girls and about 300 mg/day in boys. In children, and in adults, unrefined carbohydrates (e.g. bread, potatoes) are better than refined sugars (as in table sugar and sweets) because unrefined carbohydrates release glucose slowly, and thus sustain energy over longer periods, than do the refined sugars which release glucose rapidly for short periods only.

Nutrition in the elderly

In the elderly, the advancing years provide three reasons why energy food consumption should be reduced:

1 A reduction in physical activity results in the need for less energy-rich food.
2 The lean (protein) body mass declines, mainly protein in skeletal muscle, and this results in reduced muscle activity and therefore lower energy requirement.
3 The gradual reduction in the **basal metabolic rate (BMR)** also leads to lower energy requirement.

Table 6.6 shows an example of the energy input reduction expected with advancing years.

TABLE 6.6 Energy requirements at different ages

Male Age (years)	Kilocalories per day	Female Age (years)	Kilocalories per day
19–24	3000	19–24	2100
50–74	2300	50–74	1800
75+	2000	75+	1500

Diet containing high-energy foods continued into older age would result in chronic positive energy intake and this could lead to weight increase, even obesity. However, protein requirements in adults of all ages remains about the same, i.e. about 57 g/day for men, 41 g/day for women. Fat gradually increases as stored adipose tissue with age, e.g. around the abdomen in men, and on the buttocks and thighs in women. Adipose deposited around internal organs in either sex may increase the risk of cardiac problems. Vitamin and mineral requirements remain about the same in all adults, the two exceptions being in women, where *less* iron but *more* calcium is required after menopause:

- **Iron**: pre-menopause (especially during menstruation) = 14 mg/day, post-menopause = 7 mg/day; since no further menstrual blood loss after menopause means less iron loss.
- **Calcium**: pre-menopausal requirement = 700 mg/day; post-menopausal requirement = 800–1000 mg/day, to help prevent thinning of the bone mass (**osteoporosis**), which otherwise may lead to fractures.

Reduced digestive enzymes, gastric acidity and bowel movements all occur with age, but not normally enough to cause any degree of malnutrition provided the diet is adequate. Absorption of all the major nutrients from the bowel is good well into old age. If malnutrition is occurring in an older patient, it may be caused by poor diet. If so, this could be due to a diet of high carbohydrate and low protein, because carbohydrate foods are cheaper to buy than protein. However, some simple observations may reveal other factors involved, such as dental losses, poor salivation (which can be due to dehydration, see Chapter 5), and mouth infections due to poor oral hygiene (see Chapter 5). General ill health may also be a cause, especially when patients are unable to get out for shopping or they lack the fitness or motivation to cook. Constipation, which is often common in the elderly, may be an important, but relatively easily treated, cause of loss of appetite.

Disorders of nutrition

Weight loss

Weight loss may be due to dehydration in the first instance if the patient does not drink enough. Additional weight loss can initially involve body fat losses, followed later by protein reduction in the form of **muscle wasting**. However, not all weight loss is due to poor dietary intake. Sometimes pathological changes in the body metabolism result in reduced body mass from muscle wasting, severe weight loss, weakness and fatigue, anorexia, immobility, and anaemia. The term **cachexia** refers to this moribund state of metabolic malfunction and it is usually found in terminally ill patients or those who fail to absorb nutrients. Cachexia puts the patient's life at great risk, and it cannot easily be reversed, even by giving nutrition, either by mouth or other route. It therefore most often becomes a terminal state, and it is usually seen in diseases such incurable cancer or acquired immune deficiency syndrome (AIDS). This is not the same as **starvation**. Cachexia patients tend to respond poorly, or not at all, to the administration of nutrition, while giving nutrition will reverse starvation and restore health in most cases. In starvation, the immediate problem faced by the body is to get energy nutrient to the cells and tissues before they malfunction and die. Glucose and glycogen stores are quite quickly used up (i.e. within 24 hours), and the body starts to use other stored energy sources, notably fatty acids and glycerol from triglycerides stored in adipose tissue (see p. 6). Both ketone production (see **ketoacidosis**, Chapter 7) and fatty acid levels in the blood become increased (i.e. **hyperlipidaemia**) as stored fats are mobilised by enzymes to provide energy. If the patient reaches the point where all the fat has been used, the body is now at crisis point, and must then turn to using amino acids from proteins for energy. The process of using amino acids for energy first involves using up the stored amino acids in the liver (the amino acid pool), then finally releasing amino acids from both skeletal and smooth muscle, a **catabolic** process (see p. 133) causing muscle wastage and organ dysfunction.

Anorexia and **bulimia** are two eating disorders that often result in nutritional problems. Anorexia is a failure to consume adequate nutrients and is seen most often in young women. They starve themselves and therefore lack many of the vital nutrients, especially energy and protein. Recent work has shown that there is an important element of chronic stress involved in the cause of this disorder, although this may not always be identified or admitted by the patient. Bulimia is an eating disorder where the patient has food binges during which they eat all they can. This is followed by a period of guilt feelings during which they make efforts to recover the food by inducing vomiting or by using laxatives. There are often periods of normal eating between bouts of binge eating. The biology of food intake regulation is very complex and not entirely understood, consequently not much is known about the pathophysiology of these eating disorders, especially bulimia (Blows 2011a, 2011b). The two best-known control mechanisms, both involving the hypothalamus, are shown in Figure 6.7.

Weight gain: obesity

Described as an epidemic in some countries, obesity appears to be on the increase, particularly in the Western world. Anyone having a **body mass index** (**BMI**) greater than 30 (see p. 7) is considered as having clinical obesity. It is the result of chronic consumption of excess calorific food coupled with inadequate energy expenditure (i.e. a state of long-term positive energy balance, see p. 91). The biological causes of obesity have been largely unknown because the biology of food intake regulation and the eating–satiety cycle have been poorly understood until relatively recently. Now these cycles are gradually getting better known (Figure 6.7), we have some limited understanding of the possible genetic causes, i.e. the gene mutations that upset the feeding–satiety cycle and thus promote eating (Blows 2011b). Table 6.7 lists the genes and their possible role in promoting weight gain.

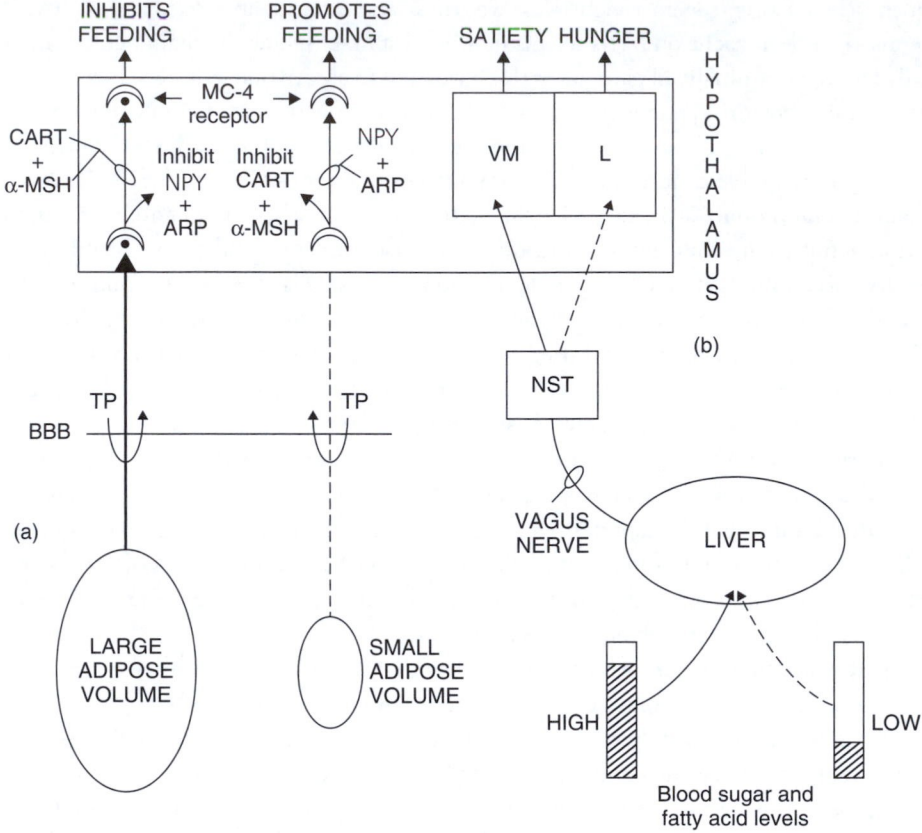

FIGURE 6.7 Two of the major pathways for regulating food intake.

(a) Large adipose mass produces bigger volumes (thick arrow) of a hormone called **leptin** than small adipose volumes (broken arrow) in the body. Leptin must be transported across the blood–brain barrier (BBB) by a transport protein (TP) before entering the hypothalamus. Leptin binds to the leptin receptor in the hypothalamus. If a substantial quantity of leptin is available for binding, this will cause the production of two hormones – cocaine-and amphetamine-regulated transcript (CART) and alpha-melanocyte-stimulating hormone (α-MSH) – which bind to the MC-4 receptor and this inhibits feeding. At the same time two other substances – neuropeptide Y (NPY) and agouti-related protein (ARP) – are inhibited. If there is very little leptin to bind, this will cause the production of ARP and NPY, which bind to the MC-4 receptor and these promote feeding. At the same time CART and α-MSH are inhibited. This is a long-term regulator of feeding behaviour, acting over a period of months or years.

(b) The liver monitors the blood fatty acid and glucose levels, and sends this information via the vagus nerve to the nucleus of the solitary tract (NST) within the brain stem. If the blood levels are high (as after a meal), the NST sends this information to the ventromedial nucleus (VM) of the hypothalamus (solid line), and this nucleus causes satiety (a feeling of fullness). If the blood levels are low (as before a meal), the NST sends this information to the lateral nucleus (L) of the hypothalamus (broken line) and this nucleus causes hunger. Hormones such as **orexin** act in the lateral nucleus to cause hunger and thus feeding. This is a short-term regulator of feeding behaviour acting over a period of minutes or hours.

TABLE 6.7 Gene mutations possibly involved in weight gain. This table should be viewed in conjunction with Figure 6.7

Gene	Possible role for gene mutation in obesity
Leptin gene (Ob gene)	May produce a leptin type that does not activate the leptin receptor very well
Leptin receptor gene (Db gene)	May produce a receptor that does not respond to leptin very well
Leptin transporter gene	May produce a transporter protein that does not transport leptin across the blood–brain barrier
MC-4 receptor gene	May produce MC-4 receptors that do not function properly
Orexin gene	May cause orexin to stimulate increased amounts of food intake
UCP2 gene	May cause malfunction of energy production and thus contribute to obesity

The problems and complications associated with obesity are:

- *Increased mortality* due to the serious medical conditions linked to being overweight. These are **hypertension**, **myocardial infarction**, **angina pectoris** and **congestive cardiac failure (CCF)**. Obesity puts a lot of strain on the heart. Obesity carries a 20% increase in sudden death when compared with those of normal weight.
- *Increased metabolic disorders* such as diabetes and gout.
- *Musculo-skeletal problems* such as joint disorders (**osteoarthritis**) and flat feet.
- *Respiratory problems*, as the ribs may be impeded, thus making breathing more difficult.
- *Accidents* are more common due to balance and movement co-ordination difficulties.
- *Poor surgical risk*, which means obese patients carry a greater risk of dying under anaesthesia and may suffer more complications following surgery.

Nutritional deficiencies

For the most part, normal diets will supply all the nutrients required by the body for its daily needs. However, apart from areas of the world where food is in short supply, deficiencies of all kinds in the diet can, and sometimes do, occur in hospital patients for many reasons. The patient may be nil by mouth (NBM) for quite some time, and dextrose or saline intravenous infusions provide very few nutrients, and certainly no amino acids. Vomiting (see p. 138) and pain will reduce the appetite, and digestive disorders may make feeding or digestion difficult. Some hospital patients, especially the frail, may suffer a mild degree of kwashiorkor (see p. 93), i.e. a lack of protein accompanied by stress. Inadequate food intake and the stress of admission, pain, investigations and surgery all contribute to this condition. It is important that the nurse recognises that vitamin and mineral deficiencies (Tables 6.3 and 6.4), dehydration (see Chapter 5) and a lack of fibre can also occur in hospitals.

Observations of the nutritional state

More than 50 published screening tools are now available for nurses to assess the patient's nutritional status (Bell 2007; Perry 2009). While at home or in hospital, the simplest observations are often the best, e.g.

- Ensure that the patient is physically able to eat, e.g. they can hold and use cutlery adequately, can they can chew properly or do they need assistance?
- Ensure that the patient eats adequately and drinks enough to sustain fluid balance, including if required, a measurement of the calorific and protein intake per 24 hours.
- Observe the patient's mouth daily to assess the state of cleanliness and to identify any oral infections or dry, cracking of the mouth corners or lips that may cause pain on eating, and may therefore reduce the appetite. Poor mouth hygiene not only contributes to poor nutrition, it can also lead to throat, chest, ear and even brain infections. Mouth dryness, and therefore risk of oral infections, increase if the patient is nil by mouth for any significant period of time (Wilson 2011).
- Check that false teeth are clean, well-fitting and that the patient uses them.
- Check hair, nails and skin (see Chapter 9) for abnormalities (e.g. hair loss or cracked nails) which may be linked to poor nutrition.
- Daily weighing recorded on a weight chart will permit weight loss to be detected.

Body weight

Weighing the patient is the standard measurement of assessing their general nutritional status, i.e. it is a guide indicating if the patient has been in positive, neutral or negative energy balance over the last few weeks or months (see p. 91). *Weight loss* programmes to combat overweight or obesity usually require appropriate adjustments to the diet, i.e. typically involving lower fat and carbohydrate intake. This is coupled with an increase in physical activity within the patient's ability. These measures should be aimed at putting the patient into a slight negative energy balance so the body must mobilise stored energy to make up the shortfall, and weight is therefore lost. *Weight gain* programmes, as in anorexia, involve increasing energy-rich foods in the diet, i.e. a positive energy balance, so the body can replace the energy stores such as adipose tissue. Promoting weight gain in anorexia, however, is not an easy task since the patient's negative approach to eating creates a psychological barrier that is difficult to circumvent. It becomes a major challenge for both the nurses and the patient's family.

Basal metabolic rate (BMR) and body mass index (BMI)

BMR measures the rate of energy expenditure required to maintain cellular metabolism *at rest* after fasting for 12 hours. This means that the BMR will increase with activity, as cells need and create extra energy as activity increases, especially muscle cells, e.g. BMR increases four-fold during a brisk walk. Calculating the BMR is complicated and involves special clinical conditions that are not always available; therefore this observation is not undertaken regularly. The results also vary according from one patient to another, and are therefore specific to the individual involved.

The BMI is more widely adopted as it is easy to calculate at home as well as in the clinical setting. It estimates body fat by comparison of body weight with height. The BMI is calculated by the formula:

BMI = body weight in kilogrammes (kg) ÷ (height in metres)^2

After measuring the person's body weight in kilogrammes, and their height in metres, it is just a matter of multiplying the height by the height (i.e. height^2), then dividing this result into the weight. As an example, if a man weighing 78 kg is 1.8 metres tall, then:

Height^2 = 1.8 × 1.8 = 3.24 (warning: *do not* convert the metres to centimetres!)
BMI = 78 ÷ 3.24 = 24 (there are no units).

It can also be done easily on BMI calculators that do the arithmetic for you. They can be downloaded from the Internet or obtained from health care product suppliers. The results are usually interpreted in this manner:

- BMI below 18.5 = underweight
- BMI 18.5–24.9 = normal weight
- BMI 25–30 = overweight
- BMI more than 30 = obesity.

Bioelectrical impedance analysis (BIA)

Bioelectrical impedance analysis uses a piece of equipment that passes a safe, low-voltage electrical current through the body. This current is not enough to be felt by the subject. Because electrical currents flow faster through water-rich areas of the body (e.g. muscle), fat tissue (which has low water content) will impede the flow. These variations in flow rates are measured by the machine, which, together with information on the subject's height, weight, age and gender, allows the instrument to calculate the percentage of body fat (Haroun *et al.* 2010).

Total parenteral nutrition (TPN)

Total parenteral nutrition (TPN) is a treatment regime that is used to replace oral food intake in those patients who are unable to take any food or fluid by mouth. The nutrition and fluids are administered by intravenous cannula directly into a main venous blood vessel, usually a central vein. Smaller veins are not recommended as they may get blocked as a result of the fluid administered. The nutrition provided must be in the same form that would be absorbed from the digestive tract, i.e. glucose, fatty acids, amino acids, vitamins and minerals. It gives the staff the opportunity to measure and record nutritional and fluid intake very accurately, and thus to work out the nutritional and fluid balances. Very careful mouth observations and management must be made to prevent dryness and infection since a major part of normal mouth cleanliness comes from drinking fluids.

Key points

Energy

- Energy balance is the energy intake compared with the energy used.
- Neutral energy balance means the intake equals the energy used.
- Positive balance, i.e. greater energy input than used, can lead to overweight.
- Negative balance, i.e. less energy input than used, can lead to weight loss.

Proteins

- Amino acids are the components of proteins; they contain an amino group (NH_2), a carboxyl group (COOH) and a radical that differs between the various amino acids.
- Proteins in the body function as structures (e.g. muscle), hormones, antibodies, plasma proteins, enzymes and other important elements.
- Proteins are not used for energy except as a last resort.
- Some hospital patients may be subject to a mild form of kwashiorkor and this should be considered when assessing patients in hospital.

Fats

- Fats (notably fatty acids) are our secondary energy source.
- It is the healthier option to reduce the intake of saturated fats.

Carbohydrates

- Carbohydrates (notably glucose) are our primary energy source.

Vitamins

- Vitamins are organic nutrients required in small quantities.
- Vitamins A, D, E and K are fat-soluble, and their presence requires some fat in the diet. Other vitamins are water-soluble.

Minerals

- Minerals are inorganic chemical elements required in the diet.
- Electrolytes are charged particles in solution.

Fibre

- Fibre remains unchanged in the digestive system; it is not absorbed and provides no direct nutritional value.

Nutrition in the young and the elderly

- Adequate nutrients to sustain growth are essential throughout childhood.
- Energy food consumption should be reduced as people get older.
- Women after menopause require less iron but more calcium.

Disorders of nutrition

- Cachexia is a moribund state of critical malnutrition caused by a metabolic malfunction.
- Starvation is a lack of food that, if it continues, results in weight loss, muscle wasting and possibly death.
- Anorexia is starvation due to an eating disorder more often seen in young women.
- Bulimia is an eating disorder where eating binges are followed by periods of guilt during which the patients try to retrieve the food by vomiting and the use of laxatives.
- Obesity causes multiple long-term complications to health and shortens the life span.

Observations of the nutritional state

- Simple observations of nutritional status include the dietary history, observing the patient eat and ensuring they are able to eat adequately.
- Other observations include body weight, the body mass index (BMI) and bioelectrical impedance analysis (BIA) to measure fat percentage.

References

Bell J. (2007) Nutritional screening during hospital admission: 1. *Nursing Times*, 103(37): 30–31.

Best C. (2004) How 'nil by mouth' instructions impact on patient behaviour. *Nursing Times*, 100(39): 32.

Blows W. T. (2011a) *The Biological Basis of Mental Health Nursing*, 2nd edition. Routledge, London.

Blows W. T. (2011b) The physiology of food intake regulation and eating disorders. *Journal of Gastrointestinal Nursing*, 9(6): 40–45.

Haroun D., Taylor S. J., Viner R. M., Hayward R. S., Darch T. S., Eaton S., Cole T. J. and Wells J. C. (2010) Validation of bioelectrical impedance analysis in adolescents across different ethnic groups. *Obesity*, 18(6): 1252–1259.

Perry L. (2009) Using nutritional screening tools to identify malnourished patients. *Nursing Times*. Available at: http://www.nursingtimes.net/nursing-practice/clinical-specialisms/nutrition/using-nutritional-screening-tools-to-identify-malnourished-patients/1958881.article?referrer=RSS (accessed April 2011).

Wilson A. (2011) How to provide effective oral care. *Nursing Times*, 107(6): 14–21.

Chapter 7 Elimination (I)
Urinary observations

- Introduction
- Urine formation
- Urinary observations
- Urinary volume
- Colour, smell and deposits
- Specific gravity
- Urinalysis
- When to test urine
- Key points
- References

Introduction

The eliminatory systems, the bowel and kidneys, are the body's principal excretory pathways for many surplus and toxic substances produced from a wide variety of tissues. Their functions are crucial in the maintenance of the body's tissue and blood contents at permanently optimum levels essential for life. It is natural that the body should excrete products generated not only in health but as a result of pathology, and the nurse must be familiar with the normal and abnormal states of the eliminated product. Urine, for example, a seemingly waste material, offers a unique insight into the physiological workings of many body systems. Accurate observations of urine can reveal much about the individual at that time, both the factors affecting the system and the underlying metabolism.

Urine formation

The formation of urine is the role of the **nephron** (Figure 7.1), of which there are about one million in each of the two kidneys. Urine production takes place in three distinct steps.

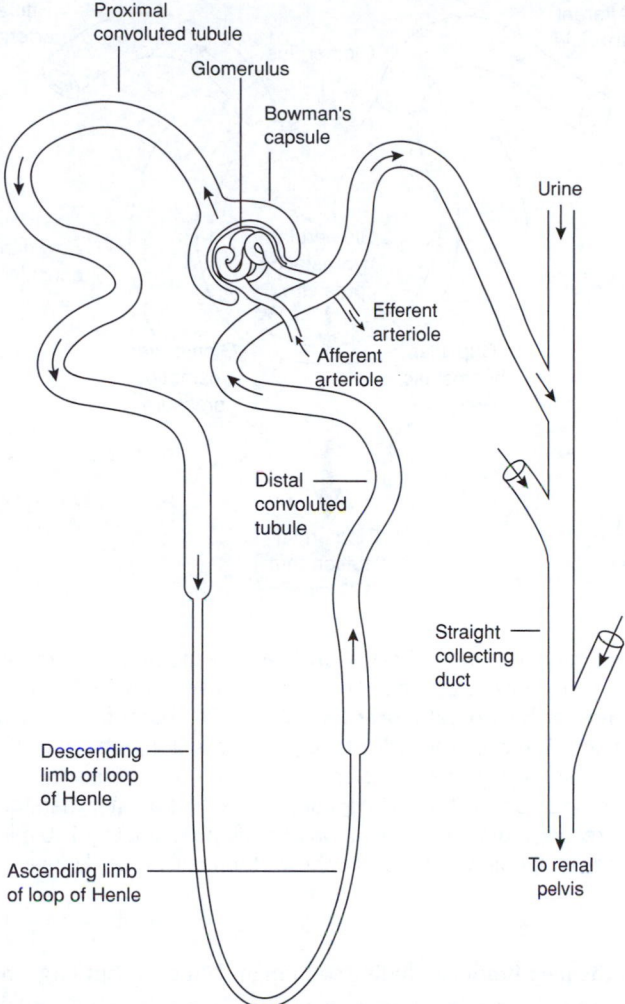

FIGURE 7.1 The renal nephron. The glomerulus, inside the Bowman's capsule, is formed from a tuft of arterioles; the blood enters via the afferent arteriole and leaves via the efferent arteriole. Filtrate flows along the proximal convoluted tubule to the loop of Henle, passing down the descending limb and up the ascending limb. The distal convoluted tubule conveys filtrate to the straight collecting duct, where, as urine, it flows to the renal pelvis and to the bladder.

- *Step 1* is **filtration under pressure** in the **glomerulus,** which is surrounded by the **glomerular (Bowman's) capsule** (Figure 7.2). Blood plasma passing through the glomerular arterioles is subject to **hydrostatic pressure** (i.e. blood pressure as it occurs in the glomerular arterioles), causing filtration by forcing water and other substances through the **glomerular membrane.** The resulting filtrate is collected in the capsule at a rate known as the **glomerular filtration rate (GFR),** which is about 120 ml per minute, measured as a total of all two million nephrons. Water and other small molecules may

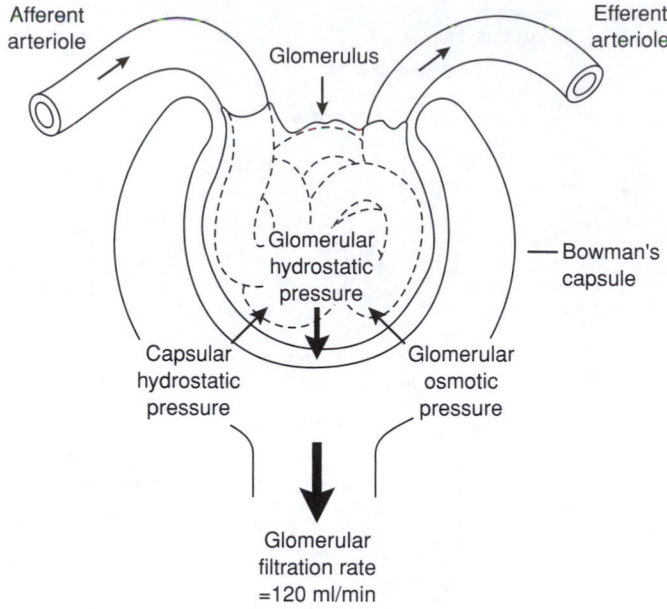

FIGURE 7.2 The glomerulus and Bowman's capsule. The glomerulus is covered by a filtration membrane. Water is pushed out of the blood and into the Bowman's capsule by the **glomerular hydrostatic pressure (GHP)**. Two other forces are returning water to the blood. The capsular hydrostatic pressure is the pressure of the fluid within the capsule, and the glomerular osmotic pressure is the force exerted by the proteins within the blood to attract water back. The GHP is greater than the sum of the other two, creating a glomerular filtration rate of approximately 120 ml/min, measured as a sum total for all two million nephrons (one million per kidney).

pass through the membrane, including sodium and glucose, but large molecules, such as most proteins and blood cells, cannot pass through and remain in the blood.

- *Step 2* is the re-absorption of required substances, including much of the water, back into the circulation from the **proximal convoluted tubule** (Figure 7.3). Water returns to the blood at a rate of about 105 ml per minute, measured as a total of all two million nephrons. Other substances returned include some sodium and all of the glucose. The remaining filtrate passes into the **loop of Henle**, which has the effect of causing an osmotic gradient across the renal cortex that becomes important to water re-absorption from the straight collecting ducts (Figure 7.4). Filtrate then passes into the **distal convoluted tubule,** where further re-absorption of substances takes place, some of which is under hormonal control. The re-absorption of water is controlled by **antidiuretic hormone (ADH)** and that of sodium by **aldosterone** (Figure 7.5). ADH is also active along the straight collecting ducts controlling water re-absorption in response to the osmotic gradient mentioned earlier.
- *Step 3* involves the addition of certain substances, notably hydrogen ions (H^+) (see p. 62), ammonia (NH_3) (see p. 62) and potassium ions (K^+) into the filtrate from the

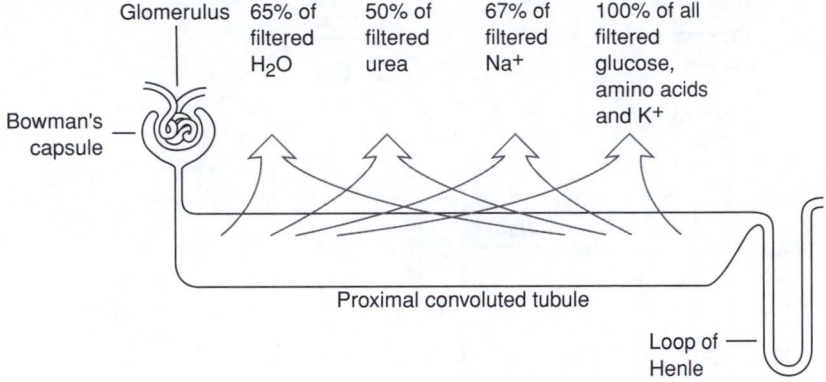

FIGURE 7.3 The proximal convoluted tubule, between the Bowman's capsule and the loop of Henle, re-absorbs water, urea, sodium and other substances. The percentage shown is that of the amount filtered by the glomerulus.

blood by means of **tubular secretion**, which takes place in the **straight collecting ducts**. The resultant filtrate is now urine, which then passes to the renal pelvis and into the bladder for elimination.

Urinary observations

Urinary observations are made on the volume, colour, smell, deposits and specific gravity of the urine and chemical tests are performed for glucose, pH, protein, blood, bilirubin, urobilinogen, ketones, nitrite and leucocytes. Collecting urinary specimens and the use of reagent testing strips are described by Simerville *et al.* (2005). The correct technique cannot be over-emphasised, since the reagent test strips are calibrated to perform accurately within precise limits, and they will give false results if used wrongly. These limits include using the strips before the expiry dates, storage in a dry environment and reading the results at the specified time limit (usually 60 seconds). Holding the strip the correct way round when comparing the reactive pads with the colour chart is another vital point so often overlooked by those who are new to the procedure. Testing freshly voided urine is another critical point, since urine constituents change with time when left standing, especially when exposed to the air. Again, false results occur when testing old urine. The accuracy of the reagent strips is discussed by Simerville *et al.* (2005).

Urinary volume

Between them, the two kidneys produce urine at the average rate of 1 ml per minute given an average oral intake of fluids. Variations in oral intake will change this output volume by adjusting the levels of ADH in the blood. ADH is produced by the hypothalamus of the brain and moves to the posterior pituitary gland. From here it is released into the

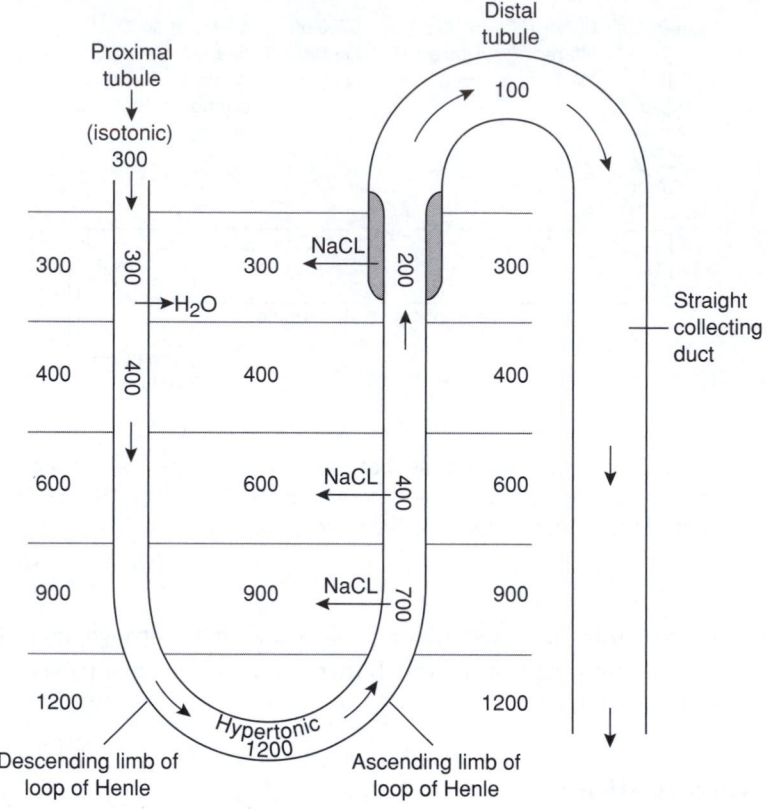

All figures in mosmol/l
(milliosmoles per litre)

FIGURE 7.4 The loop of Henle passes through a sodium concentration gradient outside the loop caused by blood capillaries called the vasa recta, which follow the loop closely (not shown). The concentration gradient is shown from 300 to 1200 mosmol/l. Water can pass out of the descending limb but not the ascending limb, and sodium is unable to pass out of the descending limb but is actively transported out of the ascending limb. The filtrate passing down the descending limb is isotonic to begin with but becomes more concentrated in sodium (i.e. hypertonic) as water is lost. As the filtrate returns up the ascending limb, sodium is lost and it becomes less concentrated. The resultant dilution of the filtrate in the distal convoluted tubule (100 mosmol/l) allows the kidney to excrete urine more dilute than body fluids (hypotonic) when necessary. The gradient along the straight collecting duct allows the kidney to reclaim water (under antidiuretic hormone control) and therefore excrete urine more concentrated than body fluids (hypertonic) when necessary (see Figures 7.5–7.7).

circulation and acts on the straight collecting ducts leading from the nephrons. The role of ADH is to facilitate the return of water from the urinary filtrate back to the blood, thus controlling the concentration of urine, and it is therefore a major influence on fluid balance in the body. It works by binding to ADH receptors on the surface of cells lining the

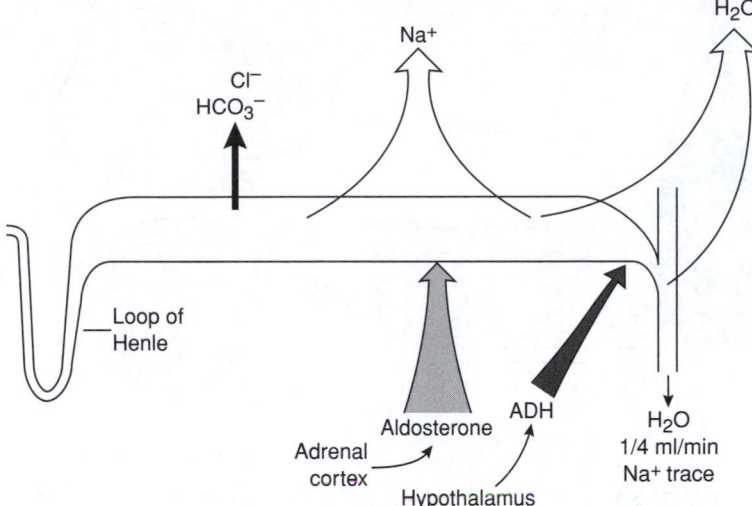

FIGURE 7.5 The distal convoluted tubule. After the loop of Henle, the distal tubule absorbs chlorine (Cl^-) and bicarbonate (HCO_3^-). Sodium (Na^+) is reabsorbed under aldosterone control from the adrenal cortex, and water (H_2O) is re-absorbed under the control of antidiuretic hormone (ADH) from the hypothalamus. The amount of water returned to the blood allows an average of one-quarter of a millilitre per hour as urine production.

straight collecting duct, cells that also have a surface close to the local blood circulation. Binding of ADH activates intracellular systems that open channels specific to water on the cell surfaces facing the filtrate. Water passes down these channels into the cell, driven by the osmotic gradient set up by the loop of Henle. From there, water passes back into the blood. After the GFR of 120 ml per minute and the re-absorption of water from the proximal convoluted tubule, the remaining filtrate has a water volume of about 15 ml per minute. Average ADH levels, as found in those who are drinking normal amounts daily, return about 14 ml per minute to the blood, leaving an average of 1 ml per minute as urine. But let us consider the extremes of ADH activity as seen in those persons with very different oral intakes of fluid.

Mr Wet is in the pub drinking multiple pints in quick succession (Figure 7.6). His high oral intake of fluid (mostly water) sends stimuli to the hypothalamus to reduce ADH production and release, and it thus lowers the amount that is active on the kidneys. A minimum of ADH release can be achieved if the oral intake is high enough. Less water is returned from the collecting duct as a result, i.e. little or no post-loop re-absorption occurs, and the urine output increases to a maximum of 15 ml per minute, the **renal maximum** (causing a large urine output called a **polyuria**, or **diuresis**). Outputs higher than this suggest that the kidneys have lost control of fluid balance, a feature of **chronic renal failure**. Failure here means failure to control fluid balance. As Mr Wet's drink contains alcohol, this will have a further dehydrating effect during the following few hours by suppressing ADH production. Dehydration is said to be one of the causes of the hangover. Meanwhile, poor Mr Dry is crawling

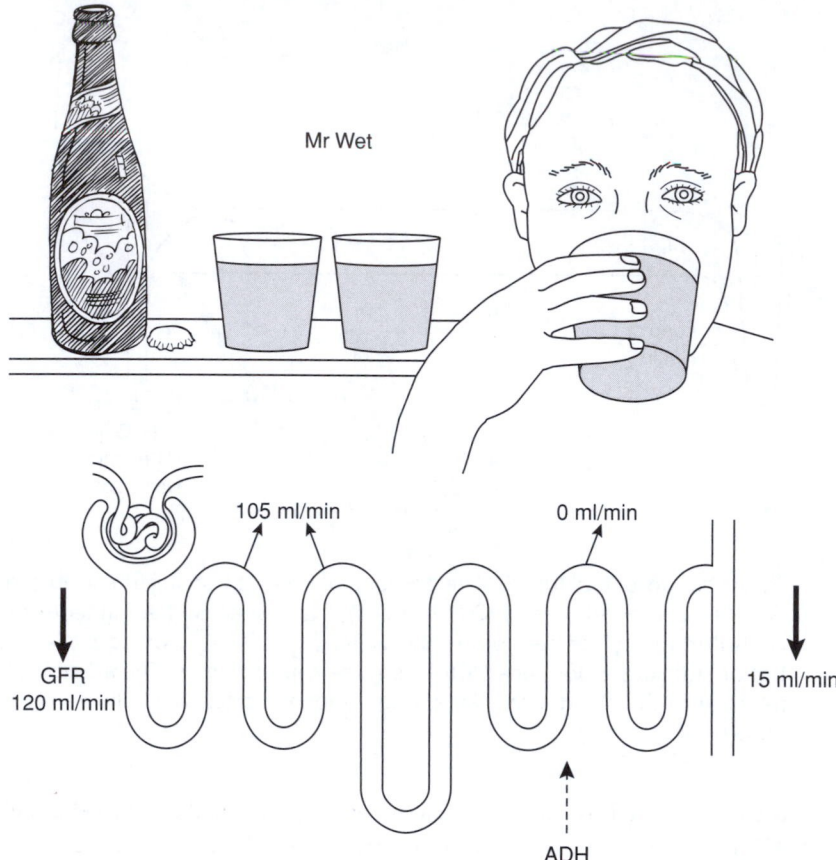

FIGURE 7.6 Mr Wet physiology. If a large volume of fluid is drunk, the kidney can compensate by excreting more urine. The figures are totals for the two million nephrons (one million per kidney). The glomerular filtration rate (GFR) is approximately 120 ml/min, and the first tubule re-absorption rate is approximately 105 ml/min. The variations begin in the distal tubule because of very low levels of antidiuretic hormone (ADH). Signals to the brain have caused a shutdown of ADH production and release, as little or none of the water in the distal tubule can be returned to the blood, giving a urine output of 15 ml/min, the renal maximum.

through the desert, with no oral fluids, and he is losing a great deal of water through his skin by sweating in the hot sun (Figure 7.7). The fizzy drinks machines he sees are, unfortunately for him, all mirages. His low oral intake of fluid causes stimuli to pass to the hypothalamus causing an increase in the production and release of ADH, therefore boosting his ADH activity on the kidneys.

Up to 14.75 ml per minute of the post-loop 15 ml per minute filtrate can be returned, leaving a urine output of about 0.25 ml per minute, the **renal minimum** (causing a very low output called an **oliguria**). Zero output (anuria) is not possible in normal renal physiology as this would cause retention of wastes, especially urea, a feature of **acute renal failure**. Here,

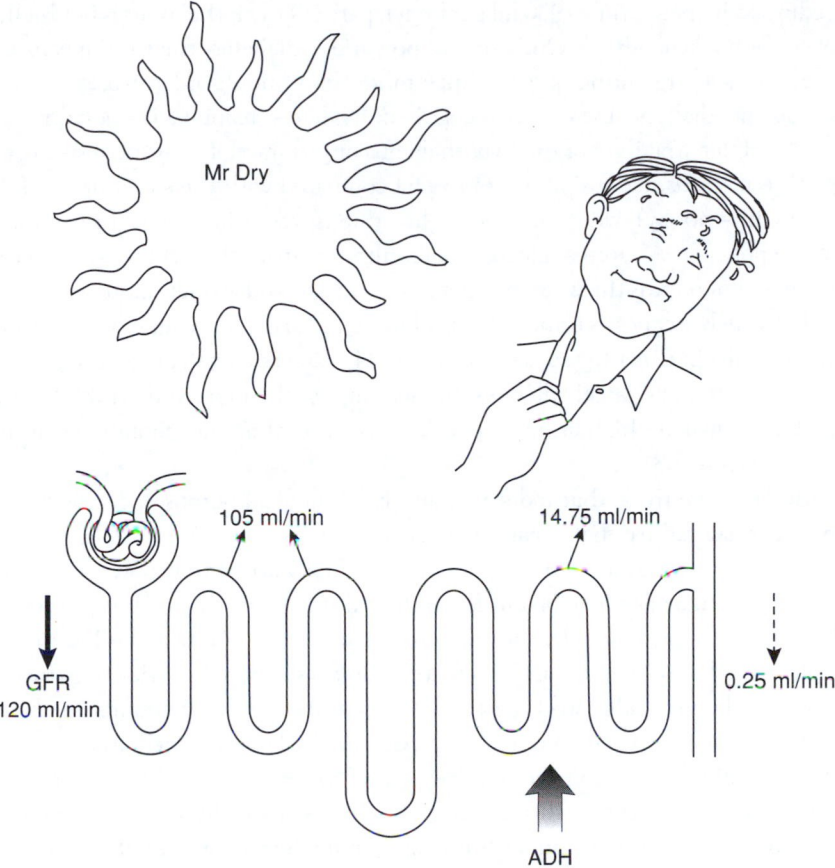

FIGURE 7.7 Mr Dry physiology. If the oral intake of fluids is very low, the kidney can compensate to prevent unnecessary water loss. The figures shown are totals for the two million nephrons (one million per kidney). The glomerular filtration rate (GFR) is approximately 120 ml/min; the reabsorption rate from the first tubule is about 105 ml/min. The difference begins in the second tubule when large amounts of antidiuretic hormone (ADH) are active, returning up to 14.75 ml/min water to the blood and creating a urine output of only one-quarter of a millilitre per minute, the renal minimum.

the word 'failure' means failure to produce urine, otherwise known as **renal shutdown**. Observations of urine output volume are made in relation to total fluid balance in those patients at most risk of imbalance, i.e. those who are nil by mouth or are not drinking well; those on intravenous infusion; those with excessive fluid losses from sweating, over-breathing, bleeding or drains; and those with renal disease or children with diarrhoea and vomiting (see Chapter 5). Outputs falling below 1 ml per minute (60 ml per hour) should be monitored closely and medical advice sought if the output reaches 30 ml or less per hour. High outputs should return to normal as fluid balance is restored, but outputs remaining consistently high, or exceeding 15 ml per minute (900 ml per hour), particularly if the input is not high, should be referred for medical advice. One cause of polyuria is **diabetes**; the word means a disease characterised by a large urine output. Since more than one disorder causes a polyuria, at least two distinct diabetic diseases are recognised. **Diabetes insipidus** is a polyuria caused by a lack of ADH due to failure of the hypothalamus or pituitary. The urine tests negative for glucose (thus *insipidus*, i.e. insipid = not sweet) compared with the sweet urine of **diabetes mellitus** (melli = honey), where glucose in the urine (glycosuria) is a major feature and the cause of the polyuria. Abnormal glucose-laden filtrate within the nephron tubule exerts an osmotic force that retains the water present in the filtrate and attracts more water out of the blood, all of which escapes as urine. The resultant large urine loss causes a state of dehydration which results in thirst to replace this water. This is a reversal of the normal condition, i.e. normally oral intake largely dictates urinary output (the more you drink, the more you urinate), but in diabetes high urine output dictates the oral intake amount (i.e. it increases oral intake) (Figure 7.8).

Diuretic drugs are those that induce a diuresis for medical purposes, e.g. to treat **hypertension** or **cardiac failure** that is causing **oedema** (see Chapter 5). Several groups of drugs achieve a large urine output, and the patient should be warned that they will be passing a lot of urine. The **thiazides** (e.g. **bendroflumethiazide**) prevent the re-absorption of sodium from the distal parts of the tubule. The sodium remains in the filtrate and is lost in the urine. Water follows sodium, so a sodium loss creates a diuresis. **Loop diuretics** (e.g. **furosemide/frusemide** and **bumetanide**) work by preventing re-absorption of sodium at the loop of Henle. They are the most potent diuretics, producing the largest urine outputs but with the greatest potential for causing unwanted reactions. They may promote the loss of potassium as well, and this can be a complication. The **potassium-sparing** diuretics (e.g. **amiloride** and **spironolactone**) conserve potassium while causing mild diuresis as a result of sodium loss. In addition, spironolactone is an aldosterone **antagonist**, i.e. it reduces the activity of aldosterone and this promotes further sodium and water loss.

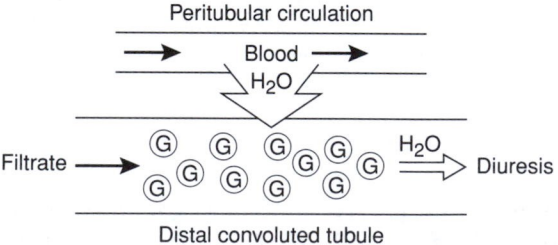

FIGURE 7.8   Mechanism of the large urine loss (diuresis) in uncontrolled diabetes. Glucose is not normally present in the distal convoluted tubule, so if glucose molecules (G) do get through to this part of the nephron, they cause a return of water (H_2O) from the peritubular blood circulation to the filtrate. This osmotic increase in filtrate water causes the large urine loss (diuresis) that is seen in uncontrolled diabetes.

Colour, smell and deposits

The normal colour of urine is a clear pale yellow with no clouding or deposits. Urine density affects the colour: the more dilute the urine is with water, the weaker the colour. Concentrated urine becomes darker, depending on how much pigment is present. This is normal, but the colour can also change when unusual substances are present (see Table 7.1 and Plate 1).

Bilirubin will stain the urine a strong yellow colour, and when seen in bulk in concentrated urine, it can appear to be black. Bilirubin is the end product of the breakdown of haemoglobin from erythrocytes (red blood cells) in circulation (see bilirubin and urobilinogen, p. 126). Whole blood will change the colour according to the amount present and how long it has been mixed with urine. Small amounts of blood added to the urine during formation, i.e. well mixed with the filtrate in the nephron, may give a grey smoky appearance, whereas larger amounts of blood added lower down the renal tract, especially in the bladder, will appear as true blood colour, i.e. red urine (haematuria, see p. 125). Red urine may also be a feature of excessive beetroot consumption in the diet, and some drugs may affect the colour, e.g. **anthraquinones** in laxatives such as **senna** may turn urine yellow, brown or orange. Simerville *et al.* (2005) give a comprehensive list of urine colours and the causes, including some drugs (see also Table 7.1).

Both **urea** and **ammonia** are nitrogenous (i.e. containing nitrogen) wastes of protein metabolism, normally produced by the liver from excess protein. Ammonia is more toxic that urea and gives a more powerful smell. The ammonia smell associated with some urine specimens is due to infective organisms in the urinary tract (a **urinary tract infection**, or **UTI**) that split the urea molecules present in urine into ammonia. Urine can smell of **acetone** (see below) if left to stand for some hours, the result of collecting organisms from the environment and a good reason for testing only fresh samples. **Ketones** (such as acetone) are waste

TABLE 7.1 Urine colour

Urine colour	Possible causes
Dark yellow	Concentrated (inadequate fluid intake, i.e. dehydration); jaundice (bilirubin) from hepatic disease
Neon yellow	Excessive vitamin B group intake
Orange	Excess carotene (carrots); vitamin C, blackberries, beetroot or rhubarb in the diet; some drugs (antibiotics, laxatives, some chemotherapy agents)
Brown	Jaundice (bilirubin); excess fava beans in diet; copper poisoning; melanoma; laxatives
Red/pink	Blood (haematuria) due to trauma, renal calculi (stones), urinary tract infections (UTIs), neoplasms, excess beetroot, blackberries, rhubarb in diet; red food dye in sweets and medication
Black	Severe jaundice (bilirubin) from hepatic disease
Very pale	Very dilute urine from excessive fluid intake
Green	UTIs; bilirubin; excess vitamin B intake; artificial food colouring
Blue	*Pseudomonas* urinary tract infection; excess calcium in urine; dyes in some drugs; artificial food colouring
Cloudy	UTIs; excess calcium in urine; renal calculi (stones) debris

products of fat (lipid) metabolism. Acetone is the main ketone produced and gives the urine a pear-drop or nail-polish remover smell. This is usually present in association with glycosuria in diabetes mellitus (see p. 123). Deposits are another indication of a potential problem with urine. Cloudy urine in UTIs is caused by the presence of inflammatory cells (leucocytes), bacteria (both live and dead), pus, mucus and cellular debris. Alternatively, excessive calcium excretion can give a cloudy effect and leave a chalky deposit on standing. This may be due to excessive calcium in the diet or to any of the decalcifying bone diseases, such as **osteoporosis**. Here, too much calcium leaves the bone and passes to the kidneys via the blood and is excreted in the urine; patients are said to be *urinating their skeleton*. Excessive calcium lost in urine also increases that person's risk of forming renal stones (Arshad and Shar-Baloch 2007). Phosphates and **urates** (salts of **uric acid**) can produce cloudy effects in urine. Uric acid is the excretory product from the breakdown of nucleic acids such as **deoxyribonucleic acid (DNA)** and **ribonucleic acid (RNA)**. **Casts** can also leave a visible deposit when urine is left to stand. Casts are made from a matrix of a mucoprotein produced by the distal tubular epithelium that fills and takes the shape of the tubule lumen. Cells get incorporated into this matrix, which can then be washed out by the urine. When excreted, these casts indicate a potentially high protein content and a low urinary pH. When cloudy urine is observed, a sample should be collected for laboratory analysis to determine the exact component and its cause.

Specific gravity

The **density** of urine identifies how much **solute** there is present. Solutes are chemical substances that are dissolved in the water component, such as sodium chloride (found in trace quantities in urine). Specific gravity is the measure of urine density compared with the density of pure water (see Plate 2). By using water as a baseline density, the specific gravity of urine states just how much more dense than water a certain urine sample is. Since the fluid component of urine is water, the specific gravity measures the volume of dissolved solutes in that water. The baseline density of water is 1000 (or 1.000, labelled 0 on some hydrometers), and a particular urine sample will measure greater than this, e.g. 1010, (or 1.010) if the hydrometer reads 10. The normal range of specific gravity for urine is 1002 (or 1.002) for dilute urine, to 1035 (or 1.035) for concentrated urine (see p. 115). The **hydrometer** (or **urinometer**) floats in the urine sample with the large bulb downwards, and measurement is made from where the urine surface crosses the stem scale (see Plate 3). How high (in dense urine) or how low (in dilute urine) the urinometer floats is an indication of how much the urine is pushing back against the weight of the instrument, and this is the effect of the solute content. Think of the difference between a body floating in the swimming pool (low solute density) and floating in the Dead Sea (high solute density).

The specific gravity is affected by both the water concentration and the solute concentration in the urine sample. The water concentration varies as described (see p. 115). Solutes vary in concentration, depending on several factors because many different solutes are involved. **Sodium (Na^+)** is naturally excreted from the kidneys in amounts according to blood levels of sodium and its controlling hormone, **aldosterone**. A high oral intake of sodium chloride (NaCl) increases the blood level, which promotes removal of more sodium by glomerular filtration. The majority of the filtered sodium will return to the blood from the

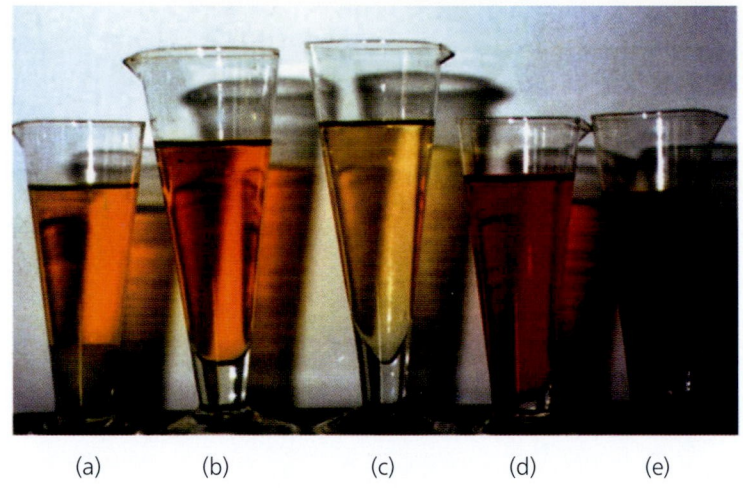

(a)   (b)   (c)   (d)   (e)

PLATE 1   Different colours of urine and sedimentation. (a) chalky sedimentation, which may indicate the excretion of too much calcium; (b) concentrated urine, as may be passed on a hot day or because of reduced fluid intake; (c) dilute urine, as may be passed when fluid intake is high; (d) blood in the urine (frank haematuria); (e) dark urine seen in jaundice, when the urine is rich in bilirubin.

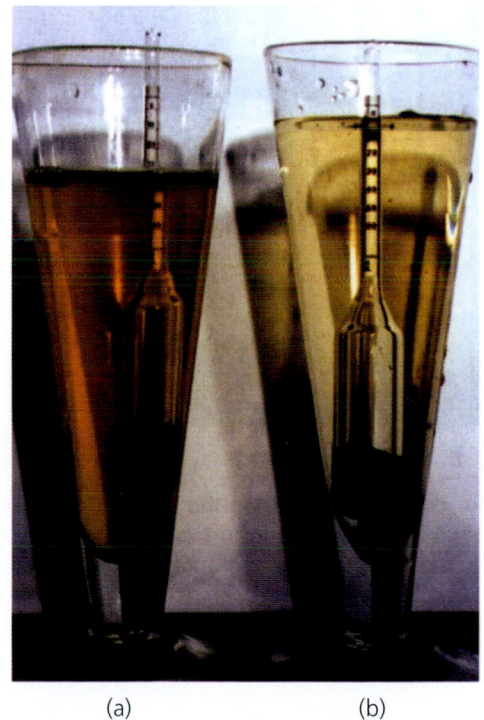

(a)   (b)

PLATE 2   Different densities of urine and specific gravity. (a) denser (darker) urine, which indicates less water is lost through the kidneys, as occurs on a hot day and when dehydrated; (b) dilute urine, as may be passed when fluid intake is high. Note the hydrometer (urinometer) floats lower in (b) than in (a) and deeper urine is needed to keep the hydrometer from touching the bottom. The hydrometer is a measure of the density observed.

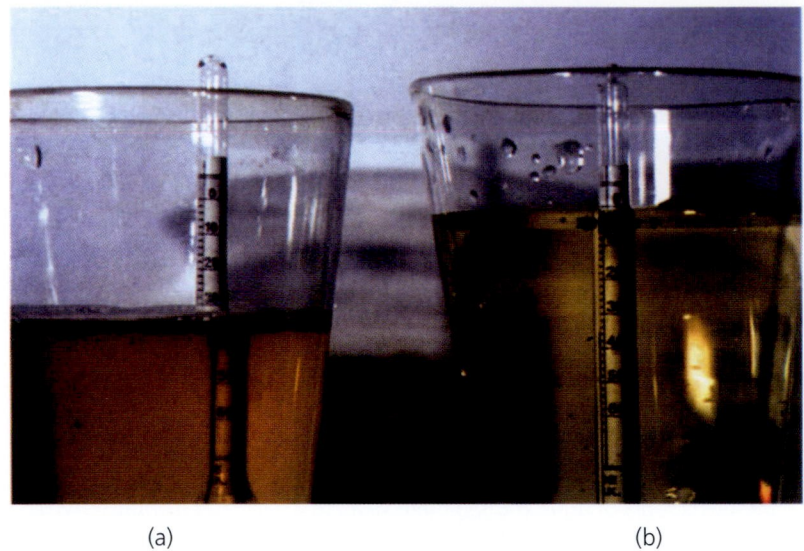

(a)   (b)

Plate 3 Different densities of urine and the hydrometer scale. (a) denser urine that measures between 30 and 40 on the hydrometer scale (where the urine level crosses the scale); (b) dilute urine that measures close to 0 on the scale. Zero is the specific gravity of pure water, so (b) is not much denser than pure water. Note that the hydrometer appears 'broken' in (a) owing to the different refraction (bending) of light seen through denser urine.

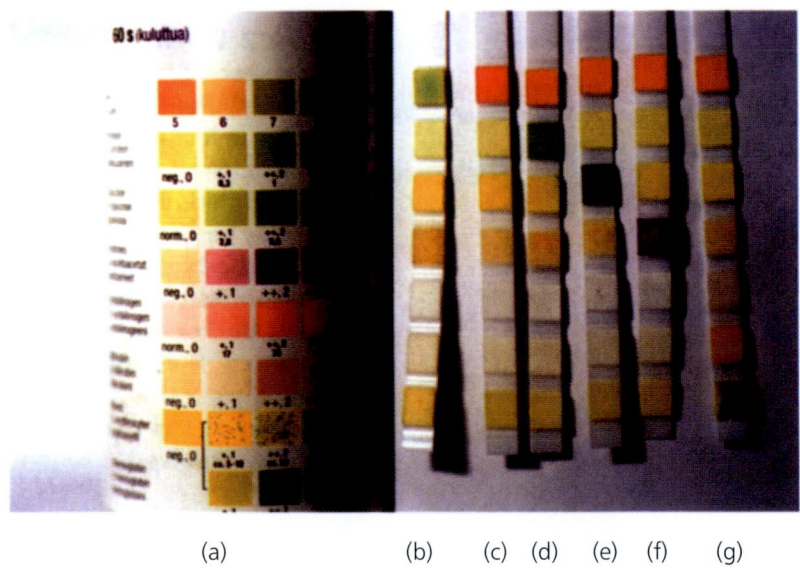

(a)   (b)   (c) (d) (e) (f)   (g)

Plate 4 Urine testing strips. (a) the colour chart for comparing the colour changes seen on the strips after immersion in urine. The tests are, from top to bottom, pH (measuring the acidity or alkalinity of urine), protein, glucose, ketones, urobilinogen, bilirubin, blood and haemoglobin. (b) a stick essentially normal with pH approximately 7; (c) a stick with pH 5 (acidic); (d) protein is present; (e) large amounts of glucose; (f) positive for ketones; (g) positive for blood.

proximal convoluted tubule; most of the remainder will be re-absorbed from the distal convoluted tubule under aldosterone control. Aldosterone comes from the adrenal cortex, and is released according to blood sodium levels: higher levels reduce aldosterone release; lower levels increase its release. Aldosterone acts to facilitate sodium reabsorption back into the blood. In high blood sodium levels (hypernatraemia), less aldosterone allows more sodium to escape in the urine and reduce the blood level. In low blood sodium levels (hyponatraemia), the higher aldosterone release allows more sodium to return to the blood and thereby increase the blood level. Aldosterone release is also facilitated by the **renin–angiotensin–aldosterone cycle**, whereby the kidney emergency hormone renin is produced under low blood pressure or low blood sodium conditions. Renin activates the blood protein angiotensin (a vasoconstrictive agent that raises blood pressure), which in turn also stimulates aldosterone release to conserve sodium. Sodium is filtered and re-absorbed under aldosterone control very much like water and ADH (Table 7.2).

Calcium (Ca^{2+}), phosphates and other solutes are eliminated in the filtrate and contribute to the specific gravity. However, some solutes, such as potassium, are also excreted using a different process. **Potassium (K^+)** is largely added to urine by tubular secretion using a cellular mechanism that also transports hydrogen (H^+) (Figure 7.9). This occurs at the straight collecting duct, eliminating the exact amount of these substances required to maintain normal blood levels.

Urinalysis

Eight different chemical tests have been developed to measure the amounts of important solutes in urine that may indicate disease. These are impregnated into pads and mounted on plastic strips in a convenient manner for urine testing (see Plate 4).

Glucose in urine

Glucose is filtered via the glomerulus and absorbed back into the blood from the proximal convoluted tubule. Under normal circumstances, this return to circulation is total, leaving no glucose in the filtrate or urine. The process of absorption involves glucose transport molecules within the cells that line the tubule, and these molecules move glucose from the filtrate back into the blood. A set amount of transport molecules means that glucose movement is finite, but this is adequate for the average volume of glucose found in the filtrate under normal conditions. It is possible, sometimes, for glomerular filtration to exceed

TABLE 7.2 Water and sodium in urine

Substance	Glomerular filtered	Proximal tubule	Hormone	Distal tubule	Amount in urine
Water	Yes	Most is re-absorbed	ADH	Average 14 ml/min	Average 1 ml/min
Sodium	Yes	Most is re-absorbed	Aldosterone	Most is re-absorbed	Trace

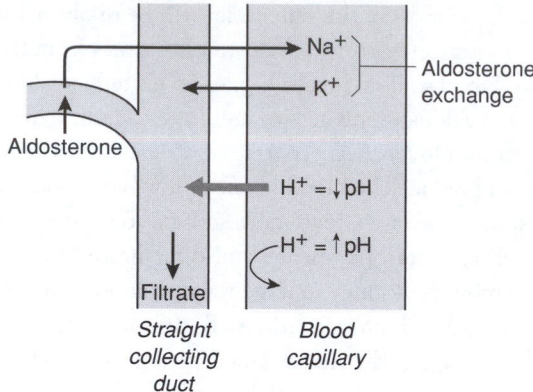

FIGURE 7.9 **FIGURE 7.9** Mechanism of aldosterone action. The return of sodium (Na^+) to the blood by aldosterone in the distal convoluted tubule is accompanied by the return of potassium (K^+) to the filtrate (aldosterone exchange). Thus aldosterone influences the potassium balance. In addition, hydrogen ions (H^+) can be returned to the filtrate from the straight collecting duct or retained in the blood, according to the need to maintain the blood pH balance at pH 7.4. Under low-pH conditions (e.g. acidosis) hydrogen ions are excreted, and under high-pH conditions (alkalosis) hydrogen ions are retained.

this **renal threshold** for glucose, and the surplus glucose remaining in the filtrate passes through the remaining nephron and into the urine. This will happen mostly when excess glucose occurs in the blood (hyperglycaemia), as in diabetes mellitus. More appears in the filtrate than the transport mechanisms can return to circulation and the renal threshold is exceeded. Glycosuria can also occur during pregnancy, but it is usually of no significance, or in individuals with naturally fewer transport molecules but who do not have diabetes. Glucose is, of course, sweet, and glycosuria makes urine sweet, a fact that was all too obvious to doctors and nurses before the days of chemical tests. They had to test urine by tasting it. Now, health and safety regulations would not allow this, and sophisticated tests such as those described here have, for many years, made the tasting method of testing urine unnecessary. Modern chemical tests provide a more reliable and accurate alternative. However, keen observation still remains important, as with the case of the psychiatric charge nurse who noticed that one patient's urine, when accidentally dripped on the floor, attracted ants. Further investigation revealed that the patient had glycosuria and diabetes.

Protein in urine

Protein does not normally appear in the urine. Blood proteins include **albumin**, which occurs in larger quantities than all the others, and **globulin, fibrinogen** and **prothrombin** (the last two are also clotting factors). Protein molecules are, at 7–9 nm, too large to pass through the glomerular membrane pores (about 3 nm). Albumin could pass through the pores but is mostly repelled back into the circulation by the strong negative charges associated with the glycoproteins of the glomerular membrane. What few proteins do appear in the filtrate can be reclaimed by **pinocytosis** (a process similar to phagocytosis) of the urinary cells. Protein in the urine (**proteinuria**, or more specifically **albuminuria**) can be caused by damage to the glomerular membrane, resulting in a larger pore size, such as in glomerular infections (glomerulonephritis), and nephrotoxic agents. Systemic hypertension raises the intraglomerular blood pressure and forces more protein into the filtrate. The presence of blood in urine also means protein is there as well (since blood is rich in protein), and therefore urine with blood added will show some positive result for protein. **Nephrotic syndrome** is a condition recognised by a persistent protein loss in the urine (3.5 g or more of protein lost per day) and can result in a reduced blood protein level with the consequence of tissue oedema (see p. 84).

Blood in urine

Blood in the urine (haematuria) may be normal in some circumstances (e.g. blood contamination of urine during menstruation), or may be expected (e.g. immediately after bladder or prostate surgery) but is often a manifestation of a pathology that requires investigation. Blood in the urine can occur as a result of trauma to any part of the renal system (Pfitzenmaier *et al.* 2008), or can be caused by the effects of renal stones damaging the urinary tract wall (Arshad and Shar-Baloch 2007). Blood can also occur as a result of infections or new growths within the bladder, kidney or prostate gland. The test pad for blood on clinical sticks is sensitive to haemoglobin, ensuring a positive result even when red blood cells have been broken down. Haematuria is often a post-operative feature of bladder, prostate or renal surgery, and it appears as bright red urine (frank blood), diminishing in intensity over several post-operative days until the urine appears normal and blood can only be detected by testing. Eventually, uncomplicated recovery, aided by good fluid input, results in a blood-free urinalysis.

Ketones in urine

Ketones are the end product of excess **adipose** (fat) breakdown in the body. Adipose stores fats in the form of **triglyceride**, which has three fatty acids attached to a glycerol molecule (see Figure 1.4). Normally, fatty acids are repackaged for return to the circulation by the liver. In diabetes mellitus, when a lack of insulin prevents cells from using glucose as an energy source, or in starvation, when glucose is in short supply, adipose is broken down (lipolysis) to release more of the fatty acids. Fatty acids can be used as an additional (secondary) energy supply by entering the tricarboxylic acid (Krebs) cycle (see Figure 1.1), and in the presence of oxygen they are used to create energy in the form of **adenosine triphosphate (ATP)** (see Chapter 1). Massive release of fatty acids into the circulation results in the liver converting the excess (that which cannot be metabolised to energy), through an anaerobic route, into any of the three human ketones, mostly **acetone**, but also **acetoacetic acid** and **beta-hydroxybutyric acid**. Acetone, being the largest amount produced, is excreted via both the kidneys and the lungs, giving a sweet pear-drop smell to the urine and breath, as noted in diabetes mellitus (see Chapter 1).

Bilirubin in urine

Bilirubin and urobilinogen are products of the breakdown of haemoglobin when it is released from old destroyed red blood cells (Figure 7.10). **Erythrocytes** (red blood cells) degrade and release haemoglobin after about 120 days in circulation. Haemoglobin is first split into a *haem* and a *globin* portion. Globin, a protein, can be reduced to amino acids, and the iron

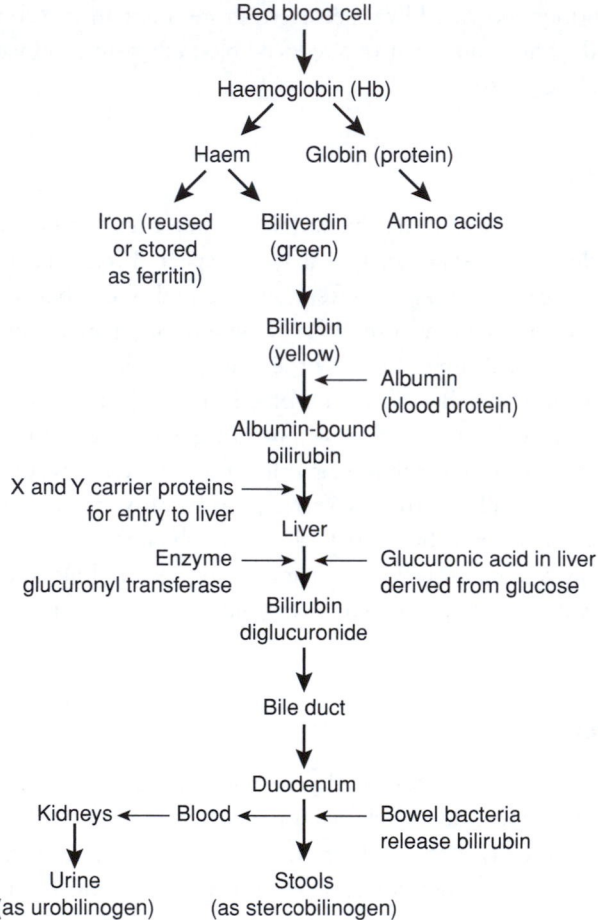

FIGURE 7.10   The natural history of bilirubin. Red cell breakdown causes the release of haemo-globin, which quickly breaks down into a haem group and the protein globin. Globin can be further reduced to amino acids; the haem group (containing iron) releases the iron, which can be stored or re-used. The remainder is biliverdin, which is green, and this is converted to yellow bilirubin. Albumin, a blood protein, binds bilirubin, and other proteins called X and Y help to transport the bilirubin to the liver. Here the enzyme glucuronyl transferase causes the bilirubin to combine with the glucuronic acid to form bilirubin diglucuronide, which becomes one component of bile. Bile arrives in the duodenum, where further conversion to bilirubin creates stercobilinogen, a component of stools. Some bilirubin is re-absorbed into the blood and filtered in the urine as urobilinogen.

is removed from the haem for storage in the liver. What is left of the haem component is **biliverdin** (which is green), which is further converted to bilirubin (which is yellow). Unconjugated bilirubin (i.e. fat-soluble) binds to blood albumin for movement to the liver. Fat-soluble substances cannot blend into a water medium like blood without first binding to a transport protein. With the aid of two carrier proteins known as X and Y, bilirubin enters the liver, where it combines with **glucuronic acid** (which is derived from glucose) to form **bilirubin diglucuronide**. This conjugated form (i.e. water-soluble) becomes a component of bile produced in the liver, and thus drains into the digestive system. Some bilirubin in the colon is acted on by bacteria, creating urobilinogen, which will be absorbed back into the blood and excreted in the urine. The remainder will be incorporated into the stools (sometimes referred to as **stercobilinogen**, sterco = of the faeces). Normal urobilinogen levels in urine are small (0.09–4.23 µmol per 24 hours), but levels will increase in **jaundice**. This condition occurs if the liver is no longer able to accept or handle bilirubin adequately (i.e. **hepatic jaundice** as in **liver failure**, **cirrhosis** or **hepatitis**) or if the bile drainage is obstructed (i.e. **post-hepatic jaundice**, caused by an impacted **biliary stone** or **pancreatic cancer**). **Pre-hepatic jaundice** can also occur when the breakdown of red cells, or **haemolysis**, is happening too quickly, as in **haemolytic anaemia**, and bilirubin is produced faster than the liver can accept. The surplus is removed by the kidney and lost in the urine, but not before the excess bilirubin colours the skin and **sclera** (the white of the eyes) yellow. Bilirubin, being not normally found in urine, will appear to make urine very dark (see p. 121) along with the raised urobilinogen.

Acid–base measurement of urine

pH is the acidity or alkalinity of a substance. It is a measure of the **hydrogen ion (H$^+$)** concentration (written [pH], where the square brackets mean 'concentration of'). Strong concentrations give an acid solution (low pH 1–6) and a weak concentration gives an alkaline solution (high pH 8–14). pH 7 is neutral and is the value found in most water samples tested, especially distilled water. In urine, the hydrogen ion concentration varies according to the diet and tissue metabolism from pH 5 to 8. Hydrogen ions are the end waste product of energy (ATP) production by the cells, from glucose or fatty acids (see Chapter 1), and also from ketone production (see p. 125) and from acids taken in the diet. Because hydrogen ions cause acidity, they are potentially hazardous; they have to be transported in the blood and need to be excreted. Blood pH is critical at pH 7.4, and it must be stabilised at this value. Hydrogen ions entering the blood must be buffered, then removed by the kidneys for excretion. **Buffers** are a means of 'tying up' hydrogen ions into compounds so that they are unable to contribute to the hydrogen ion concentration. This allows them to be carried safely in the blood without affecting the blood pH. Examples are bicarbonate, proteins, haemoglobin and phosphate buffers. Of these, haemoglobin (Hb) is very important for buffering hydrogen ions in the blood (Hb+H$^+$$\rightarrow$ HHb), followed by blood proteins, which have a nitrogenous component (NH$_2$) able to take up surplus H$^+$ (NH$_2$+H$^+$$\rightarrow$NH$_3$$^+$), and then bicarbonate. Bicarbonate (HCO$_3$$^-$) is filtered from the blood in the glomerulus and serves to buffer urine in the proximal tubule (HCO$_3$$^-$+H$^+$$\rightarrow$H$_2CO_3$$\rightarrow$H$_2$O+CO$_2$), where CO$_2$ is removed from the blood via the lungs, and H$_2$O is excreted through the kidneys. Phosphate (HPO$_4$$^{2-}$) is a major buffer in the renal filtrate of the distal tubular cells ($HPO_4^{2-}+H^++Na^+\rightarrow NaH_2PO_4$). Phosphate prevents urine from becoming too acidic or alkaline, which would otherwise damage the tract lining and cause great discomfort, especially when passing urine (micturition). Increased urinary pH (above pH 8, i.e. alkaline urine) occurs in **alkalosis** (high blood pH, as may occur in a vegetarian diet). It occurs naturally soon after a meal. Low urinary pH (below pH 5, i.e. acidic urine) appears in **acidosis** (low blood pH as in diabetic ketoacidosis or aspirin overdose) or after the consumption of prunes or cranberries, or as a result of starvation. Disturbance of blood pH (and thus urinary pH) can happen in various therapies that influence the fluid balance of the body. Since H^+ and K^+ share the same excretory mechanism in the distal tubule and collecting duct cells, the excretion of large quantities of K^+ (as may be the case with excessive intravenous potassium chloride (KCl) treatment or diuretic therapy) may cause retention of H^+.

Nitrites in urine

Nitrites can be tested for as an indicator of the presence of a urinary tract infection (UTI). Nitrites are the result of the breakdown of nitrates in the urinary system. Nitrates are a component of our diet and are excreted normally in the urine. The presence of nitrites, however, indicates that there is a bacterial infection by a type of organism that is capable of producing an enzyme, **nitrate reductase**, necessary for converting nitrate to nitrite. Ninety per cent of UTIs are caused by organisms of this type (e.g. Gram-negative bacteria such as *Escherichia coli*), and therefore the nitrite test stick is of increasing clinical importance as a quick, accurate means of detecting UTIs. The remaining 10% of urinary infections include staphylococci, *Pseudomonas* species and enterococci. These are organisms that do not produce the enzyme and therefore the test is not sensitive to them. Chemical stick reagent tests can often replace the more expensive laboratory tests, and give quicker results. Urine cultures and microscopy are the largest numbers of requests made to pathology departments for laboratory examination, and it is possible that this workload, and the cost to the health service this causes, could be reduced by incorporating some laboratory tests within the stick format. The nitrite and leucocyte test strips (see p. 129) are an attempt to identify those urines with infection before laboratory culture, and they therefore reduce the time and cost involved in the analysis of negative samples. The problems have centred on the accuracy of the chemical test strip. If they are used routinely for the identification of UTIs before laboratory cultures are taken, the risk is that they may miss some clinically significant infections. Some authors, however, are already convinced that stick analysis of urine for infection is now accurate enough to be used to identify only those urines that need laboratory culture and analysis (Doley and Nelligan 2003).

Leucocytes in urine

Leucocytes of the granulocyte type (especially neutrophils) produce another enzyme, **leucocyte esterase**, that can be detected in urine. This test will identify the presence of intact and lysed (broken-down) granulocytes in the urine either with or without infection. The presence of leucocytes indicates an inflammation, either with organisms (infection) or without (sterile).

When to test urine

Urinalysis has become a standard routine test carried out on admission to hospital and in the doctor's surgery, and it is often expected regardless of whether or not it is required for the patient's assessment. It is easy to see why these tests have become so widespread. The tests are quick, cheap and non-invasive, with on-the-spot results, and they can provide a wealth of information by virtue of there being multiple tests on one stick. The alternative is laboratory analysis of urine, which is time-consuming and more expensive and on average the results take a few days to return. For reagent strip analysis, all that is required is a very small quantity of fresh urine, one stick and a few minutes of time. If the results are recorded as NAD (nothing abnormal detected), then it is known that the renal system appears to be functioning normally, the chance of trauma is less, and there is probably no diabetes, ketoacidosis, bleeding or jaundice. For these reasons, methods for putting other urine tests on a reagent strip are being considered so that the test can be ward-based rather than laboratory-based. The nitrite and leucocyte tests are two of the results of these initiatives; previously urinalysis for UTIs took about three days of laboratory work for a result. Although this is still necessary to identify the organism and the antibiotic required for treatment, a quick reagent strip test that can identify the presence or absence of UTI will cut down the number of sterile specimens sent to the laboratory and in many cases provide instant reassurance to the patient. By making it possible to do a test in the clinical area, the test itself becomes far less labour-intensive, more cost-effective and reduces the time factor to minutes, an important point for patient comfort and recovery. No doubt other stick-mounted tests will be developed, which, by reducing the laboratory input, allows more laboratory time for other things.

As a standard screening device, reagent strip urinalysis can be carried out as routine almost anywhere, and certainly on admission to hospital, pre-operatively, post-operatively, and in the outpatient clinic and the accident centre, where it can be used to help eliminate trauma to the kidneys (Worrall 2009). In the community, it can be used in the doctor's surgery or in the patient's own home by visiting nurses. Being simple to use, it can also be taught to the patient to do for themselves or by the patient's carer. Chemistry has come to the aid of the health care professional and has allowed the test to be taken to the patient rather than the patient (or at least their urine) to be taken to the test.

New and potential urine tests include identifying disorders not directly affecting the urinary system:

- Testing for a distinctive metabolite pattern in urine produced by the bacteria *Streptococcus pneumoniae*. This is an important organism causing community-acquired pneumonia (CAP), a serious lung disease. Early detection of this organism can result in rapid treatment and the saving of many lives (Watt *et al.* 2010).
- The possibility of testing for the protein biomarker called leucine-rich alpha-2-glycoprotein (LRG), which, if present, indicates the presence of appendicitis in young children's urine (Kentsis *et al.* 2010).
- The levels of 4-(methylnitrosamino)-1-(3-pyridyl)-1-butanol (NNAL) can be measured in urine. NNAL is a metabolite of 4-(methylnitrosamino)-1-(3-pyridyl)-1-butanone

(NNK), a component of tobacco smoke. Both NNK and NNAL are potent pulmonary carcinogens, and the presence of raised NNAL in urine can suggest a higher risk of lung cancer (Hecht *et al.* 2001).

- A simple urine test that can detect for four different RNA (ribonucleic acid) molecules that are indicative of prostate cancer with an accuracy which does away with the need for the standard blood test and prostatic biopsy investigations (Laxman *et al.* 2008).

Key points

- The functional unit of the kidney is the nephron. About one million nephrons exist in each of the two kidneys.
- Urine forms in three steps: filtration from the glomerulus; reabsorption from the convoluted tubules; and secretion from the straight collecting ducts.
- Urine is formed at an average rate of 1 ml per minute.
- For accurate results, urine must be tested when fresh using the correct technique.
- Normal urine is a pale straw colour, clear with no deposits.
- On testing, normal urine should show negative results for glucose, blood, protein, ketones and bilirubin.
- Urinary pH ranges from 5 to 8 with an average about 6.
- The specific gravity measures the density of dissolved solutes in urine compared with water, normally about 1010 (water = 1000).
- Nitrite and leucocyte test for infection or inflammatory cells in urine.
- Diuretic drugs induce a large urine output as a treatment for hypertension, oedema or cardiac failure.

References

Arshad I. and Shar-Baloch K. (2007) Renal stones. *Annals of the Royal College of Surgeons of England,* **89**(3): 926.

Doley A. and Nelligan M. (2003) Is a negative dipstick urinalysis good enough to exclude urinary tract infection in paediatric emergency department patients? *Emergency Medicine Fremantle WA,* **15**(1): 77–80.

Hecht S. S., Ye M., Carmella S. G., Fredrickson A., Adgate J. L., Greaves I. A., Church T. R., Ryan A. D., Mongin S. J. and Sexton K. (2001) Metabolites of a tobacco-specific lung carcinogen in the urine of elementary school-aged children. *Cancer Epidemiology Biomarkers Prevention,* **10**(11): 1109–1116.

Kentsis A., Lin Y. Y., Kurek K., Calicchio M., Wang Y. Y., Monigatti F., Campagne F., Lee R., Horwitz B., Steen H. and Bachur R. (2010) Discovery and validation of urine markers of acute pediatric appendicitis using high-accuracy mass spectrometry. *Annals of Emergency Medicine,* **55**(1), 62–70.e4.

Laxman B., Morris D. S., Yu J., Siddiqui J., Cao J., Mehra R., Lonigro R. J., Tsodikov A., Wei J. T., Tomlins S. A. and Chinnaiyan A. M. (2008) A first-generation multiplex biomarker analysis of urine for the early detection of prostate cancer. *Cancer Research,* **68**(3): 645–649.

Pfitzenmaier J., Buse S., Haferkamp A., Pahernik S., Djakovic N. and Hohenfellner M. (2008) Kidney trauma. *Der Urologe Ausg A,* **47**(6): 759–767; quiz 768. Retrieved from http://www.ncbi.nlm.nih.gov/pubmed/18478197.

Simerville J. A., Maxted W. C. and Pahira J. J. (2005) Urinalysis: a comprehensive review. *American Family Physician*, **71**(6):1153–1162.

Watt J. P., Moïsi J. C., Donaldson R. L. A., Reid R., Ferro S., Whitney C. G., Santosham M. and O'Brien K. L. (2010) Use of serology and urine antigen detection to estimate the proportion of adult community-acquired pneumonia attributable to Streptococcus pneumoniae. *Epidemiology and Infection*, 1–8. Retrieved from http://www.ncbi.nlm.nih.gov/pubmed/20334727.

Worrall J. C. (2009) Emergency department visual urinalysis versus laboratory urinalysis. CJEM *Canadian Journal of Emergency Medical Care, JCMU Journal Canadien de Soins Médicaux d'Urgence*, **11**(6), 540–543.

Chapter 8   **Elimination (II)**
Digestive observations

- Introduction
- Faeces
- The mechanism of defecation
- Disorders of faecal elimination
- The mechanism of vomiting
- Observations regarding vomiting
- Drugs affecting vomiting
- Key points
- References

Introduction

Although generally thought of as a distasteful subject, abnormal elimination, such as diarrhoea or vomiting, indicates that changes have occurred in the patterns of physiology within the digestive system, changes of which health care professionals must be aware. The presence of these phenomena alone is an important observation, but additional data can be obtained from further observation, testing and questioning to ascertain any associated evidence. An understanding of the facts gained from observation, combined with a knowledge of the underlying pathophysiology, allows greater opportunities to make accurate decisions, for example when to involve the medical staff.

Faeces

Faeces is waste material obtained primarily from ingested food. It normally contains **fibre**, a collective term for several indigestible components of the diet that provides the bulk of the stool. Fibre is derived mostly from the plant substances in the diet, i.e. fruit and vegetables, but less is found in meats. The varieties of fibre include **cellulose**, hemicellulose, pectins, gums and **lignins** (see p. 102). These are mostly large-molecular **polysaccharides** that form the walls of plant cells. These particular polysaccharides are complex carbohydrate molecules that are indigestible by any of the digestive enzymes in the small bowel (ileum), but some can be broken down (catabolised) to a certain extent by digestive bacteria present in the large bowel (colon). These bacteria are **commensals**, that is they survive in the human bowel without causing any harm. In fact, human bowel commensals actually produce important vitamins from their activity on bowel contents, i.e. **niacin**, which is also known as **nicotinic acid**; **thiamine**, which is **vitamin B_1**; and **vitamin K**, which we can absorb and use (see p. 98). Fibre has several properties; in particular, it absorbs and holds water, **electrolytes** and bile salts. Holding water makes it soft normally so that the stool is easy to pass. However, the action of the colon in absorbing water from the bowel contents prevents the faeces from being too wet normally. The absorption of electrolytes and bile salts into the fibre itself aids the elimination of these substances. **Refined foods** are those in which the fibre is largely removed or cooked sufficiently to break it down to digestible carbohydrates and provide a greater degree of nutrient efficiency with less waste material. The refining of foods, as is common in the Western diet, has resulted, however, in an increase in bowel disorders such as colon cancers and **diverticular disease**. The latter is a condition in which the mucous lining of the bowel is pushed through the muscular wall into pouches that can become inflamed. Clearly, fibre has a greater role to play in human digestion than was at first thought, being vital for correct bowel function and, as such, is protective against bowel disease.

The mechanism of defecation

The rectum is normally empty. Bowel wall movements push faecal matter into the rectum, stretching the rectal wall. This stretching triggers the **defecation reflex** (Figure 8.1), an automatic action involving afferent sensory pathways from stretch receptors in the rectal wall to the spinal cord, and efferent motor pathways from the cord to the rectal muscles.

Activation of this pathway results in the muscular walls of the sigmoid colon and rectum contracting, pushing the contents further along, and the anal sphincters to relax. Relaxation of sphincters causes them to open, and here this means opening the escape route for faeces. However, whereas the internal anal sphincter is autonomic (smooth muscle), the external requires voluntary control (skeletal muscle), thus allowing the time needed for the sphincter to be opened appropriately. It is this last aspect that is important in childhood, for control of the external sphincter is a skill that has to be learnt. Expulsion of faeces is achieved by contraction of the rectal wall, depression of the diaphragm and contraction of abdominal muscles, the last two causing an increase in the intra-abdominal pressure, aided perhaps by holding the breath. Although this is a spinal reflex, achieved by the **parasympathetic nervous system** from the sacral outflow (Figure 8.1), the medulla is involved in co-ordinating the various muscle activities. It is useful to think of the parasympathetic nervous system as being the neurological control of all three normal emptying mechanisms of the body, i.e. urination, defecation and (in males) ejaculation.

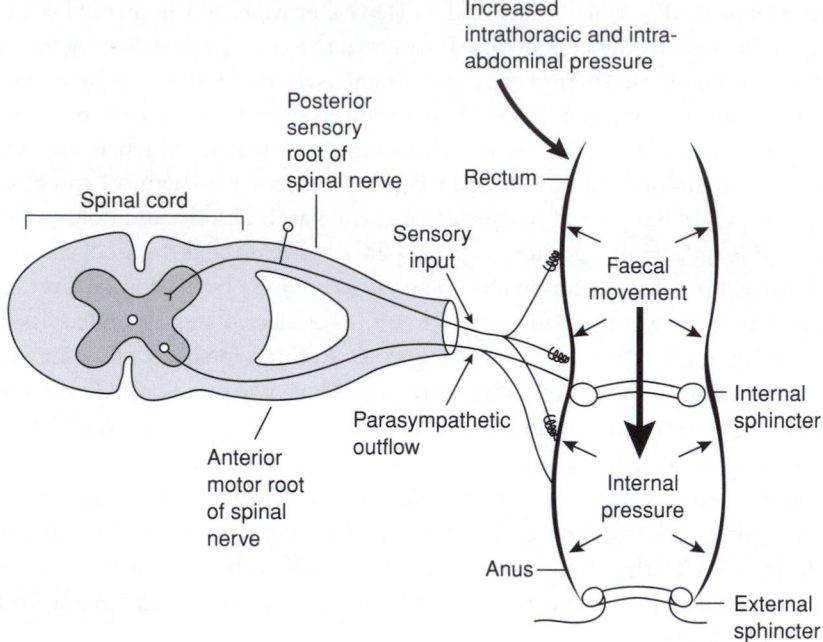

Figure 8.1 Physiology of defecation. Internal pressure from descending stools into the rectum stretches the rectal wall. Sensory input from stretch receptors trigger a parasympathetic output from the spinal cord which relaxes the internal sphincter and contracts smooth muscle in the bowel wall. This puts pressure on the external sphincter to open, but being voluntary skeletal muscle this sphincter opens under conscious control. Increasing intrathoracic and intra-abdominal pressure pushes the bowel contents forward.

Disorders of faecal elimination

Diarrhoea

The word **rrhoea** arises at the end of several words such as diarrhoea and steatorrhoea, and it means 'flow'. **Diarrhoea** is a flow of faeces in fluid form, since the water content is paramount and the fibre bulk is minimal. Diarrhoea has numerous causes, and some basic observations are needed to establish a possible **aetiology**. These observations are for quantity and number of bowel evacuations that occur per day. This will give an estimate of the fluid loss the patient is experiencing, and fluid balance records may be necessary. Identification of any abnormal content, e.g. the presence of blood or mucus, is important.

Blood in the stools

Blood in the stools may be fresh and red, indicating a bleed somewhere within the colon or rectum itself. Otherwise it may be a darker red-brown (or even black, and is then called **melaena**), suggesting that the blood has undergone some degree of digestion. In this case it must come from higher in the digestive system: a bleed within the stomach or ileum. Digestive bleeds can arise from mucosal ulcerations or growths that erode blood vessels, ruptures of varicose veins within the oesophagus or rectum, or abdominal trauma. Being a liquid itself, blood can provide the necessary water to prevent colonic contents from being converted to solid stool, and blood therefore can become thoroughly integrated with the faecal matter. Of course, heavy digestive bleeds are likely to be accompanied by other symptoms of blood loss, notably pallor, increased and weakened pulse rate, low blood pressure, and even shock.

Mucus in diarrhoea

Mucus is the natural secretion of the mucous membrane and acts as a lubricant in the bowel for the passage of food and faecal content and dissolves some nutrients before it is itself re-absorbed. Mucus in diarrhoea is an indication of excessive inflammatory changes within the mucous membrane that result in overproduction of mucus. **Inflammatory bowel disease (IBD)** is a term that encompasses at least two bowel disorders, **ulcerative colitis** and **Crohn's disease**, both characterised by inflammation of the mucous lining of the bowel with blood and by mucus present in the diarrhoea.

Other causes of diarrhoea

Diarrhoea can also be caused by overstimulation of bowel movements by the parasympathetic nervous system, which promotes digestive activity. Normally, bowel contents are propelled along by waves of muscle contraction (called **peristalsis**) at a speed that allows water to be absorbed and therefore faeces to be well formed. If this rate of propulsion is speeded up (known as increased bowel **motility**), the contents reach the rectum before all the water is absorbed and liquid faeces results. This speeding up of peristalsis also causes the other symptom associated with diarrhoea, that of very frequent bowel evacuations and abdominal pain that occurs during peristalsis (known as **colic**). A patient suffering from a severe form of IBD, for example, 40 or more diarrhoea bowel evacuations in 24 hours, may sometimes experience sleep loss and severe restriction of activities. Such a patient could also experience dehydration and electrolyte imbalance and distressing pain and tenderness around the anal ring. Infections such as *Shigella*, an organism that causes **dysentery**, or food-poisoning organisms such as *Staphylococcus* or *Salmonella* can have similar effects. Non-infectious causes include the overuse of **purgatives** (or **laxatives**, see below), **malabsorption syndromes**, certain foods in the diet that increase bowel propulsion, treatments like radiation therapy involving the digestive tract and even anxiety ('nervous diarrhoea').

Drug-induced diarrhoea is an important cause of the problem, especially in elderly people because they often require more medication than younger people and therefore suffer more side effects (Ratnaike and Jones 1998). **Antibiotic drugs** can cause diarrhoea as a side effect because their activity against living organisms may also involve killing the natural colonic commensals, bacteria we need for normal bowel function. Drugs of the laxative kind fall into four main groups: the bulk-forming agents (e.g. **ispaghula husk**, such as **Fibrogel** or **Isogel**); the stimulants (e.g. **senna**, such as **Senokot**); the faecal softeners (e.g. oils, such as **arachis oil**); and the osmotic laxatives (e.g. **lactulose**).

Constipation

Constipation is the failure to evacuate the bowel adequately, often totally, leading to an increasing collection of faeces in the colon. Perhaps as many as 10% of the Western population suffers varying degrees of retained bowel content. Unlike diarrhoea, constipation provides few external clues to its presence, and the nurse usually relies on a history of bowel activity over the previous few days to identify the problem. It is important to recognise the patient who is *at risk* of constipation: notably the patient with reduced mobility, altered levels of consciousness, inadequate fluid intake or any combination of these. The case of one elderly lady illustrates this point. She was immobile, drowsy, hypothermic and not drinking well with a degree of dehydration. After several days on the ward she developed abdominal pain. Nobody on the ward knew if this lady had passed any faeces since she had been admitted. The doctors discovered she was constipated and ordered an enema, which was given by the nurses, and this solved her problem. The relatives were very pleased with the nurses' actions since her pain had been relieved, but in fact the nurses had failed to recognise that this lady was at risk of constipation from the moment of admission. Her pain was *preventable*, not just *curable*, by the identification of her risk status, by the monitoring of her bowel movements and by the correction of her dehydration. In some patients, improvements in their mobility also contribute to the prevention of constipation, as well as the many other complications of immobility.

One bowel evacuation each 24 hours is the average, but considerable variation does occur, with some individuals claiming that bowel evacuations of only once or twice per week is normal for them. Others may pass faeces more than once a day. What *is* abnormal is a total absence of any bowel evacuation, and what *may* be abnormal is a significant change in a person's bowel habit, especially if this change is persistent. If once a day is normal for an individual, then three days without evacuation is a potential for constipation. Additional signs to aid the diagnosis of constipation include the presence or absence of **anorexia** (loss of appetite), abdominal pain and distension, nausea, and confusion. This last symptom is particularly important in elderly people, when the brain becomes especially susceptible to the toxic effects of constipation, i.e. waste products in faeces that are normally excreted are reabsorbed into the blood; confusion as a result of constipation must be identified, as families can think that their elderly relative is becoming demented when all that is required is an enema. Diet is also important to note, since a lack of oral fluid or fibre in the diet is an important factor leading to constipation. Lack of exercise, especially complete immobility, reduces bowel movement, which, in turn, causes the contents to remain longer in the colon. During this longer stay in the colon more and more water is absorbed from the contents, which then get drier and harder to propel and evacuate. Total obstruction of the bowel with hard, solid faeces can follow on from this in some extreme cases, made worse by any condition that narrows the bowel lumen, for example, new growths. Some drugs that have a constipating side effect include **morphine** and its derivatives. High dosage, as in the management of some terminal disorders, may cause this unwelcome side effect, which then requires additional management. Assessing the risk of constipation requires keen observation of diet and fluid input, mobility, attempts at defecation, abdominal pain, and mental alertness, and these are sometimes put together in risk assessment scales, which may be useful in some clinical areas (Duffy and Zernike 1997). Elderly people are always said to be at highest risk because of reduced mobility and a decline in the health status of the bowel with age (Bouras and Tangalos 2009).

Stomas

A **stoma** is an artificial opening in the bowel to allow the excretion of bowel contents into a collection bag on the abdominal wall when normal defecation is not possible. Stomas are made into the ileum (ileostomy) or colon (colostomy), depending on the nature of the problem. Stomas are sometimes used in the management of bowel cancers, ulcerative colitis, diverticular disease or after permanent **bowel resection** (removal of part of the bowel). A colostomy opening made into the *proximal* half of the colon (on the right side of the abdomen) will, at first, result in a more liquid stool than an opening into the *distal* half of the colon (on the left side of the abdomen). This is due to the water extraction function of the colon. The proximal half contains liquid stools from the small intestine, whereas the distal half contains stools that have travelled nearly the entire length of the bowel and are therefore much drier. Stoma bags require changing, which the patient can often do themselves after recovery from surgery and after being taught about their stoma. Observation is important during the changing procedure, when the stoma itself should be examined for a healthy red (the natural colour of mucous membrane that is well supplied with blood) with no bleeding. Pallor or cyanosis (blue coloration) may indicate reduced blood supply, which can cause complications, and must be reported to the doctor. The skin around the stoma must be inspected for soreness and inflammation plus any broken areas and infection. This is important since some collection devices work by sticking to the skin, and this could become problematic. The bag contents are observed for the same constituents as faeces, i.e. for diarrhoea, blood, bile or mucus, and also colour and quantity. Some drugs may affect the function of stomas or change the colour of the bag contents. These drugs include laxatives and antacids (both of which are best avoided for most stoma patients unless prescribed and monitored carefully). **Narrow-spectrum antibiotics** are preferable to **broad-spectrum antibiotics** when such drugs are necessary, since their narrow spectrum means they will have less effect on the normal bowel commensals with less risk of diarrhoea. Diarrhoea in a stoma patient is very difficult to manage since it requires numerous and frequent changes of the collection bag, which disrupts normal daily activities and results in complications of the skin at the stoma site. Skin irritation and breakdown around the stoma are particularly unfortunate and should be avoided if possible. The broad-spectrum antibiotics, like penicillin, not only can cause diarrhoea but also can directly irritate the skin at the stoma site. Antibiotics can also change the faeces to a grey-green colour. Other colour changes caused by drugs include **iron** (black), **tetracycline** (red), **heparin** (pink or red), **indometacin** (green) and **aspirin** (pink or red). This last drug, aspirin, is acidic and therefore may cause mucosal and skin irritation at the stoma site. It also contributes to anticoagulation of blood, i.e. helps to stop blood clotting and promotes bleeding, and is therefore best avoided for these reasons. Stoma care is a specialist nursing subject and nurse practitioners train specifically in this subject. Stoma patients will be referred to the care of such a specialist nurse, who should be consulted on all matters concerning these patients.

The mechanism of vomiting

Vomiting can be regarded generally as a normal physiological response to an abnormal condition affecting either the digestive system or its neurological control. Stomach and sometimes bowel contents are driven the wrong way up the oesophagus back into the mouth. This usually only happens as a result of a pathological state, and accurate observations can provide important clues about the nature of this pathology.

The brain stem medullary **vomit reflex centre** co-ordinates what is a relatively complex process involving a range of different stimuli (Figure 8.2). Also in the brain, and closely associated with the vomit centre, is the **chemoreceptor trigger zone (CTZ)**. This is in the floor of the fourth ventricle (in an area called the **area postrema**), and this receives impulses from chemical stimuli in the blood. These chemicals include various drugs (e.g. cytotoxic agents) and other toxins from perhaps food or infectious organisms. Such stimulation of the CTZ causes stimulation of the vomit reflex centre, and vomiting can then occur. The chemoreceptor trigger zone also receives impulses from the **cerebellum**, part of the brain that co-ordinates muscle activity and balance. The cerebellum obtains sensory information on balance (**vestibular** information) from the semi-circular canals in both ears via the vestibular branch of the eighth cranial nerve (the **vestibulocochlear nerve**). These canals register changes in balance and head movement as nerve impulses that are transmitted first to the **vestibular nuclei** in the medulla, then to the cerebellum (Figure 8.3).

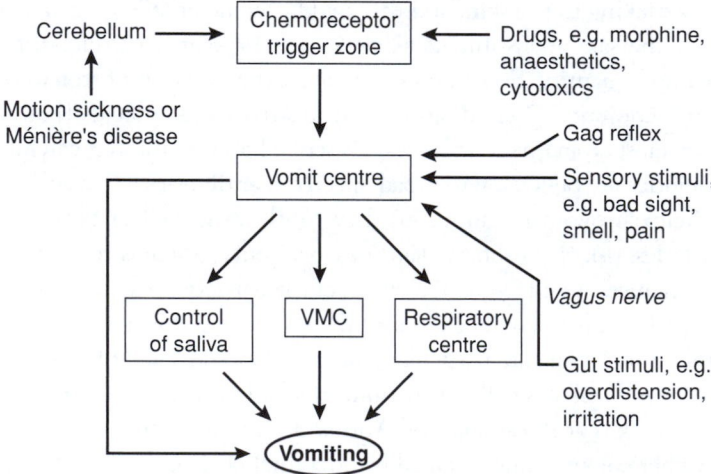

FIGURE 8.2 Stimulation of the vomit centre is often via the chemoreceptor trigger zone, which itself is stimulated by motion or drugs, or sometimes directly by bad sensory stimuli (e.g. an unpleasant smell or sight) or by vagal stimuli from the gut. The vomit centre output is via the vasomotor centre (VMC), which influences the blood pressure, via the respiratory centre, which regulates breathing throughout vomiting; the vomit centre controls saliva production.

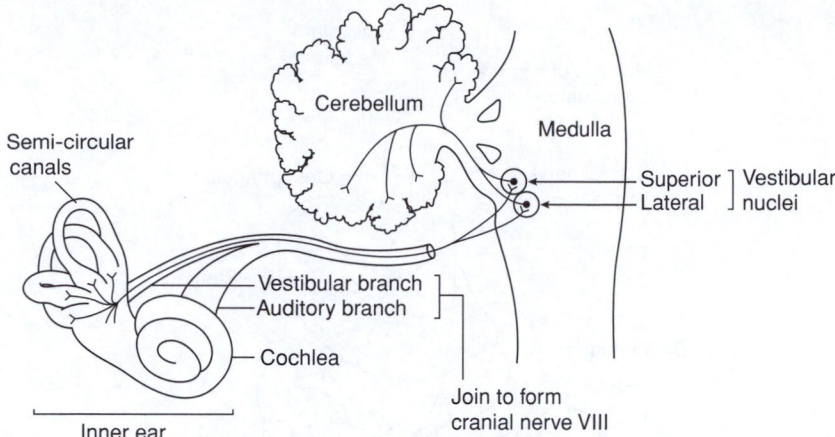

FIGURE 8.3 Vestibular stimulation of the cerebellum. Impulses from the semi-circular canals of the inner ear pass via the vestibulocochlear nerve (cranial nerve VIII) to the vestibular nuclei of the medulla and then on to the cerebellum.

Any disturbing movements or upsets in balance, as in motion sickness, can produce adverse nerve impulses that pass through the vestibular nuclei, the cerebellum and on to the chemoreceptor trigger zone. From here the vomit reflex centre is stimulated and vomiting occurs. A disease that causes vomiting via this route is **Ménière's disease**, a chronic disorder of the inner ear where the amount of the fluid called endolymph becomes excessive. This causes sudden attacks of **vertigo** (dizziness), nausea and vomiting, progressive deafness, and **tinnitus** (continued internal sounds in the ear). It is interesting that the word 'vertigo' has become commonly associated with dizziness caused by heights. However, the word simply means dizziness linked to a whirling-round sensation; it is not especially related to heights, and in reality people can suffer from vertigo at any height, often at ground level.

Some stimuli can cause vomiting without affecting the chemoreceptor trigger zone, i.e. affecting the vomit reflex centre directly. These include the **gag reflex**, a feeling of retching when the back of the tongue is touched with a finger or tongue depressor. Bad sights or smells stimulate the vomit reflex centre via the **cerebral cortex**, our conscious part of the brain, and stimuli from the digestive tract itself, such as over-distension or inflammatory irritation, arrive at the vomit centre via the **vagus nerve** (the tenth cranial nerve) (Figure 8.4).

The result of initiating activation of the vomit reflex centre is to first induce **nausea,** a feeling of sickness without actual vomiting, followed by retching and then finally vomiting. The person will inhale deeply as peristalsis is reversed. **Peristalsis** is the propulsive intermittent waves of smooth muscle contraction that pass along the bowel to push the contents forwards. Reversal of the direction of this contraction wave ensures that the digestive contents will be driven towards the mouth during vomiting. Just as with swallowing, the airway must be protected against inhalation during vomiting. Inhalation of vomit would involve not only obstructing the airway, but gastric acid and digestive enzymes would severely damage the delicate lung tissues and death would occur. To pre-

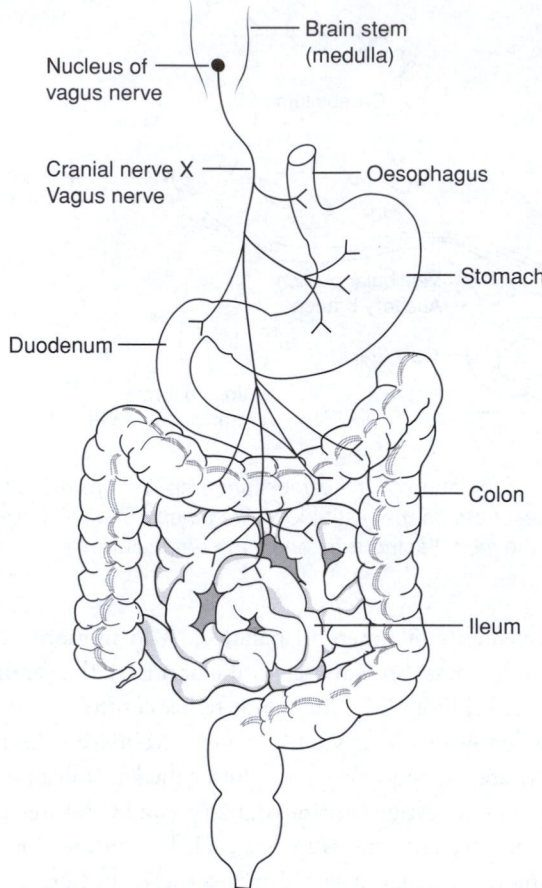

FIGURE 8.4 Vagus innervation of the digestive tract. The vagus (cranial nerve X) is the primary visceral sensory nerve. Branches to the stomach increase gastric acidity and the parasympathetic component promotes digestion generally.

vent this, the glottis is closed by lowering the epiglottis and raising the hyoid bone and larynx. The **glottis** is the narrowest part of the airway opening and is found inside the larynx. The **epiglottis** is a flap of cartilage above the glottis that acts as a lid for the glottis by folding downwards at the same time as the **larynx** (voice box) is raised. In this way the glottis is closed and vomit cannot pass into the lungs. The **soft palate** is raised to close the **nasopharynx**, the passage from the nose to the throat, to prevent vomit entering the nose. If this is not achieved properly, vomit may come from the nasal passages as well as the mouth. The top opening into the stomach (called the **cardiac sphincter** because it is close to the heart) is dilated, and the lower opening (the **pyloric sphincter**) is closed. The gastric muscles (smooth type) and abdominal muscles (skeletal type) both contract, forcing the stomach contents upwards towards the mouth. The **diaphragm** (skeletal muscle) also flattens to aid in this process, helping to increase the intra-abdominal pressure. The process leaves the person a little breathless because energy is used (the generation of which requires oxygen, see Chapter 1) and breathing has been temporarily suspended. It is also accompanied and preceded by increases in both salivation and heart rate, the onset of pallor, sweating, pupillary dilation and distress, much of which is caused by **sympathetic nerve** stimulation of the sweat glands, the heart and the pupils.

Nausea, which is simply feeling sick, acts as an early warning that vomiting may happen. It is an unpleasant sensation that may persist alone or quickly result in the act of vomiting. It can occur under all the same pathological conditions that cause vomiting. However, nausea, and sometimes vomiting, can occur in non-pathological conditions, e.g. they are often features of early pregnancy (i.e. **morning sickness**). This is probably due to hormonal changes occurring at that time, especially the introduction of hormones from the placenta, such as **human chorionic gonadotrophin (hCG)**, or hormones from the **corpus luteum**, and the gradual decline in these pregnancy-related hormones is associated with the relief of sickness (Coutts 1998). Approximately one-quarter of people coming into hospital for treatment of cancer feel nauseated on arrival, before the therapy has begun. It can happen before second or subsequent treatments where side effects experienced from the first treatment are anticipated. This is termed **anticipatory nausea and vomiting (ANV)** and can sometimes be relieved or prevented in susceptible patients (Aapro *et al.* 2005).

Observations regarding vomiting

It is important to take into account how much is vomited, what the contents are and when vomiting occurs. The quantity is important because the gastric volume is limited, and the stomach may not have been full originally. Vomiting should stop once the stomach has been emptied if this was the purpose of the phenomenon. When this happens, it suggests that a cause lies within the stomach itself or its contents. But if vomiting persists beyond this point, it is likely to become unproductive once the stomach is empty, or produce only small volumes of gastrointestinal fluid. **Retching** is an attempt to vomit but with no gastric or duodenal content produced. At this point it is possible to say that the process of vomiting is not solely to empty the stomach but is caused by factors outside the digestive system continuously stimulating the vomit reflex centre in the brain. This in turn is affecting what is quite possibly a normal stomach.

In all cases, the nurse should ascertain some basic facts by asking questions, when possible, e.g. how long has the vomiting persisted? It should also be established if the vomiting is associated with:

- pain (e.g. abdominal or migraine) (see Chapter 11);
- the intake of food in general, or specific foods, drugs or alcohol;
- exposure to motion, as in spinning round, sea or travel sickness;
- exposure to obnoxious substances or emotionally disturbing experiences, e.g. the sight of blood, someone else vomiting or a foul smell;
- persistent coughing, since coughing itself can trigger the vomit reflex. This is a phenomenon mostly seen in children, in whom prolonged coughing may stimulate the vomit reflex centre. The cough and vomit centres both occur close together in the medulla, part of the brain stem.

How long the vomiting has persisted is vital to confirm because prolonged and persistent vomiting results in fluid and electrolyte losses leading to imbalance and of course various degrees of malnutrition. This is especially the case for children, especially small children, who will become ill rapidly if the fluid and electrolyte imbalance is not corrected quickly and vomiting is not brought under control. It may be the case that the vomiting can be traced back to the start of a new medication. In addition, observations are made on the content of the vomiting to identify whether it is food (digested or not), blood, bile or other gastrointestinal fluids.

Food in vomit

Food when vomited indicates that the time span between eating and vomiting is relatively short, i.e. within 4 hours of each other, and generally the shorter the time span, the less digestion has occurred. In this case, either the stomach cannot tolerate the food, or the food itself causes a vomit reaction. The former happens often as a result of infection or inflammation of the stomach (gastritis), or if the food was accompanied by large quantities of alcohol, or due to the inability of the stomach to pass food into the bowel because of an obstruction. One example of obstruction is **pyloric stenosis**, as seen in young children. This is a restriction of the flow of gastric contents through a tight or closed pyloric sphincter. Pyloric stenosis can be associated with **projectile vomiting**, when peristalsis attempts to force food through the obstruction but actually ejects it under pressure. Bowel obstructions are also caused by **neoplasms** ('new growths') or compression of the bowel by abdominal muscle contractions, as seen in **strangulated hernias**, both conditions found in the older adult. Some degree of obstruction can occur in torsions of the bowel such as **intussusception** (telescoping of the bowel) or **volvulus** (twisting of the bowel), both of these being conditions found usually in younger children.

Where the food itself causes the vomiting, it occurs as a result of infections or toxins in the food (food poisoning). A number of different organisms cause food poisoning of varying degrees, some more dangerous than others, e.g. *Clostridium botulinum*, the cause of **botulism**. This is a rare but potentially fatal form of food poisoning often contracted after eating contaminated canned meat products. Such contamination results from failure of the can-sealing process, or ruptured seals on cans during transport. All the seals at the joints in the metal of canned meats should be inspected before purchase, and any breaks in these joints reported to the shop staff. A less dangerous, yet very unpleasant, food poisoning is caused by *Staphylococcus aureus*, usually implanted on food by those preparing the food. This gives 24 hours of vomiting and diarrhoea, leaving the person feeling debilitated and very unwell.

Blood in vomit

Blood appears in different forms in vomit, depending on where the bleeding is occurring. Fresh bright-red blood in the vomit means it has not been in the stomach for very long, perhaps only minutes, and may indicate a possible gastric bleed, known as a **haematemesis**, from an ulceration or neoplasm. However, swallowed blood, often from an **epistaxis** (nose bleed), can be vomited back since the acidic stomach cannot tolerate large quantities of

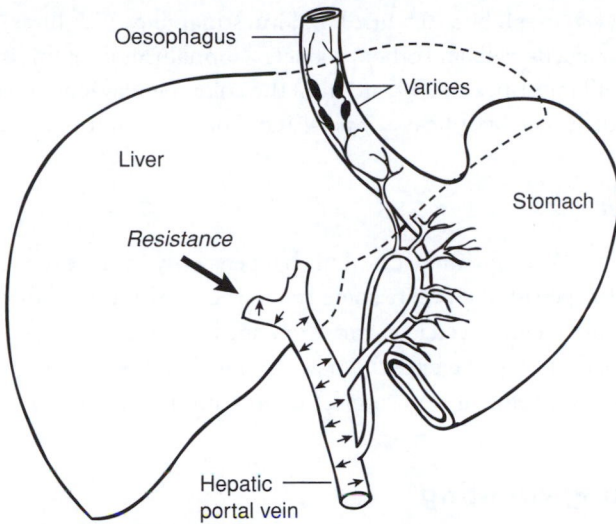

FIGURE 8.5 Oesophageal varices caused by portal hypertension. High blood pressure inside the portal vein (shown by small arrows inside the vessel) is due to some resistance to blood flow within the liver, often the result of liver disease. Back flow of blood to the lower end of the oesophagus causes venous dilations, which can rupture and bleed severely.

blood. This is a good reason for holding the head forward when treating nose bleeds, to prevent posterior bleeding, which will otherwise be swallowed and cause vomiting. Vomiting blood can continue for some time, i.e. until the patient collapses from shock, and requires urgent intervention. Sudden massive quantities of vomited blood are sometimes seen in ruptured **oesophageal varices**, varicose veins of the lower oesophagus caused by congestion of hepatic portal venous blood as a result of obstructive liver diseases (Figure 8.5). An important cause of liver obstruction is **cirrhosis**, a gradual loss of liver cells that are replaced by scar tissue, and which is usually accompanied by **hepatic failure**.

Blood that has been in the stomach for an hour or more before being vomited has been subject to changes caused by digestion and the hydrochloric acid conditions. In this case it is described as **coffee grounds**, a reference to its appearance. This type of bleeding indicates low-grade blood loss, which the stomach can tolerate for a while, possibly from an ulceration.

Bile in vomit

Bile and other gastrointestinal fluids do occasionally appear in vomit, especially if persistent vomiting has emptied the stomach and has forced duodenal or even ileal contents up into the mouth. About 500 ml of bile comes from the liver each day into the duodenum (see Chapter 7), and it gives a strong unpleasant alkaline burning taste in the mouth and throat when vomited. The digestive system as a whole produces 7 litres of fluid secreted into the bowel lumen over 24 hours, which consists of saliva (1.5 litres), gastric juice (2 litres), pancreatic juice (1.5 litres), bile (0.5 litre) and intestinal juice (1.5 litres), which contains digestive enzymes, mucus, cells and other products. Normally most of this is re-absorbed (6.5 litres from the small intestines and 350 ml from the colon per day), but it can be vomited as a watery fluid, usually seen after heavy or persistent bouts of vomiting.

Faeces in vomit

Vary rarely it is possible to vomit faeces. This happens only in the event of a severe bowel obstruction that has persisted for quite some time, when any form of bowel evacuation has stopped. The actual time involved may vary from one patient to another. Under these conditions it becomes necessary to empty the bowel as much as possible while supporting fluid and electrolyte balance before urgent surgical intervention.

Drugs affecting vomiting

Vomiting can be caused or prevented by various drugs. They can cause vomiting by irritating the mucosal lining directly or by stimulating the chemoreceptor trigger zone (CTZ) once in circulation (see also Chapter 14). Some **emetics**, such as **apomorphine** (derived from **morphine**), are drugs that can cause nausea and vomiting by stimulating receptors on the CTZ (see Figure 8.2). The list of drugs that act in this way includes **cytotoxic agents** (used in cancer therapy), some of the **opioid analgesics** that act on the brain stem (such as morphine), some **anaesthetics** and **ipecacuanha**, a substance that is both a digestive irritant and a CTZ stimulant. This has been used with good effect in emergency departments to cause vomiting in children suspected of an accidental oral overdose of drugs. **Pilocarpine** is a drug that can cause vomiting by stimulating the cerebellum directly, thus bypassing the CTZ.

Drugs with the opposite effect are the anti-emetics, which prevent vomiting in several ways. **Anticholinergics** (e.g. **hyoscine**) block stimuli from the vestibular system and are therefore useful in the treatment of motion sickness. Try checking the ingredients of several brands of travel sickness tablets to see which ones contain hyoscine. The side effects are sometimes troublesome, notably a dry mouth, blurred vision and drowsiness. Drowsiness is dangerous if driving, and a warning against combining these drugs with driving should be on the pack. The **antihistamines** are also used in motion sickness therapy; they are less effective than hyoscine but produce fewer side effects. They include cyclizine, promethazine and dimenhydrinate. These drugs block receptor sites for **histamine** (the H_1 receptor), but it is not clear how they prevent sickness. **Cannabinoids**, such as the drug **nabilone**, act on the chemoreceptor trigger zone and are useful in treating sickness during cytotoxic therapy, but they do cause drowsiness, dizziness and a dry mouth. The **dopamine antagonists** work by blocking the dopamine receptors (**type D_2 receptors**) in the area postrema, reducing the CTZ stimulation of the vomit reflex centre. They are therefore less useful in treating motion sickness. Included in this group are the non-phenothiazines metoclopramide and domperidone. Metoclopramide can also act on the stomach, promoting its emptying via the normal pyloric route. The side effects are sedation, **hypotension** (low blood pressure) and some problems of movement involving the **extra-pyramidal tract system** of the brain.

Key points

- Diarrhoea and vomiting are indications that changes have occurred in the patterns of physiology within the digestive system.
- Fibre has an important role to play in human digestion, being vital for correct bowel function and protection against bowel disease.
- Blood in the stools may indicate a bleed somewhere within the colon if fresh, or a bleed within the stomach or ileum if darker.
- Mucus in diarrhoea is an indication of excessive inflammatory changes within the mucous membrane that result in overproduction of mucus, as in inflammatory bowel disease.
- Diarrhoea can be caused by excessive bowel movements that can occur in bowel infections or food poisoning, the overuse of laxatives, malabsorption syndromes or treatments such as radiation therapy.
- Signs of constipation include anorexia, abdominal pain, distension, nausea and confusion.
- Lack of fluid or fibre in the diet and lack of exercise are important factors leading to constipation.
- A stoma is an artificial opening in the bowel. Stomas open into the ileum (ileostomy) or colon (colostomy).
- In the event of vomiting, checks are important to assess how long it has persisted, whether the vomiting is associated with any pain, food intake, drugs, alcohol, exposure to motion, obnoxious substances or an emotionally disturbing experience or whether there is any persistent coughing.
- Observe and report any food, blood, bile or faeces in vomit.
- Prolonged vomiting results in fluid and electrolyte losses, especially in young children, who will become ill rapidly if the fluid and electrolyte imbalance is not corrected quickly and vomiting is not brought under control.
- Emetics are drugs that can cause nausea and vomiting, and the anti-emetics prevent vomiting.

References

Aapro M. S., Molassiotis A. and Olver I. (2005) Anticipatory nausea and vomiting. *Supportive Care in Cancer*, **13**(2): 117–121.

Bouras E. P. and Tangalos E. G. (2009) Chronic constipation in the elderly. *Gastroenterology Clinics of North America*, **38**(3): 463–480.

Coutts A. (1998) The 'minor' problems of pregnancy: a review. *Professional Care of Mother and Child*, **8**(4): 95–97.

Duffy J. and Zernike W. (1997) Development of a constipation risk assessment scale. *International Journal of Nursing Practice*, **3**(4): 260–263.

Edwards S. L. (1998) Malnutrition in hospital patients: where does it come from? *British Journal of Nursing*, **7**(16): 954–974.

Ratnaike R. N. and Jones T. E. (1998) Mechanisms of drug-induced diarrhoea in the elderly. *Drugs-Aging*, **13**(3): 245–253.

Scorza K., Williams A., Phillips J. D., and Shaw J. (2007) Evaluation of nausea and vomiting. *American Family Physician*, **76**(1): 76–84.

Chapter 9 **Skin**

- Introduction
- The structure and function of skin
- Skin observations
- Skin trauma
- Important skin diseases
- Key points
- References

Introduction

The skin, also known as the **integumentary system,** can be regarded as the largest organ of the body. It accounts for 16% of the body weight, it is between 1.5 and 2 square metres in area and it mostly averages between 2 to 3 mm thick. In some specific places, such as the soles of the feet, it is often thicker to sustain weight bearing. As with all organs, the skin has it own unique structure and set of functions.

The structure and function of skin

Figure 9.1 shows the structure of the skin in cross-section form. There are two major divisions of the skin: the outer **epidermis** and the deeper **dermis**.

Epidermis

The epidermis is made up of five layers of cells, which are, in fact, the same cells that started life in the deepest of the layers and are migrating slowly towards the surface. The five layers, starting with the deepest layer, are (Figure 9.1):

1   The **stratum germinativum** is the deepest of the five epidermal layers, which lies directly on top of the dermis. The basal cells of this layer, next to the dermis, are constantly

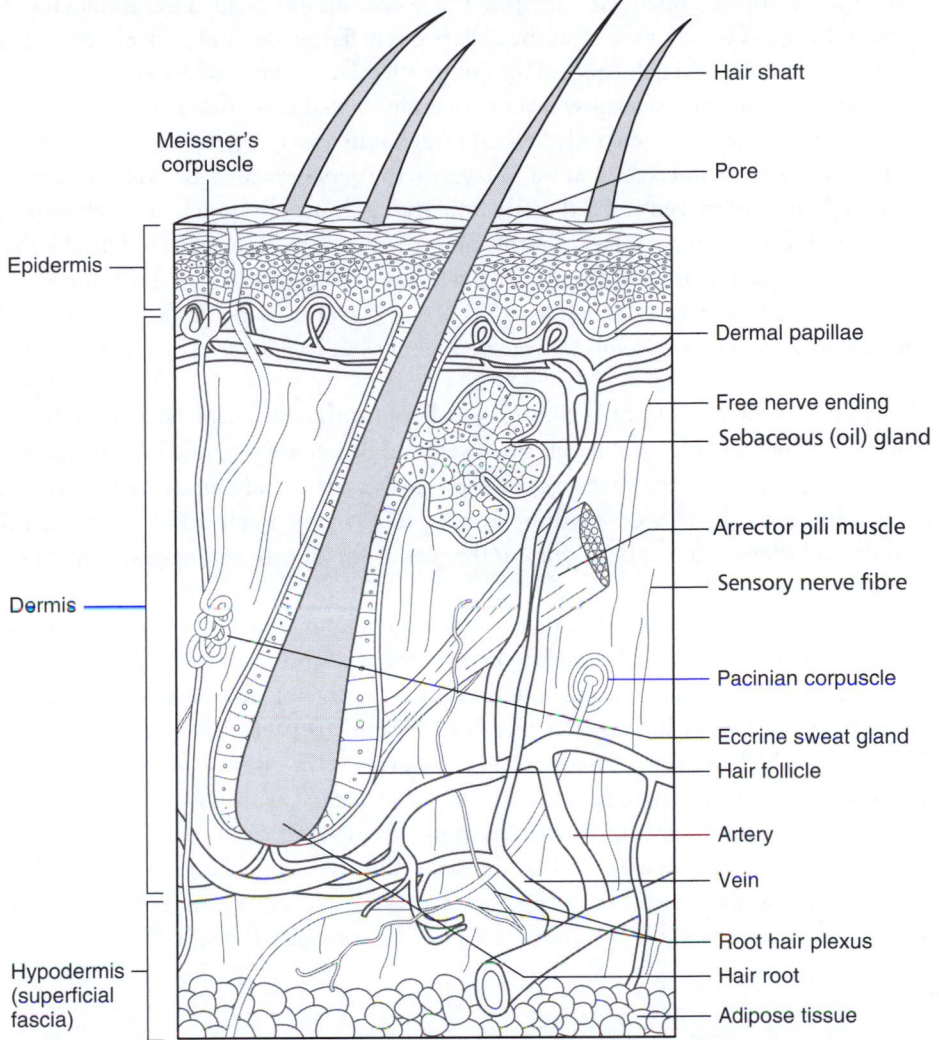

Hair shaft

Meissner's corpuscle

Pore

Epidermis

Dermal papillae

Free nerve ending

Sebaceous (oil) gland

Arrector pili muscle

Sensory nerve fibre

Dermis

Pacinian corpuscle

Eccrine sweat gland

Hair follicle

Artery

Vein

Hypodermis (superficial fascia)

Root hair plexus

Hair root

Adipose tissue

FIGURE 9.1 Section through the skin showing the epidermis, dermis and hypodermis. Sweat glands, hair roots and sebaceous glands are shown originating in the dermis. Nerve endings are listed and described in Table 9.1.

    dividing by mitosis (i.e. standard cell division). From here, cells migrate upwards away from the dermis. As they do, they enter the next layer.

2   The **stratum spinosum** ('spiny layer') is where the cells from the stratum germinativum develop shrinking cytoplasm but many can still continue to divide.

3   The **stratum granulosum** ('grainy layer') is where cells migrated from the stratum spinosum show no further cell division. Instead, they produce considerable amounts of a fibrous protein called **keratin** (a process called **keratinisation**). The cell membranes get thicker and the passage of substances through these membranes becomes difficult and declines. Eventually the nucleus and organelles of the cells disintegrate and the cells

die; their cytoplasm filled with keratin. These cells are now called **keratinocytes**. Towards the upper limits of the layer the cells begin to flatten out and pack closer together as they lose water and dehydrate. This is now effectively a layer of dry keratin.

4 The **stratum lucidum** is a glassy layer of densely packed keratinised cells derived from the stratum granulosum and only found in thick skin areas (e.g. the sole of the foot).

5 The **stratum corneum** is the outermost layer on the very surface of the skin. These keratinised dead cells derived either directly from the stratum granulosum or via the stratum lucidum form a protective layer for the deeper parts of the skin. Flakes of dead keratin are being shed from the surface all the time (about 30,000 flakes shed per minute). In the hair this is referred to as **dandruff**. This outer layer is therefore dead tissue, which means when you look at someone you are looking at a layer of *dead tissue*.

The epidermis can be thought of as a cell 'escalator', with newly evolved cells in the stratum germinativum moving up through the layers and becoming flat, dead, keratinised cell remnants as they arrive in the stratum corneum. This way, the epidermis is constantly being replaced with new cells. It takes anything from 15 to 30 days for cells to move through the epidermis, and they remain as dead cells on the surface for a further two weeks before being shed into the environment.

Other important cells exist at specific layers of the epidermis, particularly **melanocytes** in the stratum germinativum and **Langerhan cells** in the stratum spinosum.

Melanocytes (Figure 9.2) are pigmentation cells producing the dark brown pigment **melanin** from the dietary amino acid **tyrosine**. Melanin is packed inside vesicles called **melanosomes**, which are transported into keratinocytes. This protects vital cell structures (e.g. the nucleus) against harmful exposure to ultraviolet (UV) light in sunlight as the keratinocytes migrate towards the surface. Eventually the melanosomes are destroyed and the keratinocyte nucleus degrades and the cells die. The differences between light and dark skin is that dark-skinned people have larger melanosomes and the melanin levels are higher and persist for longer than in light-skinned people. The concentration of melanocytes in the

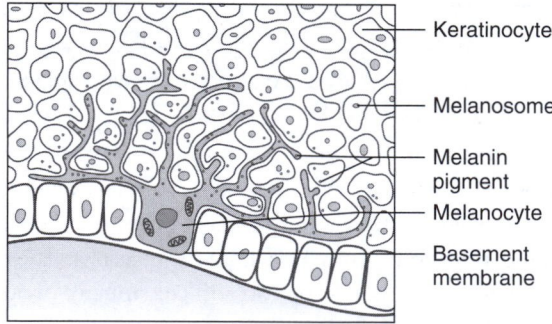

FIGURE 9.2 Melanocytes occur in the deepest layers of the epidermis. They produce the pigment called melanin, which is packaged in melanosomes. These melanosomes infiltrate into the keratinocytes and help to protect them from sunlight during the early stages of their migration towards the surface.

epidermis is about 1000 per mm², but this doubles in more heavily pigmented areas of the body such as the nipples, labia and scrotum.

Langerhan cells are immune cells that fight invasion from micro-organisms from the environment that have penetrated deep into the epidermis. The skin surface has its own ecosystem of micro-organisms consisting of bacteria, yeasts and viral agents. Each square inch (6.5 cm²) has approximately 50 million bacteria, a figure that rises to 500 million in areas of skin subjected to rich oily secretions. On the surface they are harmless to the skin because they are incapable of causing harm to the dead keratinised outer layer, but should they penetrate deeper, they may cause infection. Langerhan cells are an important part of our protection against these deeper organisms.

Epidermal growth, i.e. the growth of new cells in the stratum germinativum, is promoted by the production of a hormone called **epidermal growth factor** (**EGF**). It has a wide range of functions throughout the body, but in the skin it promotes growth by increasing cell division and keratin production, and is an important factor in wound healing (see p. 158).

Dermis

The 'true skin' layer beneath the epidermis is the dermis. This is subdivided into two main layers. The *outermost* layer is called the **stratum papillare** made from **areolar** connective tissue. Areolar connective tissue is common in the body, not just the skin, acting as a loose packing material between other structures. It contains random collagen fibres, elastic fibres (called **elastin**) and reticular fibres, with small blood vessels, nerve endings and some open spaces. The junction between the epidermis and the dermis is folded into **dermal papillae**, i.e. extensions of the stratum papillare that push upwards into the basal area of the stratum germinativum (Figure 9.1). Dermal papillae contain blood vessels that mark the closest extension of the blood supply to the skin surface (i.e. the epidermis is mostly blood-free, a good reason why epidermal cells are largely dead). Dilation and constriction of the blood vessels within the papillae, being so close to the skin surface, affect heat loss (dilation) or heat conservation (constriction), part of the body's temperature control mechanism (see Chapter 1). Some dermal papillae contain Meissner's corpuscles; sensory nerve endings for the purpose of touch. Below this layer, i.e. the *innermost* of the two layers, is the **stratum reticulare**, which is made from **collagen** fibres in bundles (for strength) and elastin. Cells embedded within this matrix are **fibroblasts** (cells for the production of protein fibres), **macrophages** (specialised cells of the immune system) and small patches of **adipocytes** (fat cells).

There are some additional embedded structures within the dermis (see Figure 9.1). These are:

- **Sweat glands**, which produce sweat from blood plasma, and this is released onto the skin surface. Sweat contains water and salts, and some urea (see Chapter 7). Sweating occurs either in response to high body temperature as part of temperature control mechanism (see Chapter 1) or in response to overactivity of the sympathetic nervous system.
- **Hair follicles** containing hairs, which grow and protect various body areas and provide some, albeit minimal, insulation against heat loss. They are made from hard keratin (outer layer) and soft keratin (inner core). There is an average of 5 million human hairs,

most of which (98%) are not on the head! Hair shafts (which are part of the follicle) pass from the dermis to the epidermis. They have **sebaceous glands** attached, which secrete **sebum**, an oily fluid that lubricates the hair shaft.

- **Nails**, which are made from the same dead keratin protein as epidermal keratinocytes but more densely packed for strength. Nails grow slowly from a nail bed and they provide protective and functional appendages at the ends of the digits (fingers and toes).
- **Nerve endings**, making the skin a vital sensory organ. Table 9.1 explains the various nerve endings found in the skin and their role.

Beneath the dermis is the **subcutaneous** tissue (also called the **hypodermis**), which is, strictly speaking, not part of the integument. It is made from some areolar connective tissue with a large but variable amount of **adipose** (fat) tissue, which is made from adipocytes. Here the dense adipose areas act as an energy store, they provide insulation against heat loss and they have a protective role against skin impacts, i.e. a shock-absorbing function. Within the outermost section of the hypodermis (immediately below the dermis), there is a network of larger arteries and veins, the **cutaneous plexus**, that supplies blood to the dermis above.

The functions of skin

When asked in an examination question 'What are the functions of skin?', a student wrote: 'It keeps insides in.' It would have been better if the student had turned this statement back to front and written: 'It keeps outsides out.' There is an element of truth in the second

TABLE 9.1 Nerve endings in the skin

Nerve ending in dermis	Notes
Free dendritic nerve endings	Sensitive to pain, heat, cold and pressure. Found in most body tissues, including the dermis and lower layers of epidermis.
Root hair plexus	Sensitive to hair movement. Found around hair roots.
Merkel cells with tactile discs	Sensitive to touch and light pressure. Found across the dermis–epidermis border.
Meissner's corpuscles	Sensitive to touch, light pressure and low-frequency vibrations. Found in the dermal papillae, especially over sensitive areas such as the nipples, external genitalia, fingertips and eyelids.
Krause's end bulb	A modified Meissner's corpuscle. Found in mucous membrane and some skin areas.
Pacinian corpuscles	Sensitive to deep pressure, stretching and high-frequency vibrations. Found in the subcutaneous tissues of the skin, especially on the fingers, feet, external genitalia and nipples, and also some deeper tissues.
Ruffini's corpuscles	Sensitive to deep pressure, stretching. Found in the dermis and subcutaneous tissues and joint capsules.

statement because skin is a vital barrier to most of the disease-causing organisms that inhabit our world. The full range of skin functions are as follows:

- The barrier mentioned here is a major part of our **non-specific** immune system. It is non-specific because it does not distinguish between one type of organism or another.
- Almost all organisms from the environment, i.e. bacteria, viruses and fungi, are incapable of penetrating intact skin. However, if the skin breaks down, that barrier is lost and infection can result in the body. Maintenance of this surface barrier involves the secretion of sebum from sebaceous glands attached to hair follicles (see p. 147).
- The skin is the body's vital touch sense organ. The rich supply of nerve endings in the skin provides a wide range of sensations, including touch, pain, temperature and pressure (Figure 9.1 and Table 9.1). Some areas of skin, e.g. the finger tips, are more sensitive than others to allow them to carry out their specific sensory functions.
- The skin is an important excretory organ, allowing the controlled loss of salts, water and organic wastes (e.g. **urea**) through sweat glands. Water and salt excretion are involved in fluid balance (see Chapter 5).
- Skin is also part of the temperature regulation mechanism, since heat is lost though the skin (see heat loss mechanism in Chapter 1). The deeper layers of skin often have fat present, which provides some insulation against the cold.
- Skin stores some nutrients, e.g. lipids in fat cells.
- Skin carries out synthesis of vitamin D_3 (**cholecalciferol**), which is produced when a naturally occurring substance in the skin, called **7-dehydrocholesterol** (which is derived from cholesterol), is exposed to **ultraviolet B light** (**UVB**). Cholecalciferol is also obtained from the diet. Further processing of cholecalciferol in the liver results in the active form of vitamin D, i.e. **25-hydroxycholecalciferol**.
- Skin provides physical protection to underlying structures. The skin has a remarkable shielding effect against injury from the outside that stops damage occurring to delicate structures beneath the skin.
- It is also a water-resistant barrier (but it is *not* waterproof). This resistance prevents the wetting of the skin from washing away important nutrients. However, prolonged immersion in fresh water, particularly warm fresh water (e.g. a warm bath), will cause the skin to become waterlogged as this water resistance function gradually fails and water moves in, causing the epidermal cells to swell. Alternatively, because the sea is salty, prolonged seawater immersion has the effect of drawing water out of the skin which then dehydrates the skin.

Skin observations

Because the skin is the outermost organ of the body, and therefore the most easily observed organ, it is not surprising that skin observations are paramount in understanding many abnormal changes taking place, both within the skin itself and deeper within the body systems, both acute and chronic. And the skin does a good job in reflecting many of the very important pathologies taking place in the deeper structure and systems beneath it. Skin observations involve colour, lesions, rashes, trauma and abnormal temperatures.

Colour and temperatures

Permanent skin colour varies normally between people of different races, but there are some classic temporary changes in skin colour which indicate deviation from the normal as a result of pathological processes occurring in some body systems:

- **Cyanosis** is the change of skin colour from normal to a blue-purple colour as a result of a lack of oxygen in the blood. The pathophysiology of cyanosis is explained in Chapter 4 (see p. 69). Cyanosis varies largely from mild to severe, depending on how dark and extensive the blue colour is. There is also a distinction between **peripheral cyanosis** (i.e. cyanosis of the fingers, toes, feet, hands, etc.) and **central cyanosis** (cyanosis of the trunk and face). Mild cyanosis occurs in the periphery first, but if the situation gets worse, the cyanosis becomes more central. Severe central cyanosis is the worst case scenario and requires urgent treatment, including additional controlled oxygen delivery. Causes of cyanosis include respiratory diseases of various kinds (especially pneumonia and obstructive airways diseases such as asthma), and heart failure. Local cyanosis, i.e. cyanosis of one part of the body only, will occur if there is any circulatory obstruction to that area, e.g. a tight band around a limb or some form of external compression on a limb. Relief of this compression and restoration of circulation will restore normal skin colour. Cyanosis is sometimes linked to another sign, i.e. finger and toe **clubbing**. This is where the ends of the digits expand to form bulb-like swollen ends. The cause is not fully understood, although dilated blood vessels at the ends of the fingers, growth factors and other natural biochemical agents have been suggested (Anoop and George 2011).
- **Jaundice**, the condition caused by abnormal breakdown of red blood cells, produces a yellow colour to skin. This yellow colour, which is usually widespread across the body, is due to deposits in the skin of a substance called **bilirubin** (see Figure 7.10). Bilirubin results from the breakdown of **haemoglobin** derived from red blood cells (**RBCs**, also called **erythrocytes**) (see Chapter 2). Deposits of excess bilirubin in the skin (and other tissues) is caused by abnormally high bilirubin production, far more than can be excreted through the normal channels. The cause of this excess production or accumulation of bilirubin can be attributed to any one of three possible pathological events (see also p. 127):

  1 **Pre-hepatic jaundice**, where rapid red cell breakdown takes place in the general circulation, releasing excessive amounts of haemoglobin. This serious condition is called **haemolytic anaemia**, and can be caused by some blood disorders and also as a consequence of mismatched blood transfusion.
  2 **Hepatic jaundice**, where excessive bilirubin builds up as a result of liver disease, as in **liver failure**, **cirrhosis** or **hepatitis**.
  3 **Post-hepatic jaundice**, where jaundice is caused by failure of bilirubin to get into the digestive system, and therefore the faeces. This results from obstruction of the bile duct, possibly from a biliary stone or tumour. Since there is a significant number of different causes of jaundice, the symptom needs investigation involving blood tests and hepatic function (Lock-In 2006).

- **Redness** (called **erythema**) of the skin is due to increased blood supply to the skin surface. This occurs when the arterial blood vessels in the dermis, and particularly the dermal papillae, dilate (called **vasodilation**), bringing more blood closer to the surface. The extra blood also delivers more heat and therefore the area feels warm. These effects, plus swelling of the area, are classic signs of **inflammation** (see p. 157 under wound infection). Sterile inflammation (i.e. not caused by a microorganism) can be the result of a blow or scratch to the skin surface. It can also occur if the skin is subjected to an external heat source, such as a fire, since heat causes blood vessels to dilate. Also, skin redness from vasodilation occurs often from psychological causes, for example, embarrassment, stress, anger or from excessive physical activity (i.e. the part played by skin in shedding the heat generated by exercise, see Chapter 1). Pathological causes of redness include infections of the skin (as in wound infections, see p. 159) or from the immune response to a toxin (e.g. insect stings).

- **Pallor**, where the skin becomes pale, is the opposite of redness, i.e. it is caused by reduced blood supply to the skin. The skin's blood vessels constrict (called peripheral **vasoconstriction**) or the blood pressure falls, sometimes suddenly as in **shock**, and less blood is pumped to the skin (see Chapter 1). Pallor may precede cyanosis (see p. 152) if the skin's blood supply continues to be constricted. Severe pallor indicates a very low blood pressure and poor cardiac output. In shock, efforts must be made to restore blood pressure to a point where adequate blood supply to the vital organs is maintained. Restoring normal skin colour and temperature after pallor is an indication that blood pressure has been restored sufficiently high to supply the skin, and therefore the vital organs, with blood. Low blood pressures will cause a lack of blood to the brain with reduced levels of consciousness (see Chapter 10), and this becomes a priority for treatment. **Fainting** is a good example of sudden loss of blood pressure resulting in pallor and loss of consciousness (see Chapter 10). Pallor will also occur with low skin temperatures since exposure to cold constricts the local peripheral blood vessels. Again, under these circumstances, the reduced blood supply (usually to the extremities) may well be accompanied by some degree of cyanosis.

Lesions and rashes

Lesions of the skin are usually small, discrete, localised areas of disease. Skin lesions come in many forms, identified in Table 9.2. Rashes (or eruptions) are usually more widespread than lesions, and are often composed of many individual lesions.

Skin trauma

Wounds and bruises

Skin is tough, but being exposed directly to the environment means it is subject to many types of trauma. Trauma creates breaches in the protective skin barrier, which can then easily lead to infection if care is not taken to prevent this.

Wounds may be closed or open. A closed wound is called a **bruise**. There is no actual breach in the skin but the effect of the trauma is to damage dermal blood vessels, causing

TABLE 9.2 Skin lesions

Skin lesion	Description
Bulla (blister)	Similar to vesicle (see below) but larger (greater than 5 mm diameter), filled with fluid.
Cyst	An encapsulated cavity lined with epithelium within the skin, containing semi-solid material or fluid.
Macule	Localised patch of different skin colour, either darker or lighter than the surrounding skin. Some are normal (e.g. freckles), others indicate pathological changes. Usually less than 1 cm in diameter.
Mole (nevus)	A lesion formed from melanocytes accumulating at the basal epidermal layer forming a macule. Migration into the dermis causes the area to become nodular and palpable. See also Table 9.3.
Nodule	Larger than a papule (i.e. larger than 5 mm in diameter), they can be solid or a fluid-filled raised lump within any skin layer.
Papule	Small, solid raised lump less than 5 mm in diameter (e.g. a wart).
Plaque	A palpable, slightly raised, flat-topped patch of skin, more than 1 cm in diameter but usually below 5 mm in height.
Pustule	A visible collection of pus within a blister formation on the skin surface.
Scale	A thick layer of keratin loosely attached to the skin that can detach easily.
Ulcer	An open cavity in the skin, i.e. a circumscribed area of skin loss, extending into the dermis or deeper.
Vesicle	A small blister (less than 5 mm diameter) filled with clear fluid occurring within or below the skin.
Wheal	A patch of dermal erythema, slightly raised with oedema, seen in urticaria.

bleeding into the dermis and below. In a bruise (or **ecchymosis**), the blood spreads out gradually from the traumatised area as a thin sheet. The resulting limits of the bruise are often larger than the actual area of trauma. The ecchymosis may spread downwards in response to gravity, and occur in lower areas of the body. Although the blood is not lost from the body, it is lost from circulation, and extensive bruising can lead to shock if there is enough blood loss into the dermis and subcortical tissues. The elderly are especially prone to bruising due to their fragile capillaries, and extensive bruising in the elderly, e.g. following a fall down stairs, can cause shock, which requires hospital management. Bleeding often continues for some time after the initial trauma, and this blood can be trapped and accumulate in the tissues as a **haematoma**, which can then solidify into a blood clot. This clot may form a palpable lump under the skin and takes longer to disperse than a straightforward bruise.

Resolution of a bruise can take from 5 to 20 days or more depending on the extent of the bruise and the presence of any extensive haematoma. During resolution, the red cells quickly break down to release the haemoglobin. Once released, the haemoglobin undergoes all the same changes seen in jaundice (see p. 152 and Figure 7.10). The only difference is that these changes are happening in the dermis and surrounding tissues, and the colour changes (biliverdin green to bilirubin yellow) can be seen within the skin. The final stages of the bruise, i.e. the disappearance of the yellow colour, occurs as the bilirubin is removed from the skin for transport to the liver, then excreted.

Open wounds penetrate the skin to varying levels, from superficial to deep, causing many kinds of tissue damage. The nature of the wound depends on the cause (e.g. the instrument) and the energy involved. Sharp instruments, e.g. a needle or knife point, are likely to cause wounds that are limited in width and bruising, but can go in deep, causing trauma to underlying structures. Blunt instruments, such as a hammer, do the opposite. They are likely to cause minimal depth of wound and a lot more widespread bruising. Bleeding from open wounds is dependent on the nature and extent of the blood vessels damaged. All wounds will bleed from capillaries since it is impossible to damage tissues without damaging capillaries. More serious bleeding occurs when a vein or artery is damaged. Arterial bleeding is indicated by the fact that blood is under pressure from the heart, and will spurt out or flow very quickly. This scenario requires urgent digital pressure on the wound to block the flow followed by raising the injured limb if possible, then urgent transportation to hospital. Extensive wounds may cause such large amounts of tissue disruption, with accompanying blood supply losses, that some tissue may eventually die, causing areas of necrotic tissue. **Necrosis** (tissue death) happens usually some days after the trauma, and is noted by skin tissue going gradually dark and eventually turning black in colour (sometimes called **gangrene**). This is non-viable tissue and must be surgically removed before the wound will heal properly.

Wound healing is a process that depends entirely on the provision of a number of factors, and the prevention of infection (Figure 9.3). Factors affecting wound healing are:

- *Age*, where wound healing slows with age, so healing times become longer. Younger individuals should heal their minor wounds in 5 days or so, but this may become 7 to 10 days in the elderly. This is mainly due to slower growth of tissues (i.e. slower rate of cellular division, or **mitosis**) in the elderly.
- *Nutrition*, which is essential for providing the protein to build the new tissues, and the vitamins and minerals for enzyme function, and the carbohydrates for the energy required. Water is also required for the replacement intracellar and extracellular fluid, and for removal of wastes.
- *Good blood supply*, known as good **tissue perfusion**, is required to deliver oxygen and nutrients to the wound site and to remove the wastes. Poor tissue perfusion can delay healing or be a cause of non-healing, as seen, again, quite often in the elderly.
- *Adequate immune response*, in order to keep the wound infection-free, is critical to healing success. The wound offers micro-organisms a great opportunity to gain entry to the body, and local infection of the wound slows or even prevents the healing process.
- *Existing disease*, for example, diabetes or cancer in the wound, may interfere with the healing process and may cause healing wounds to break down.
- *The extent of the wound*; some severe wounds with tissue loss may not heal without specialist surgical intervention. Apart from ensuring adequate blood supply to the tissues, the importance is to try, as much as possible, to get the wound edges together. This is achieved by suturing where possible, or by skin grafts where necessary. The results are

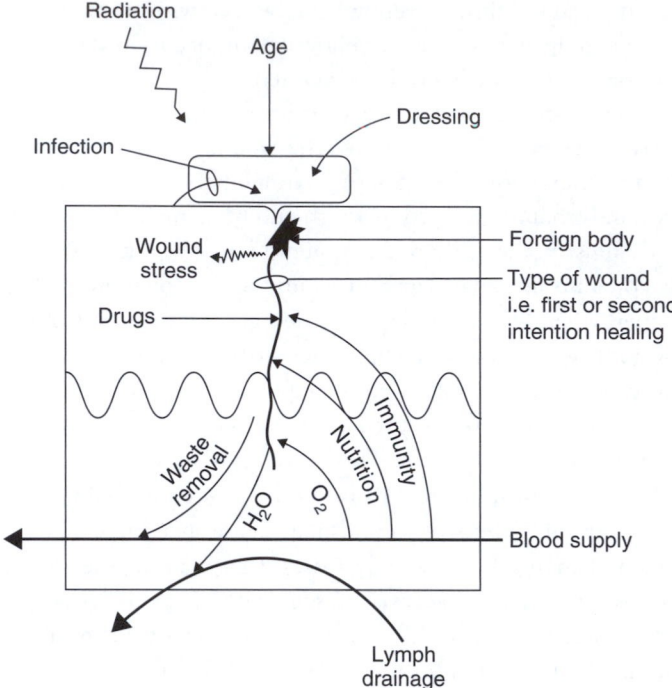

FIGURE 9.3 The factors affecting wound healing. Blood supply brings nutrients, oxygen and immune cells to the wound site, and blood and lymph removes wastes and water. The wound will heal better with first intention (primary) healing (see also Figure 9.5). Other factors include infection, age, drugs, wound stress, foreign bodies and the nature of the dressing.

proportional to the amount of skin coverage achieved. The best results will occur if 100% skin coverage can be achieved (see also the types of wound healing below).

- *Wound stress* will affect healing. This occurs if the wound edges are constantly being moved or pulled apart, as may happen in the skin over a moving joint. This wound movement disrupts healing. Stress also means any pressure placed on the wound, e.g. from a bandage or dressing that is too tight, or sutures pulled too tight. Such pressure will exclude blood from the wound site and the wound will suffer loss of oxygen and nutrients, and build-up of wastes.
- *Local factors*, e.g. a foreign body in the wound such as a splinter of wood, provides aggravation to the tissues and holds the wound open. This delays healing and increases the risk of infection. Wounds should be cleaned thoroughly of all dirt and debris initially, using a sterile technique if circumstances allow. In a first-aid situation cold running tap water is best. Dry the wound well using fresh tissues or clean cloth. However, getting the wound wet continuously or repeatedly causes delayed healing and provides the ideal environment for infection. Dressings should be sterile if available, and must always be dry for maximum healing potential and low infection risk. They should be changed appropriately, e.g. daily. They should not be too tight or made from abrasive fabrics that

will rub on the tissues at the wound site. Plasters should only be kept on minor wounds for 24 hours maximum. After this, most minor wounds will benefit from exposure to the air to keep them dry.

- *Radiation and chemotherapy*, for patients undergoing cancer treatment, will affect wound healing by causing delays in cell division.
- *General stress* causes raised levels of cortisol in circulation, and this reduces the permeability of capillary walls. Such a reduction in permeability slows the rate in which oxygen and nutrients can be delivered to the wounded tissues and this delays healing.

After any bleeding has stopped, wound healing occurs in three main stages (Figure 9.4):

1   The **inflammation phase** begins shortly after the trauma and lasts anything up to 10 days under normal healing conditions. Inflammation is often associated with infection, but the two are very different. Infection is an important cause of inflammation, but the inflammation identified here exists without infection (i.e. sterile inflammation) as a consequence of the activity by the immune system. Inflammation benefits both the immune system and the healing process, by bringing more blood to the wound site. This is achieved by the body triggering vasodilation around the wound site. This increased blood supply delivers more immune cells and proteins, more oxygen and nutrients and more water to the wound site, but it is the cause of the main symptoms we recognise as inflammation:

- redness ('rubor') due to the additional blood;
- swelling ('tumor') due to the additional fluid leaking from the capillaries into the tissues;
- heat ('calor') due to more blood bringing more heat to the site;
- pain ('dolor') due to the swelling pressing on nerve endings.

The inflammation phase gives the damaged tissues a kick start towards healing and provides a much needed immune cover to help to prevent infection.

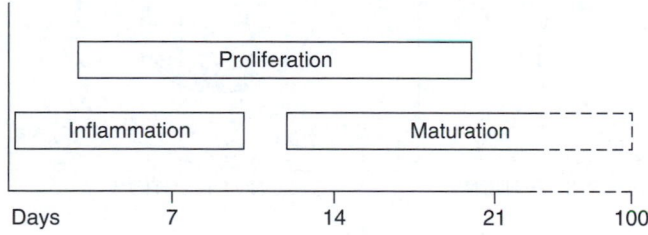

FIGURE 9.4   The stages of wound healing. Inflammation begins soon after the injury. This not only involves the immune defences, but the increased blood supply brings more oxygen and nutrients. The proliferation stage sees the growth of many new cells which heal the wound from the dermis upward. The maturation stage, which goes on indefinitely, completes the process by maturing the collagen and increasing the tensile strength (which prevents the wound from being pulled apart).

2   The **proliferation phase** begins two or three days after the trauma and continues until the wound is completely sealed over with new skin. It involves a process called **granulation**, where the structural protein collagen is produced from cells called **fibroblasts**, creating a matrix within which many blood vessels grow. This rich blood supply (i.e. highly vascular) makes granulation tissue very red in colour and it grows quickly. It fills in the dermis in the wound and is then covered by a new epidermis produced by a second process called **epithelialisation**. A new layer of stratum germinativum covers over the granulation tissue and from this a new epithelium grows.

3   The **maturation phase** is, as the name suggests, the period during which the wound matures. It starts about 12 days after the trauma, and continues indefinitely. Two main events occur in the newly healed wound during this period. The first is remodelling of the collagen, and this helps to reduce scarring (if any) to a minimum. The remodelling of collagen means it is converted from Type I to Type III collagen, a strengthening process that requires vitamin C. It is essential to strengthen collagen in this way to prevent easy breakdown of the newly healed wound (i.e. it gives the wound a *tensile strength*). The second event that takes place during maturation is **capillary regression**, i.e. the reduction of the blood supply to the granulation tissue so that further growth of this tissue stops (i.e. it prevents overgrowth). This reduction in blood also helps to reduce the impact of any scar tissue by making scars pale rather than red.

Healing of skin wounds is far more efficient if the wound edges can be held together (often with sutures) without movement for the duration of the healing process (Figure 9.5).

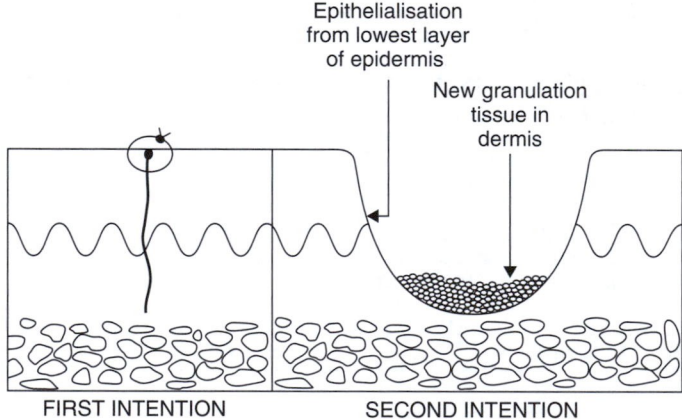

FIRST INTENTION   SECOND INTENTION

FIGURE 9.5   Different types of wound healing. First intention (or primary) means the wound edges can be held together, perhaps with sutures (as shown). This form of healing is the best process since it is the fastest, incurs the least risk of infection and heals with very little scarring. Second intention (secondary) healing involves tissue loss, leaving a wound open to the dermis or deeper tissues. Here, healing is much longer, involves a high risk of infection and scarring. Skin grafts may be needed to provide adequate skin coverage and a better outcome.

This form of healing, called **first intention** or **primary healing**, is the fastest way to heal a wound. It also carries the lowest risk of infection and other complications, and it usually heals with little or no scarring.

Secondary healing occurs when there is some tissue loss, and the wound edges cannot be brought entirely together, i.e. there is some degree of gapping. These wounds heal by processes sometimes described as **second intention** and **third intention** healing (Figure 9.5). Healing of these wounds would take much longer than by first intention, and they carry much higher risk of infection and scarring. Sometimes skin grafts, often taken from other areas on the same patient, are used to provide adequate skin coverage.

One of the worst wound complications is infection, and this should be avoided. Wound infections are mostly bacterial, and are usually caused by organisms that exist as **commensals** on the skin surface, i.e. they are harmless while on the skin surface, but they gain entry through the wound and become **pathogens** (i.e. cause disease). Infected wounds are made worse by a wet or damp wound environment, which encourages bacterial growth. It is always better to use dry dressings and to change them if they get wet. Dressings should not be kept on the wound for any longer than is necessary, as they can, after a while, encourage a wound environment that favours bacterial growth.

The symptoms of a wound infection are:

- Pain in the wound and extreme tenderness in the wound area.
- Swelling of the tissues in and around the wound site.
- Redness of the whole area, coupled with extra warmth.
- An **exudate**, which is an infected discharge coming from the wound. Non-infected wounds may leave a normal healthy yellow stain on dressings, derived from protein-rich fluid leaking from the capillaries. This fluid contains what is required to help keep the wound clean and fight infection. Infected wounds produce excessive exudate discharge called pus, a mix of fluid containing bacterial cells (alive and dead), immune cells and proteins. This infected exudate may have an unpleasant smell.
- Failure of the wound to heal properly. Such failure can be of any degree, from delayed healing to total wound breakdown.

Pressure sores (decubitus ulcers)

Pressure sores (called **decubitus ulcers**) are caused by continuous pressure on a localised skin site for many hours, or even longer. It occurs as a complication of long periods of bed rest or prolonged periods of immobility in a chair. The basic problem is that the patient is unable to move on their own and relies on their carer for frequent relief of pressure. The most common sites where persistent pressure occurs depend on the patient's position, e.g. the buttocks and shoulders in those lying on their back (Figure 9.6). The formation of a pressure sore follows a similar course to that of a closed wound, which, if left untreated, then becomes an open wound as necrotic tissues break down. They start with patches of redness (erythema, also known as a **reactive hyperaemia**) in the skin in an immobile patient. This is the first warning sign and it indicates exactly where the pressure is happening. It should also alert the carer to implement the appropriate activity to prevent the problem from getting worse. Pressure sore formation is accelerated and made much worse if the patient is lying in a bed contaminated with urine or faeces. This situation must be corrected quickly, and any acidic urine washed from the skin. Observations of the skin are best done at the time of washing or bathing the patient, since these are the times when most of the skin area is exposed and the carer can combine observations while washing the patient. Relief of pressure is paramount, usually combining change of position with pressure-relieving aids. It should not be forgotten that early ambulation out of the bed or chair, whenever possible, is the best preventative measure. If no relief of the pressure is forthcoming, the wall of capillaries in the affected area becomes disrupted and platelets aggregate, causing **microthrombi** (very small blood clots), which further block blood flow. The result is tissue **anoxia** (i.e. lack of oxygen), which leads to necrosis (dead tissue). Dead (necrotic) tissue breaks down due to the activity of **proteolytic**

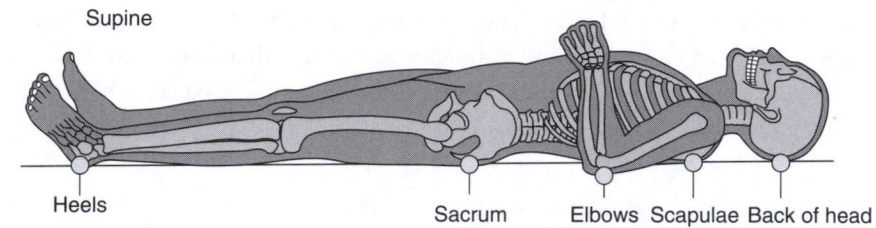

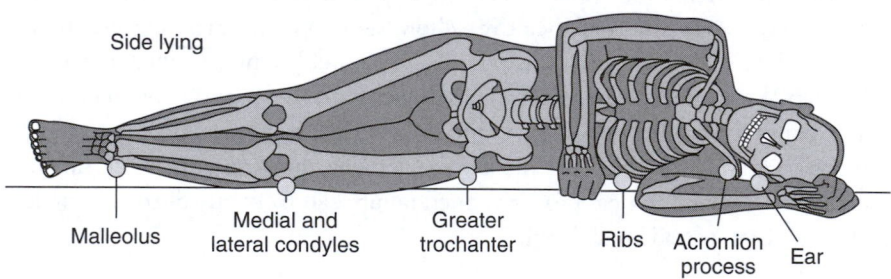

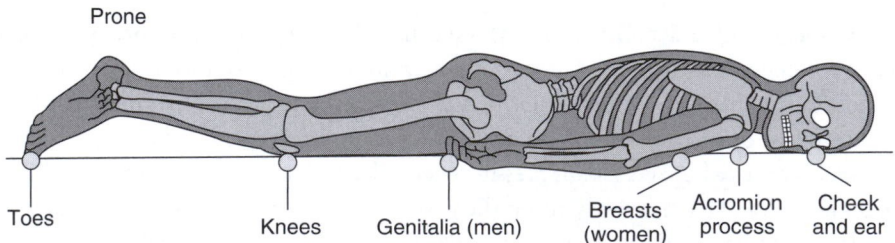

FIGURE 9.6 Sites where pressure can cause open sores. The sites are dependent on skin contact with a firm surface, usually skin over a bony prominence, thus shutting down the blood supply to that patch of skin for a significant time period.

enzymes (enzymes that break up proteins) and **macrophages** (cells that engulf and remove dead tissue). This is when the closed wound becomes open, with an increased risk of infection. The presence of infection and further pressure will ensure this particular wound will be very difficult to heal. Clearly, events should never get this far, and from the time the initial signs of erythema are identified, preventative measures must be implemented quickly.

Burns and scalds

A burn is a thermal trauma to the skin caused by contact with a source of high temperature. A variation of burns occurs as scalds, i.e. contact with a wet source of high temperature, such as boiling water or steam. Burns are sometimes classified according to skin depth, e.g. **first degree** burns (i.e. a superficial burn with damage to the epidermis only); **second degree** burns (i.e. involving the dermis, either as partial-thickness or deep partial-thickness, depending on how much dermis is involved) and **third degree** burns (i.e. involving the entire skin, subcutaneous tissues and perhaps even deeper structures) (Figure 9.7).

However, the serious nature of a burn (i.e. its life-threatening potential) depends far less on depth, but much more on the body surface area of skin actually burnt. A large body area of superficial (first degree) burn is far more serious than a small body area of deep (third degree) burn. This is because in burns of large body surface area, more skin function is disrupted, particularly control of fluid loss through the skin. Life-threatening shock from uncontrolled fluid loss through large areas of burn is a major factor in the management of those burns. The other factors that also need urgent attention when large areas of skin are involved in the burn are pain control (see Chapter 11) and reducing the risk of infection.

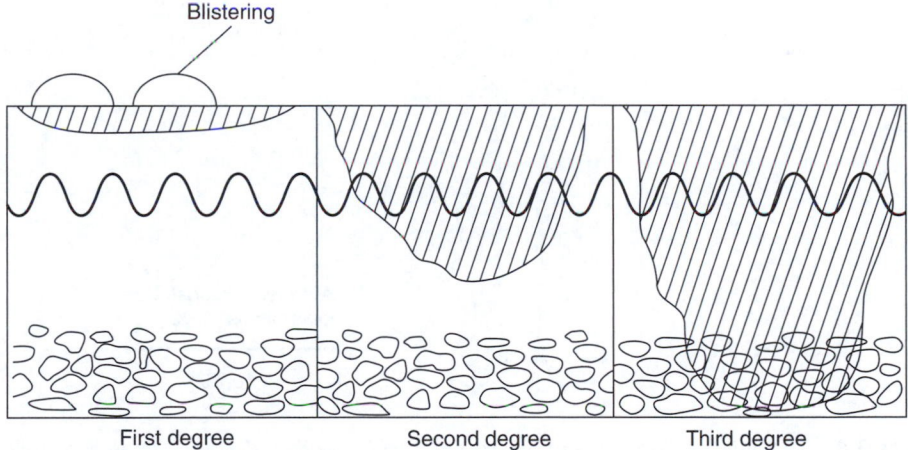

FIGURE 9.7 Degrees of burn. First degree burns are superficial, burning the top layers of epidermis only. Blistering may occur. Second and third degree burns are deeper; second degree extending the burn into the dermis, third degree extending the burn deeper into the subcutaneous tissues or even internal structures. The burn is the shaded area.

It therefore becomes a valuable tool in burns management to assess (i.e. estimate) the total surface area of the burn. Figure 9.8 shows one way to do this, called the 'Rule of Nines'.

Burns of the skin appear as red (erythema) areas, often with fluid-filled blisters forming. These blisters are caused by fluid leaking from damaged and dilated blood vessels, the fluid then getting trapped beneath the tough unbroken outer layer, the stratum corneum. As more fluid leaks out, the stratum corneum gets further stretched into a balloon of fluid, and may rupture. Blisters illustrate just how quickly fluid is lost through burns and this is why, scaled up over a large surface area, fluid loss from burns can be substantial and cause shock.

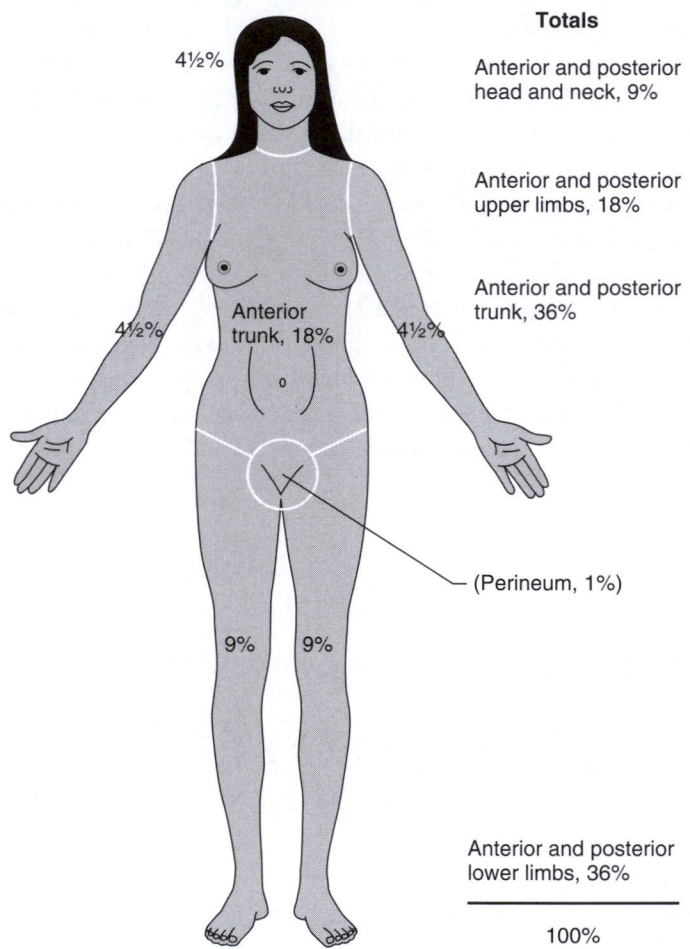

Totals

Anterior and posterior head and neck, 9%

Anterior and posterior upper limbs, 18%

Anterior and posterior trunk, 36%

(Perineum, 1%)

Anterior and posterior lower limbs, 36%

100%

FIGURE 9.8 The 'Rule of Nines' area of burn estimator. The body is divided into areas as follows: Front and back of head = 9% (4.5% front and back); trunk = 36% (18% front and back); upper limbs = 18% (4.5% front and back times 2 limbs); lower limbs = 36% (9% front and back times 2 limbs). This adds up to 99%, the remaining 1% being the perineum. The majority of the percentage area (99%) is easily divisible by 9, hence the Rule of Nines. Doctors can estimate the usual patchy nature of burns using this guide.

Burns from a fire are likely to be contaminated with blackened tissues and combustion products such as soot, or burnt clothing.

The first aid for burns is simple. Burns should be cooled rapidly in cold water only, to stop the burning process and to ease pain. In first aid, never use 'lotions, potions or mother's notions', including fats such as butter and even burn creams. Following cold water, apply a sterile (if available) or clean dressing. If no dressings are available, use freshly laundered linen. Continue to use cold water liberally to ease pain, including wetting the dressing if this helps. Seek medical advice as soon as possible. In extensive burns, urgent removal to hospital is essential to treat potential shock and pain.

The healing of burns is similar to that of other wound types. First degree burns heal by epithelialisation, which replaces the lost epidermis. Second and third degree burns heal by granulation tissue (to replace the damaged dermis) followed by epithelialisation. In addition, collagen formation may be involved. This new collagen becomes more prevalent in deeper burns (third degree) and provides strength to the new tissues. However, new collagen may sometimes be responsible for contractions and scarring, two serious disfiguring complications of burns. Infection is a major issue is burns, and again larger areas of burn are at greater risk. With any burn, there is always a chance that an infection can get into the blood and cause systemic infections. Strict sterile techniques, drugs and even isolation of the patient are used to prevent widespread infection in large area burns. As with other wounds, dead and burnt tissue (i.e. non-viable tissue) must be surgically removed as this is a potential source of infection and may delay or prevent healing. Skin coverage, even if temporary, should be achieved as soon as possible as this reduces infection risk, reduces pain and gives a better final outcome.

Important skin diseases

It is beyond the scope of this book to describe all the skin disorders that occur, as there are so many, so this text provides an overview of the pathology of five important skin disorders: acne, urticaria, eczema, psoriasis and malignant melanoma.

Acne

Teenage acne (**acne vulgaris**) is linked to hormone changes, mostly the **androgens (testosterone** and **dihydrotestosterone**) in boys. These male hormones increase both the size and activity of the sebaceous glands. It does occur in both sexes, but tends to be more severe in boys. Sebaceous glands become blocked by excess sebaceous material and keratin, and they swell as trapped sebum accumulates. They then usually get infected with the bacterium *Propionibacterium acnes*. The skin of the face, and sometimes the trunk and limbs, develops a patchy cover of inflamed spots, which form pus when infected.

Urticaria (hives)

Urticaria is recognised as patches of raised, red skin (called *wheals*), usually due to a **type I hypersensitivity** (i.e. a reaction to contact with an allergen, a foreign substance that the immune system reacts to). This allergen may be a drug, a specific food, insect or nettle stings, or exposure to heat or cold. The raised nature of the lesion is due to oedema of the upper dermis from leaking capillaries, causing the swelling. The trigger is the release of histamine from mast cells following contact with the allergen, the histamine then causing the local symptoms of inflammation. It typically lasts for less than 24 hours but may persist longer (see p. 268).

Eczema (eczematous dermatitis)

This is an inflammatory disease of the skin causing patchy areas of itchy redness, each patch showing indistinct borders. The changes in the epidermis consist of oedema forcing the keratinocytes apart and creating a spongy effect. This epidermal pathology can result in eczema patches breaking open, especially from scratching, and this allows the oedematous fluid to leak out, i.e. an oozing, which then dries to form a crust over the lesion. T-lymphocytes infiltrate the area and there is often histamine release from mast cells, which then exacerbates the irritation (Krasteva *et al.* 1998). The lesions can form anywhere, but mostly on the trunk and limbs. Acute outbreaks happen at any time, and may be related to stress. The term **eczematous dermatitis** incorporates a number of distinct conditions, all with very similar pathology but different causes. These include **contact dermatitis** (caused by skin contact with an allergen, e.g. a chemical), **atopic dermatitis** ('atopy' means prone to allergy, probably caused by an inherited gene and thus usually runs in families) and **primary irritant dermatitis** (caused by trauma to skin, such as rubbing).

Psoriasis

This skin lesion is characterised by pink, well-demarcated plaques that have a loose surface layer of silvery white scales formed from the shedding of the epidermis. The plaques commonly form over joints (especially elbows and knees), on the scalp and the lower back, but can form anywhere. It affects the nails in about 30% of cases, causing them to change colour to a dark brown and become thickened and pitted, with some degree of separation from the nail bed. Psoriasis is an **auto-immune disease**, i.e. a disorder occurring when the immune system causes disruption in a normal body system (in this case the integumentary system) (Sanchez 2010).

The immune attack on the skin involves both lymphocyte types (i.e. **B-cells** and **T-cells**), **neutrophils** and a barrage of chemical agents (including **tumour necrosis factor**, various **interleukins** and **interferon gamma**). There is evidence that at least one gene abnormality (or **mutation**) is involved in the cause, one of the HLA genes at the Cw6 allele (a gene called *PSORS1* within the 'C' region of the HLA sequence), and therefore it can be inherited, i.e. it can run in families (McCance *et al.* 2010). **HLA (human leukocyte antigen** genes on chromosome 6) code for cell surface proteins involved in immunity.

The key cellular feature indentifying psoriasis is the rapid increase in the speed in which epidermal cells are produced in the stratum germinativum and the accelerated rate at which they move through the epidermis to the stratum corneum (typically 3–4 days in psoriasis, see p. 148). These abnormalities cause the epidermis to thicken (called **acanthosis**).

Abnormally dilated blood vessels within the dermal papillae cause the erythema and they bleed easily if the skin is disturbed.

Malignant melanoma

This is a cancer of the pigment-producing cells, the melanocytes (see p. 148), mostly within the skin. The cause of melanoma is complex, and involves multiple factors, including genetics and excessive exposure to ultraviolet (UV) light, especially UVA (ultraviolet A). Those having fair or red hair and pale skin have a higher risk of developing the disease than darker-skinned people. An aggregation of melanocytes in the skin is called a **nevus** (or **mole**, see Table 9.3). Most nevi are no problem, but occasionally one may change to become malignant (cancerous). Any changes in a nevus (e.g. changes in size, colour or shape, etc.) should be reported to a doctor as soon as possible (see Table 9.3). The growth, spread and classification of melanomas are discussed in Blows (2005, p. 247).

Key points

The structure and function of skin

- There are two major divisions of the skin, the outer epidermis and the deeper dermis.
- Epidermal cells starting in the deepest layer migrate slowly towards the surface.
- Melanocytes are pigmentation cells in the epidermis.
- The dermis ('true skin') is made up of two main layers.
- The dermis contains areolar connective tissue and patches of adipose fat tissue.
- The dermis is the site for hair follicles, sweat glands, nerve endings and blood vessels.
- Subcutaneous tissues (below the dermis) contains more adipose tissue.
- The functions of skin include part of our temperature control system, a sensory organ, protection against infection, an excretory organ and vitamin D production.

Skin observations

- Skin observations involve colour, lesions, rashes, trauma and abnormal temperatures.
- Skin colour changes from normal include cyanosis (blue), jaundice (yellow), erythema (red) and pallor (white).
- Lesions of the skin are usually small, discrete, localised areas of disease.

TABLE **9.3** ABCDE of nevi changes

A	Asymmetrical in shape
B	Border irregularity
C	Colour variation
D	Diameter larger than 6 mm
E	Elevation

- Rashes (or eruptions) are more widespread than lesions, being composed of many individual lesions.

Skin trauma

- Trauma creates breaches in the skin barrier, which can then lead to infection.
- Wounds may be closed (bruises) or open.
- Open wounds penetrate the skin to varying depths, from superficial to deep, and can cause serious internal injury and blood loss.
- Arterial bleeding from a wound requires urgent compression to stop the bleeding, followed by emergency transportation to hospital.
- There are many factors that influence wound healing, and these must all be taken into account to achieve complete healing and prevent wound infection.
- Wounds must be cleaned in water (ideally sterile) but not left wet.
- Wound dressings must be sterile, or at least clean, non-abrasive and renewed often.
- Wound healing occurs in three phases: inflammation, proliferation and maturation.
- First intention or primary healing is the fastest and best way to heal a wound.
- Pressure sores (decubitus ulcers) are caused by continuous pressure on a localised skin site for a long period.
- A burn is a thermal trauma to the skin caused by contact with high temperature.
- A large body area of burn is far more serious than a deep burn. This is because large areas leak tissue fluid which can result in shock.
- The area of burnt skin can be estimated using the 'Rule of Nines'.
- First degree burns heal by epithelialisation, second and third degree burns heal by granulation tissue followed by epithelialisation.
- Keeping the burn infection free is vital to burn healing.

Important skin diseases

- Acne occurs when sebaceous glands become blocked by excess sebaceous material and keratin, causing swelling as trapped sebum accumulates, and they become infected with *Propionibacterium acnes*.
- Urticaria are red, raised patches of skin, caused by a type I hypersensitivity, a reaction to contact with an allergen.
- Eczema (dermatitis) is an inflammatory disease of the skin. It creates areas of itchy redness showing indistinct borders.
- Eczema includes contact dermatitis (skin reacting with an allergen) and atopic dermatitis (which may be a genetic disorder).
- Psoriasis causes pink, well-demarcated plaques that have a loose surface layer of silvery white scales, which is the shedding of the epidermis.
- The disease involves the rapid production and transition of cells from the lowest epidermal layers to the skin surface.
- Abnormal blood vessels in the upper dermis bleed if the skin is disturbed.
- Psoriasis is an auto-immune disease.

- Malignant melanoma is a cancer of the epidermal melanocytes, pigment-producing cells.
- Exposure to excessive ultraviolet light A (UVA) is a key risk factor in melanoma.

References

Anoop T. and George K. (2011) Differential clubbing and cyanosis. *New England Journal of Medicine*, **364**(7): 666.

Blows W. T. (2005) *The Biological Basis of Nursing: Cancer*. Routledge, London.

Krasteva M., Choquet G., Descotes J. and Nicolas J. F. (1998) Physiopathology of eczema. *La Revue du Praticien*, **48**(9): 945–950.

Lock-In I. (2006) Investigation of jaundice. *Medicine*, **30** (October): 11–13.

McCance K. L., Heuther S. E., Brashers V. L. and Rote N. S. (2010) *Pathophysiology: The Biological Basis for Disease in Adults and Children*, 6th edition. Mosby Elsevier, Missouri.

Sanchez A. P. G. (2010) Immunopathogenesis of psoriasis. *Anais Brasileiros de Dermatologia*, **85**(5): 747–749.

Chapter 10 **Neurological observations (I)**
Consciousness

- Introduction
- The cerebral cortex
- Observations of consciousness
- Major causes of unconsciousness
- The anaesthetic drugs
- Key points
- References

Introduction

To science, consciousness is a problem, referred to as the *hard problem*, simply because it cannot be explained. There is no current understanding of how brain cells can create a subjective experience like consciousness, i.e. trying to integrate the chemical activity of the cell with a concept of reality. But this understanding is so important to the medical and nursing professions, and there are some known facts. The brain area involved in consciousness is the **cerebral cortex**; and it is worth thinking of this large area as the *conscious brain*. An area called the **prefrontal cortex**, part of the **frontal lobe**, is the primary centre for consciousness; the site of the *self* and many higher intellectual functions (Carter 1998). Other areas of the cerebral cortex are conscious for special sensations: for example, the **parietal lobe** is conscious for sensations arising from the body, such as touch (known as **somatic sensations**; soma = body); the **occipital lobe** is conscious for vision; and the **temporal lobe** is conscious for hearing. All other deeper parts of the brain function at an unconscious (or subconscious) level, although many supply the cortex with essential information that makes consciousness possible. What subconscious means is that these other areas work without the individual's awareness or control; so awareness and control are qualities of the conscious state. First, *awareness* of the environment involves communication of environmental stimuli to the brain via the **sensory nervous system** and the **special senses**, such as vision and hearing. This is important since the brain is almost entirely encased within the skull, cut off from the outside world, and can only appreciate this world through sensory stimuli. It also means awareness of your own thoughts, known as the process of **cognition** (= mental activity).

Second, *control* suggests some form of meaningful interaction with the environment, mostly through the **motor nervous system**, based on an understanding of the environment and what that interaction will achieve. Sensory *input*, cognitive *processing* and motor *output* can be likened to the functions of a computer, the brain being the most advanced form of computer available. Awareness and control are lost in patients who are unconscious, i.e. the computer is *switched off*.

The cerebral cortex

When viewed from the side, the front or the top, the largest part of the human brain seen is the cerebral cortex (Figure 10.1). As the conscious brain, the cerebral cortex is responsible for the awareness and control identified above as being the components of consciousness.

The cortex is made up of nerve cells called **neurons** that have multiplied by **mitosis** (cell division) many millions of times during the embryonic development of each individual. After birth, however, in all but a few neurons, cell division effectively stops, so the cell numbers never increase again. This means that neurons lost during life cannot be replaced. The rest of the brain is also made of neurons, but they never achieve consciousness, and it is this unique function of the cerebral cortex cells that is so puzzling. Neurons have a cell body and a long process, called the **axon**, extending for varying distances away from the body (Figure 10.2).

Dendrites are shorter cell body processes connecting cells together. Dendrites are **afferent** (= towards) because they convey impulses towards the cell body; axons are **efferent** (= away from) because they convey impulses away from the cell body. The axons are mostly **myelinated**, i.e. covered by a fat (lipid) layer, the **myelin sheath**, the purpose of which is to speed up nerve impulse transmission from about 2 metres per second (unmyelinated) to as much as 120 metres per second (myelinated). In the cerebral cortex, this myelin layer is formed by cells called **oligodendrocytes** during embryonic development and childhood. Oligodendrocytes are just one type of a collection of support cells called **neuroglia** (often shortened to **glial cells**). Glial cells do not convey nerve impulses; instead, they provide other structural or chemical functions that are essential for brain activity. The human brain

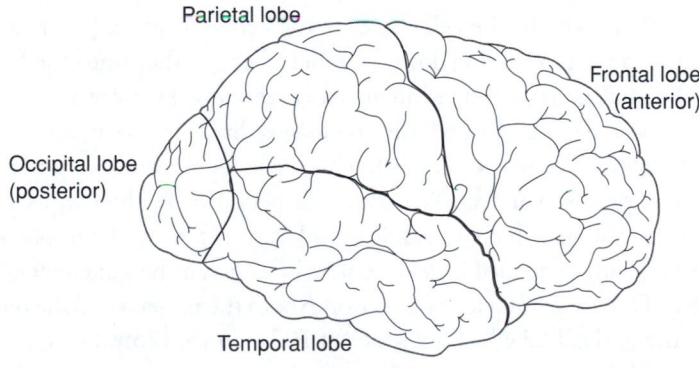

Parietal lobe

Frontal lobe (anterior)

Occipital lobe (posterior)

Temporal lobe

FIGURE 10.1 The cerebral cortex from the right side showing the major lobes.

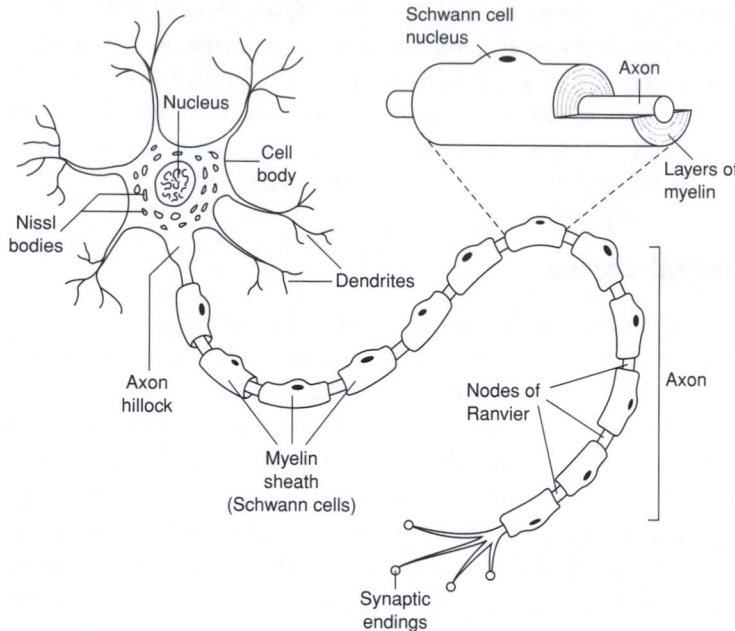

FIGURE 10.2 The neuron. The cell body shows a nucleus surrounded by Nissl bodies. The axon starts at the axon hillock and terminates at the synaptic endings. Myelin covers the axon in segments with gaps between, called the nodes of Ranvier. An enlarged myelin segment is shown. Myelin is laid down in layers by cells called Schwann cells.

has about 100 billion neurons, with about 50–80 times more neuroglia present. Of this vast number of glial cells, most are **astrocytes** (named after their star shape), which have vital chemical and nutritional roles to perform in the brain. Myelin sheaths, being made of fat from oligodendrocytes, makes the axons appear white, whereas cell bodies, being free from myelin appear grey. Hence, **grey matter** consists of cell bodies packed together, as on the surface of the cortex, whereas **white matter** consists of axons packed together as they extend deeper into the brain (Figure 10.3). Just think of a helium balloon seller at a fair; the balloons are all together up high (the cell bodies of the cerebral cortex grey matter), whereas the balloon strings are all extending down, parallel to each other, into the balloon seller's hand (the myelinated axons forming white matter extending downwards from the cortex).

The cerebral cortex has a major division, the **longitudinal fissure** along the midline running from front to back (antero-posteriorly). This separates the cortex into two halves, the left and right hemispheres, which are connected deeper down by the **corpus callosum**. It is through the corpus callosum that communication between the two hemispheres can occur. Each hemisphere is further divided by fissures into lobes given the same names as the bones that overly them. Thus the frontal lobe is anterior to both the **parietal** and the **temporal lobes**, separated from the **parietal lobe** by the **fissure of Rolando** (or **central sulcus**) and separate from the **temporal lobe** by the **fissure of Sylvius**. Posterior to all these, at the back of the cortex, is the **occipital lobe**. A **sulcus** (plural **sulci**) is a gully across the brain surface between

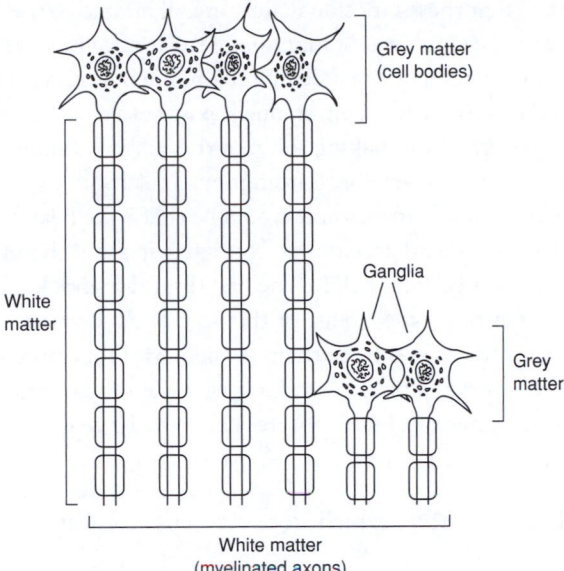

FIGURE 10.3 Neurons in clusters form grey matter (cell bodies) and white matter (axons). Ganglia are cell bodies (patches of grey matter) separated from the main group of cell bodies.

two ridges (a ridge, or up fold, is a **gyrus**, plural **gyri**). The surface is folded to increase the total surface area. In this way more grey matter can be packed into the limited skull cavity. Fissures are usually deeper divisions than sulci and mark the boundaries of the lobes.

The cells of the cerebral cortex are arranged in a strict pattern according to function; thus it becomes possible to map the brain surface (Figure 10.4).

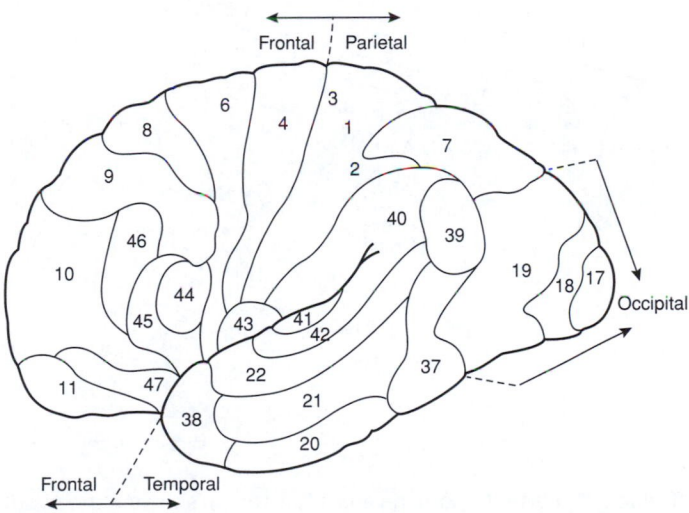

FIGURE 10.4 Map of the left cerebral cortex according to cell function. Each area has a Brodmann number.

It is not surprising that these functional areas are all related to the activities we identified with consciousness, i.e. *control* (motor function of the frontal lobe areas), *awareness* (sensory functions of the parietal, temporal and occipital lobe areas, and cognition of the frontal lobe and other **association areas**). Association areas exist between the main functional areas of the cortex and are essential for making sense of the sensory stimuli arriving at the cortex. They contain memory banks developed from previous sensory experience that are used for comparing with new stimuli. An example would be that if we hear a bell ring, we know this is a bell because we have heard previous bells ringing and can therefore make that association. A new-born child, hearing a bell for the first time, does not know what it is since there is no previous experience or knowledge of this sound. Association areas must learn these sensory stimulatory patterns and store them as memories for future use if the individual is to make sense of the world. This is one reason why the human brain is unique in taking a longer time than any other species to mature, i.e. up to 20 years or more. There are important association areas working with:

- the parietal sensory area, which receives sensations from the body, or somatic sensations;
- the occipital sensory area, which receives visual sensations from the eye (the **visual cortex**);
- the temporal sensory areas receiving sensations of hearing (the **auditory cortex**) (Figure 10.4).

Even within the main specialised functional areas of the **motor cortex** (frontal lobe) and **sensory cortex** (parietal lobe), the cells are carefully arranged in a layout that matches the body plan (Figure 10.5). Although the appropriate motor cortex cells control the muscles

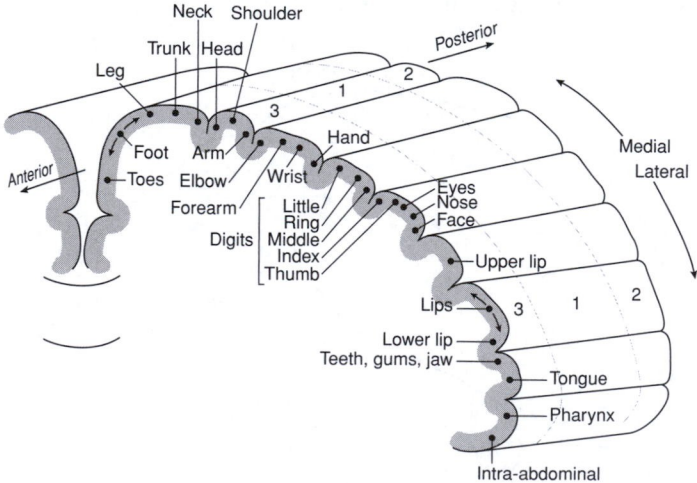

FIGURE 10.5 The sensory cortex (Brodmann areas 1, 2 and 3), showing the layout of cells according to the areas of the body that they receive transmissions from. Notice the large areas involved in sensation of the lips (a very sensitive area) and the large areas for the fingers and the hands compared with the feet and toes.

they are ultimately connected to, the delivery of somatic sensations to the relevant cells in the sensory cortex is more complex. Sensations coming into the brain from the body must first pass to the **thalamus**, a sensory relay station deeper within the brain that sorts the sensations and sends them on to the correct cerebral cells. Consider the sensory cortex as a massive company, each cell being one office. In comes a telephone call (sensory stimulus) destined for one specific office. The call must first go to an exchange (the thalamus) that connects the caller to the correct office within the company. It is important that this sorting process takes place since, for example, cells in the sensory cortex that specialise in the toes would not be interested in sensations arising from the ears, just as the occupants of one office would not be interested in taking calls destined for elsewhere. The thalamus is therefore the brain's *server* (as on a computer network), directing the *e-mails* (stimuli) to the correct *terminal computer* (sensory cell). What is amazing is that nature designed and operated human computers with server systems some four million years or so before the first computer was invented.

Neurons connect to each other through **synapses**, microscopic gaps between one axon and what lies beyond, which could be a cell body or dendrites, or another axon (Figure 10.6). Some neurons may have up to 100,000 synaptic connections each with other neu-

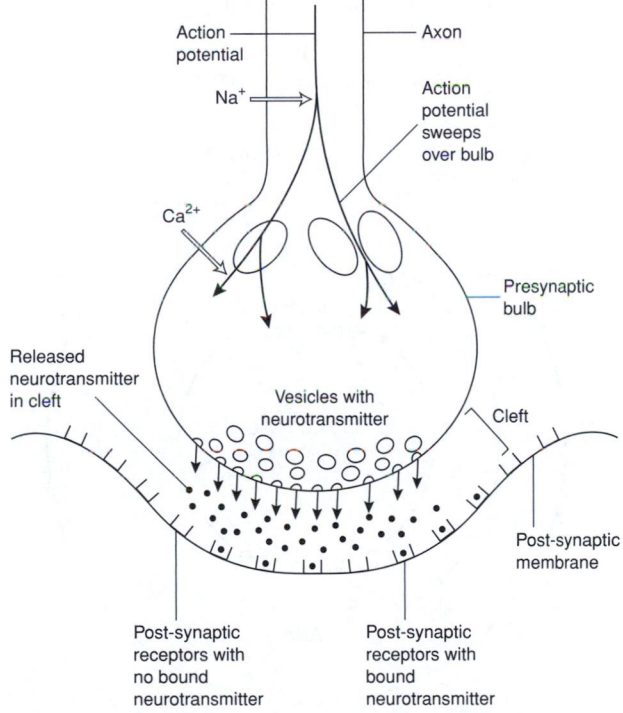

FIGURE 10.6 The synapse. As the action sweeps down the axon to the presynaptic bulb, the influxing ion changes from sodium (Na^+) to calcium (Ca^{2+}). The vesicles release a neurotransmitter into the cleft and the chemical binds to receptor sites on the post-synaptic membrane. A bound neurotransmitter will have an effect on the cell beyond the post-synaptic membrane.

rones. These tiny gaps require a bridging chemical, called a **neurotransmitter**, to fill the gaps during the passage of an impulse, and thus cause changes, like a new impulse, beyond the synapse (i.e. in the **post-synaptic membrane**). There are many different neurotransmitters, but the main chemical in the cerebral cortex is **glutamate**. Glutamate is considered to be the neurotransmitter of consciousness, although it does function elsewhere in the brain in some subconscious areas. Glutamate is **excitatory** in almost every site it is used, i.e. it generates a new increase in activity when released at the synapse, similar to the accelerator system of a car when used. Glutamate is produced as part of a chemical cycle that also generates another neurotransmitter called **GABA** (short for **gamma-aminobutyric acid**) (Figure 10.7).

This chemical is largely **inhibitory**, i.e. it binds to receptors that prevents any changes in the post-synaptic membrane and therefore acts similar to a brake in the car, i.e. it reduces (inhibits) brain activity. It should not be surprising that the brain has both excitatory (accel-eratory) and inhibitory (braking) abilities similar to a car, because this allows the brain to operate at a moderate level most of the time (as a car does at average speed), with the option of increasing or decreasing brain activity (going faster or slower) as the need arises. By care-fully regulating the chemical cycle that produces both the excitatory and inhibitory neu-

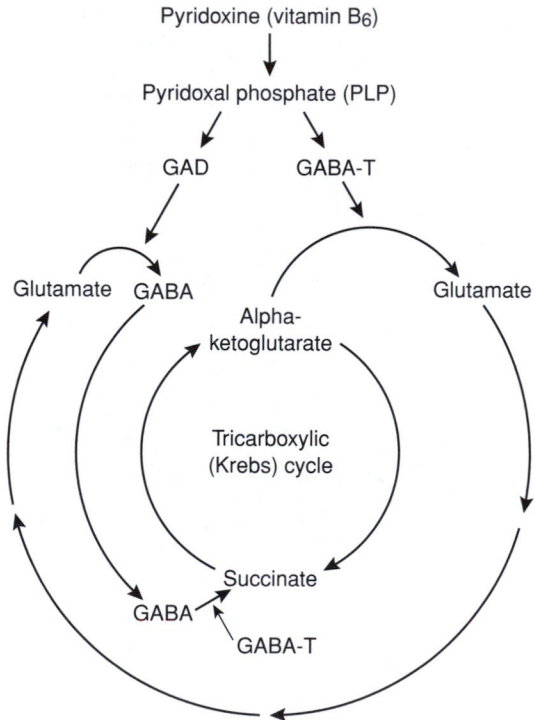

FIGURE 10.7 The gamma-aminobutyric acid (GABA) and glutamate (glutamic acid) cycle. The Krebs cycle (Figure 1.1) provides alpha-ketoglutarate as the starting point for glu-tamate, which returns to the Krebs cycle as GABA. The enzymes are GABA trans-aminase (GABA-T) and glutamic acid decarboxylase (GAD). Vitamin B_6 (pyridoxine) is important for these enzymes to function.

rotransmitters, the brain can fine-tune glutamate or GABA production to meet its activity needs (Carlson 2010).

Observations of consciousness

It is not enough to consider a person either conscious or unconscious, since there are various degrees of consciousness and changes in the levels of consciousness. It is useful to consider a spectrum from fully conscious at one end to a deep state of unconsciousness, known as **coma**, at the other. The various points on this spectrum are the **altered states of consciousness** (Figure 10.8). Notice that **sleep** does not appear on the same spectrum. Sleep is an altogether different state and should not be confused with unconsciousness. Sleep is distinguished from unconsciousness by several characteristics, notably that sleep is a natural body requirement during which the subject is rousable. Also, sleep has a typical pattern of brain activity that can be observed using an electroencephalograph, a machine for measuring and displaying the electrical output of the brain, which produces an **electroencephalogram** (**EEG**).

It becomes important to assess the level of consciousness in a patient for two reasons. First, the point that the patient occupies on the spectrum of consciousness is important since this has a bearing on the management of the patient's condition and prospects for a successful recovery (prognosis). Second, it is very important to know whether the patient is moving along the spectrum, either by regaining consciousness or more urgently to know whether the patient is deteriorating by going deeper into coma. But assessing consciousness is difficult because the patient may be unresponsive, and only close observation of specific signs can provide any evidence of the conscious state.

The **coma scale** is a series of such specific signs that can be assessed and will give some evidence of the conscious state and any changes in it. The specific signs are assessed by the nurse delivering a sensory stimulus to the patient and then observing the response. The grade recorded on the coma scale will depend on the patient's best response to that stimulus. Auditory stimuli are usually tried first. These are sounds beginning with normal speaking, e.g. asking the patient a question (e.g. *what is your name?*). If there is no response, then give a louder command (e.g. *Open your eyes*) or a clap of the hands. Such stimuli enter

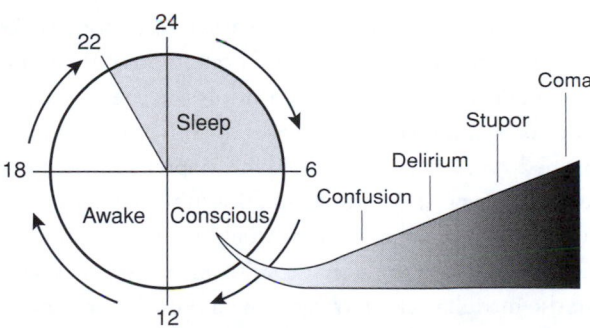

FIGURE 10.8 The consciousness–coma continuum and the sleep–wake cycle. The sleep–wake cycle is normal, but the coma continuum is due to pathology.

the brain via the **vestibulo-cochlear nerve** (**cranial nerve VIII**, previously known as the **auditory nerve**) and directly excite neurons of the auditory cortex within the temporal lobe (see p. 172 and Figure 10.4). If there is no response to auditory signals, this is noted, then **tactile stimuli** are tried. These are touch-related somatic sensations (e.g. gently shaking the patient's arm), which pass via **spinal nerves** to the **spinal cord** then on to the brain stem and upwards to the thalamus, which relays the stimulus onto the appropriate part of the parietal lobe's somatic sensory cortex. Thus speech and touch pass by different routes to different areas of the cerebral cortex. Just as we increased the auditory stimulus by raising the volume from speech to command, so we can increase the somatic stimulus from touch to pain. Almost every conscious person responds to **painful stimuli** in some form or another; it is a powerful stimulus of cerebral cortex function. However, pain is associated with injury, and it is very important to use a method of pain application that causes no tissue damage. Traditionally, rubbing the sternum with the knuckles of a clenched fist has been used, but this practice should stop since bleeding has often occurred causing large haematomas and ultimately extensive bruising over the front of the chest. It is better to apply pressure to the fingernails and toenails, which are themselves dead tissue and therefore will not be damaged. The response to pain is *motor*, i.e. a reaction from the frontal lobe's motor cortex causing the muscles to move the limbs in some manner. Even a verbal response to pain is motor in origin, albeit from the brain's specialised motor speech area (called **Broca's area**), again in the frontal lobe, but such a reaction would probably mean that the patient was fully conscious. The somatic motor responses can be called **purposeful responses** if they show limb withdrawal from the pain, or attempts to push the nurse's hand away (i.e. they show signs of trying to stop the pain, so the pain is registering as conscious). The limb movements may cross the body's midline. **Non-purposeful responses** are limb movements without any attempt to stop the pain or withdraw from it, and do not cross the midline, whereas **unresponsive** is a feature of the deepest comas. Pain is interesting because it is handled by the nervous system somewhat differently from all other stimuli. All somatic pain passes into the spinal cord and then onto the thalamus, but both the cord and the thalamus have their own ways of managing pain (see Chapter 11).

Brain stem reflexes

Being the upward extension of the spinal cord, the brain stem not only houses the vital centres of cardiac, blood pressure and respiratory function, it is also the home of several reflexes other than pain. The **pupillary reflex**, which controls the size of the pupils and their reaction to light, and the **corneal reflex**, which causes the lids to close sharply when the surface of the eyeball is touched, will both be examined in Chapter 12. The **gag reflex** occurs when a stimulus is applied to the back of the throat and this induces a sensation of retching (wanting to vomit; see Chapter 8). Such a stimulus would be a spatula or a finger placed at the back of the tongue. It is similar to the spinal cord's pain reflex arc: a sensory input passes to the vomit centre in the medulla, which triggers the motor response from the muscles of the throat and upper digestive tract; the muscles then carry out the reaction. Like all reflexes, it is protective, attempting to prevent objects from obstructing the vital passages from the mouth to the digestive system and helping to keep the airway clear at the same time.

The Glasgow Coma Scale

A coma scale is a means of identifying and recording levels of consciousness in the patient. Terminology has been developed to help in the process of positioning a patient on the consciousness spectrum using specific criteria or symptoms that may be present in any combination (see Figure 10.8; all modified from Hickey 2008):

- **Fully conscious**: awake, alert, orientated in time and place, understands spoken words, reads written words, expresses ideas verbally.

Then the altered states of consciousness:

- **Confusion**: disorientated in time, place and person; memory lapses; short attention spans; difficulty in following instructions; possibly hallucinations or false perceptions; agitation and bewilderment.
- **Lethargy**: orientated but very slow in motor activity and speech, low level of mental activity, high accident risk.
- **Obtundation**: very drowsy, arousable when stimulated, verbal responses very limited, attempts to follow only very simple commands, high accident risk.
- **Stupor**: generally unresponsive except to vigorous verbal or touch stimuli, attempts at eye opening or incomprehensible sounds may be the only response, responds to pain, minimal spontaneous movements, high accident risk.
- **Coma**: no response to verbal or touch stimuli, no verbal sounds, response to pain stimuli as follows:
  - **Light coma**: purposeful withdrawal from pain, gag, corneal and pupillary reflexes intact.
  - **Medium coma**: non-purposeful responses to pain, variable brain stem reflex responses, some being absent.
  - **Deep coma**: unresponsive to pain, brain stem reflexes absent.

Several coma scales have been developed, but the **Glasgow Coma Scale** is the most widely adopted (Figure 10.9). This assessment defines coma as three conditions: the patient is (1) unable to open the eyes; (2) unable to obey commands; and (3) unable to speak. Eye opening, motor response to both verbal commands and painful stimuli and the ability to speak are the specific signs adopted for assessment (Figure 10.9). The patient is assessed by applying various stimuli and observing a response in these areas. Reliability between different observers is good, making this a valid tool for the universal assessment of consciousness (Juarez and Lyons 1995).

Major causes of unconsciousness

Epilepsy

An abnormal pattern of electrical activity that renders the brain in some state of altered consciousness is called a **seizure**. Some seizures appear as a **convulsion** (or fit), where the

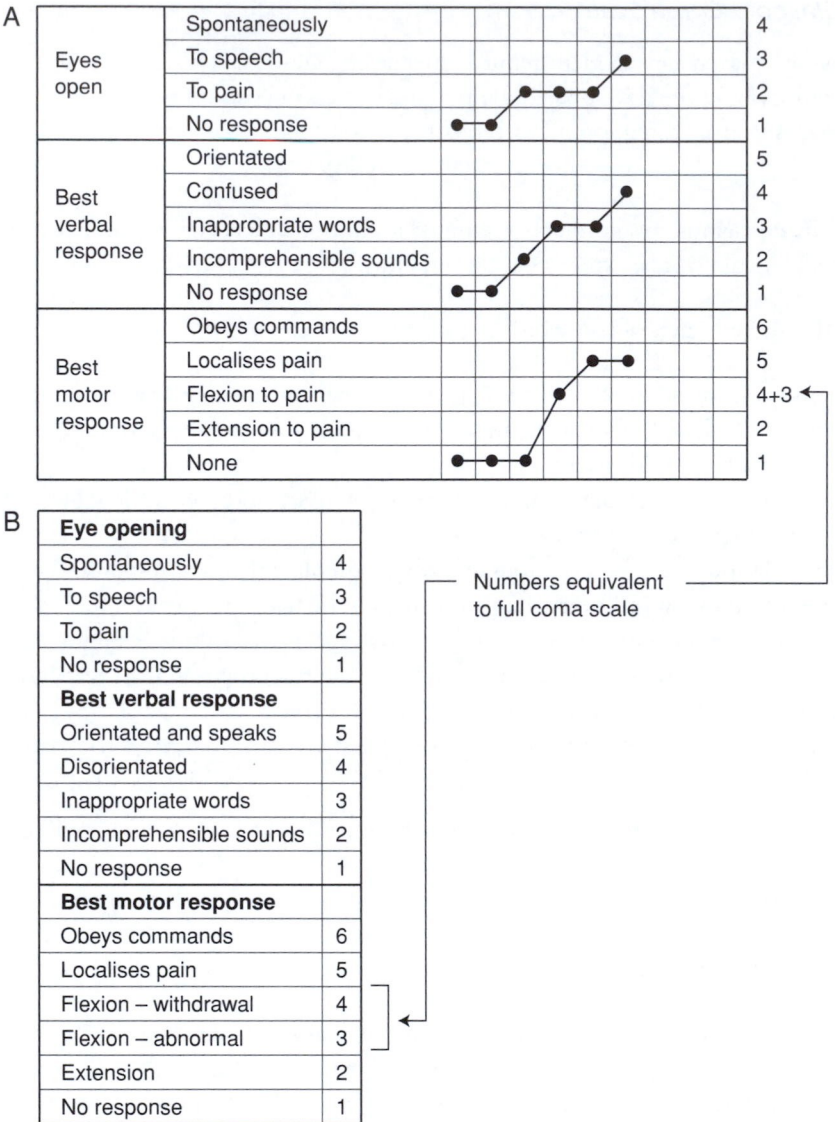

A

			4
Eyes open	Spontaneously		4
	To speech		3
	To pain		2
	No response		1
Best verbal response	Orientated		5
	Confused		4
	Inappropriate words		3
	Incomprehensible sounds		2
	No response		1
Best motor response	Obeys commands		6
	Localises pain		5
	Flexion to pain		4+3
	Extension to pain		2
	None		1

B

Eye opening	
Spontaneously	4
To speech	3
To pain	2
No response	1
Best verbal response	
Orientated and speaks	5
Disorientated	4
Inappropriate words	3
Incomprehensible sounds	2
No response	1
Best motor response	
Obeys commands	6
Localises pain	5
Flexion – withdrawal	4
Flexion – abnormal	3
Extension	2
No response	1

Numbers equivalent to full coma scale

FIGURE 10.9 The Glasgow Coma Scale, partly completed to show a patient regaining consciousness.

patients are usually unconscious and show abnormal rapid muscle activity. **Epilepsy** is a chronic disorder in which convulsions are the major feature. The affected person may go through a convulsive phase (or have a fit), but this is not always the case, since various types of epilepsy are known (Table 10.1). The cause is often a small area of damaged or disturbed brain tissue, the **epileptogenic focus**, which may or may not be detectable and therefore may or may not be operable. In any case, the focus, which is highly excitable, acts as a trigger by causing an abnormal burst of electrical impulses both sideways (laterally) into adjacent cells

TABLE 10.1 The various types of epilepsy

Type	Description
Grand mal	Major convulsive fit in several phases (see Figure 10.11). Complete loss of consciousness with no memory of the event.
Petit mal (absences)	Minor fit. Brief episode of staring vacantly (loss of touch with reality) during which objects held are dropped. Recovery in seconds.
Jacksonian	Twitching in one point in the body spreading to all other parts and causing loss of consciousness.
Focal	Twitching in one point in the body (e.g. mouth or digit) without spread or loss of consciousness.
Psychomotor	Sudden disturbance of behaviour with perhaps hallucinations. Temporal lobe epilepsy is one form.
Myoclonic	Sudden involuntary muscle jerking occurring like a shock, often in the arms of known epileptics.
Post-traumatic	After severe brain injury. It involves all epileptic types except petit mal.
Status epilepticus	Repeated epileptic fits, often one after another, before consciousness is regained and lasting for many hours.

and down the axons to all parts lower down. This is because the focus is overactive and can discharge impulses very easily. Part of the reason for this hyperactivity is a lack of GABA at the focus (see p. 174), which results in a loss of the inhibitory (braking) system, and the accelerator glutamate becomes the dominant neurotransmitter (similar to a car with no brakes). Other chemical changes at the focus also cause this area to become very excitable, such as an abnormal influx of calcium (Ca^{2+}) into the focal cells, and disturbances to glucose and protein metabolism. Impulses travelling down normal cell axons move in one direction only, away from the cell body, called **orthodromic flow**, but **antidromic flow** (backward flow of the impulse along the axon from the synapse towards the cell body) is sometimes seen in abnormal conditions such as the epileptogenic focus. Each time the axonal impulse returns to the cell body, it regenerates a new orthodromic impulse that travels down the axon. This cycle of events is repeated many times during a convulsion, causing the rhythmic thrashing of the limbs as each new impulse from this cycle passes out to the muscles (Figure 10.10). The lateral spread of the abnormal burst of impulses across the brain surface causes the other cerebral cells to stop all conscious activity, and the person becomes unconscious for the duration of the fit, perhaps about 3–5 minutes. Breathing, the heart cycle and blood pressure remain, since they are not conscious activities and are controlled by brain areas lower down in the brain stem. The course of events during a convulsion (or **grand mal** fit) involves several brief moments of collapse, rigidity (the tonic phase), convulsion (the clonic phase) and full recovery (Figure 10.11) (Blows 2011).

Minor fits (often called **petit mal** or **absences**) involve a short period of staring into space with fumbling followed by complete recovery. This is not unconsciousness as such but a kind of twilight state in which the brain is incapable of all normal conscious responses and goes into *pause* or *standby* mode. Post-epileptic complications can rarely occur, and these include

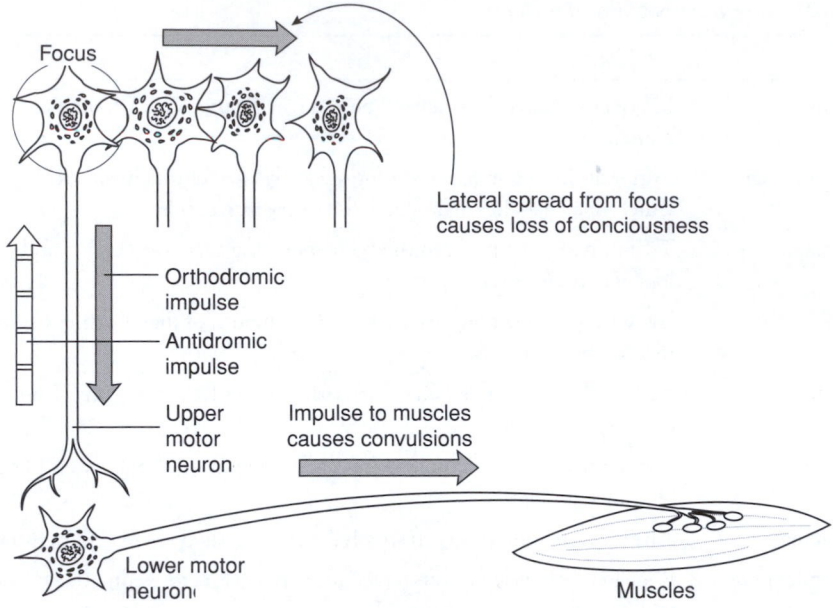

FIGURE 10.10 Events that occur during a fit. The epileptogenic focus spreads abnormal impulses laterally to cause the cerebral surface cells to lose consciousness. Impulses travelling in a normal direction down the focal axon (orthodromic) not only cause impulses to pass out to the muscles (creating seizures) but return abnormal impulses back to the focus (antidromic) as part of an impulse loop up and down the focal axon.

	Stage	Notes
1	Aura	A warning of impending fit. Not always present or recognised. May take the form of flashing lights or other hallucinations.
2	Tonic	Lasts up to 30 seconds. Full muscle tone causes gross rigidity, including respiratory muscles, causing breathing to stop.
3	Clonic	Lasts up to 45 seconds or so. The convulsion phase, with gross twitching and thrashing of limbs. Breathing is spontaneous.
4	Recovery	Clonic convulsion stops and the patient 'sleeps' off the effects for up to 15 minutes or so. Should waken with no memory of the event.

FIGURE 10.11 Stages of grand mal seizure.

status epilepticus, where the patient has repeated fits, and **twilight states**, when the patient may wander aimlessly for hours or days not knowing who or where they are (Blows 2011).

Strokes

Strokes, or **cerebrovascular accidents** (**CVA**s) are sudden, usually unpredictable, disruptions to the blood supply to the brain. The blood carries essential oxygen and glucose to the neurons and carries away the wastes of cellular metabolism, and sudden loss of these functions can cause neurons to cease functioning. In the case of neurons of the cerebral cortex, this causes unconsciousness. The disruptions to the blood supply appear in two forms: (1) bleeding into the brain itself (intracerebral bleed); and (2) sudden obstruction of the blood vessels leading to the brain (cerebral thrombosis or **embolus**).

The blood supply to the brain begins as blood leaves the left side of the heart via the aorta (see Chapter 2). A series of arteries branch off from the aorta carrying blood upwards to the head (Figure 10.12). The **brachiocephalic** and **common carotid** arteries distribute blood towards the neck; the internal carotid arteries take blood up to the **circle of Willis** in the base of the brain (Figure 10.13).

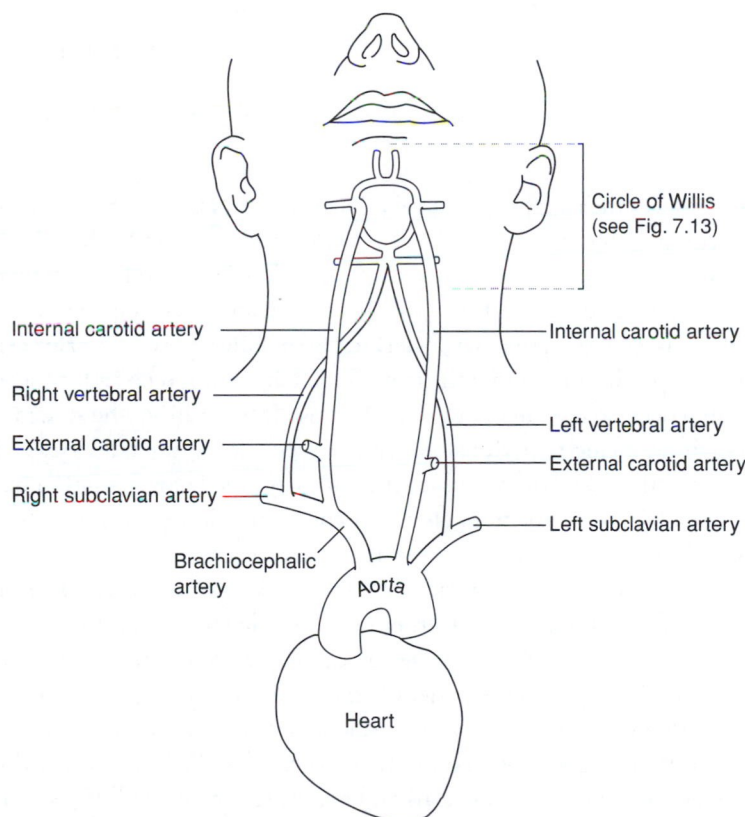

FIGURE 10.12 The blood supply to the brain from the heart.

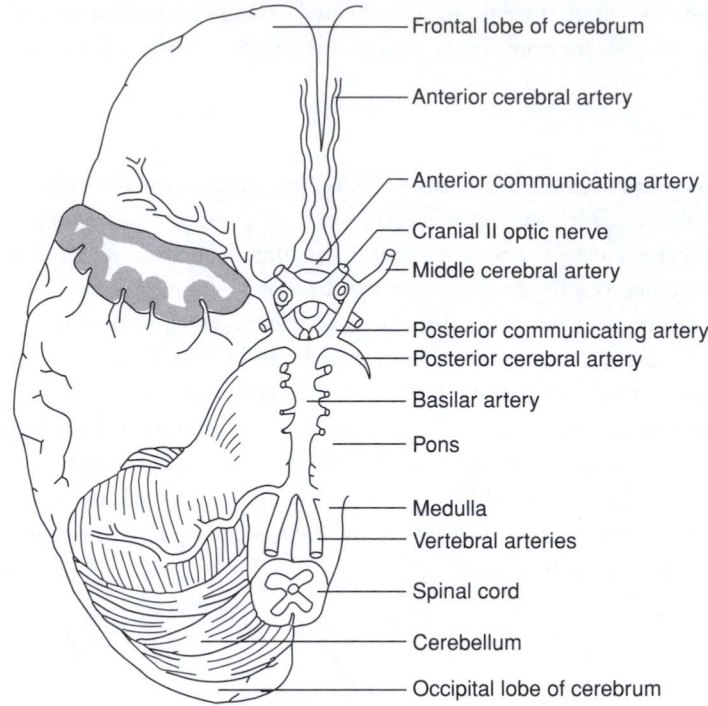

FIGURE 10.13   The arteries of the circle of Willis distributing blood to the brain.

Blood also arrives there from the **vertebral arteries**, branches of the **subclavian** arteries that pass up through the cervical (neck) vertebrae (hence *vertebral*). The bilateral nature of these arterial systems means that the circle of Willis has four blood supplies (two vertebral and two internal carotid arteries), but there are six main arteries going out of the circle. These are also bilateral pairs, the two **posterior**, two **middle** and two **anterior cerebral arteries**. The circle of Willis is therefore the major blood distribution point for the entire brain.

Strokes often occur as a result of one or both of two factors: either the systemic blood pressure is too high (**systemic hypertension**, see Chapter 3) or arterial disease, such as arteriosclerosis, narrows the vessels and leads to **thrombosis** (blood clot formation in the cerebral arteries) or **emboli** (blood clots from elsewhere in the circulation blocking the artery). The sudden loss of blood supply causes areas of the brain to cease functioning, with the loss of neurons. These areas become necrotic (dead) areas, known as **cerebral infarcts** (similar to myocardial infarcts in Chapter 3). In either case, bleeding or obstruction, the effect is rather similar, i.e. sudden collapse, varying degrees of altered consciousness, including sometimes coma, severe head pain if the patient is conscious, weakness (hemiparesis) or paralysis (hemiplegia) often experienced down one side and sometimes other signs such as loss of speech (aphasia). The signs depend entirely on where the CVA has occurred in the brain, how big the lesion is and which neurons and pathways are affected. If a small area of cerebral cortex is involved in the lesion, consciousness may be retained throughout or return quickly if lost. Alternatively, large areas of cortex involved may mean prolonged coma from which the patient may never recover. Some patients suffer brain damage to the point where they die soon after the event. Recovery is also dependent on the degree of brain damage sustained. Some survivors who regain consciousness may make a full recovery, whereas others may be left with some degree of **neurological deficit**, i.e. permanent symptoms such as one-sided weakness or speech loss that they must learn to overcome.

Head injury

Unconsciousness in head injury is caused by either shaking of the brain (known as **concussion**), damage to the brain or pressure on the brain (known as **compression**). The difference between them is critical, i.e. the difference between full recovery (as may be associated with pressure), partial or no recovery (as may be associated with brain damage). Because the brain is a soft organ inside a hard bony skull, it can suffer the *jelly in a tin* effect when the head is struck. Imagine a ready-to-eat jelly placed in a tin with the lid on. If the tin is dropped from only waist height, the tin will survive more or less intact. But will the jelly? Head injuries are either caused by a **deceleration trauma** (the head is moving but suddenly stops as it hits an immovable object) or an **acceleration trauma** (the head is stationary but is caused to move violently when struck by a fast moving object). In either case the brain movement is always slightly behind the skull movement, i.e. the skull stops suddenly but the brain carries on briefly and collides with the inside of the skull, or the skull moves suddenly and the brain lags behind and again collides with the skull. The first collision causes an injury to one part of the brain (e.g. at the front), followed by an *equal but opposite force* causing the brain to move in the opposite direction, creating a second injury directly opposite to the first (e.g. at the back), known as the **contracoup injury** (see Figure 10.14) (McCance *et al.* 2010).

The problem is that the top surface of the brain, i.e. the surface exposed to the inside of the skull, is the cerebral cortex: *the conscious brain*. So in either scenario, consciousness is

(a)   (b)

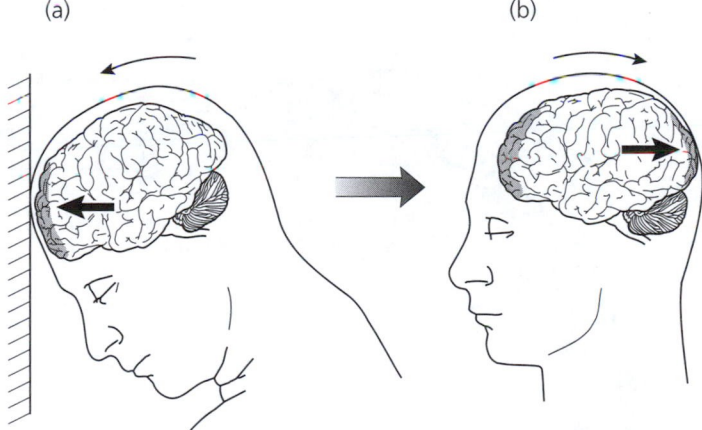

FIGURE 10.14   Contracoup trauma to the brain in head injury. (a) the initial injury to the front of the brain when the head is thrown forward and hits a solid object; (b) the secondary injury.

likely to suffer first and probably most severely. Some protection to this surface is afforded by the **meninges**, which cover the surface of the brain and cord (collectively called the **central nervous system**, or **CNS**), and by the jacket of watery fluid within the meninges (the **cerebrospinal fluid**, or **CSF**) (Figure 10.15).

The meninges are three coverings: from the inner to the outer layers they are the **pia mater**, the **arachnoid mater** and beneath the skull the **dura mater**. A small dry space, the **subdural space**, exists between the dura mater and the arachnoid mater below, but a larger CSF-filled space, the **subarachnoid space**, exists between the arachnoid mater and the pia mater below. This provides most of the cushioning effect around the brain. CSF is produced within the **ventricles** of the brain; it circulates around the brain and cord and is returned to the blood via the **arachnoid villi** extending from the arachnoid mater. Therefore this fluid is constantly being renewed, and a relatively constant pressure of CSF must be maintained. The hardness and roundness of the skull, plus the CSF cushion, all help to prevent brain injury during minor head collisions, like the many small head bumps children sustain with no ill effects. It takes a much harder blow to the skull, as is often a feature of injuries sustained while travelling at speed, to cause the involvement of consciousness. This demonstrates the need for external protection, i.e. helmets, plus seat belts and head rests, to prevent deceleration injury for various high-risk forms of transport.

The bony box we called the skull has a limited internal space, most of which is filled with the brain. This and the blood and CSF volumes circulating the brain cause an internal pressure within the skull, known as the **intracranial pressure** (or **ICP**), which is normally anything up to 15 mmHg. About 80% of this pressure is caused by the brain, and the remaining 20% is shared between the blood and CSF volumes. **Raised intracranial pressure** (or **RICP**), i.e. any pressure persistently sustained over 20 mmHg, is caused by anything that abnormally demands space inside the skull; a **space-occupying lesion** (or **SOL**). SOLs can be many things, such as brain tumours, excessive CSF volume (called **hydrocephalus**) and bleeding inside the skull from trauma. After brain shaking (**concussion**, see p. 183), small

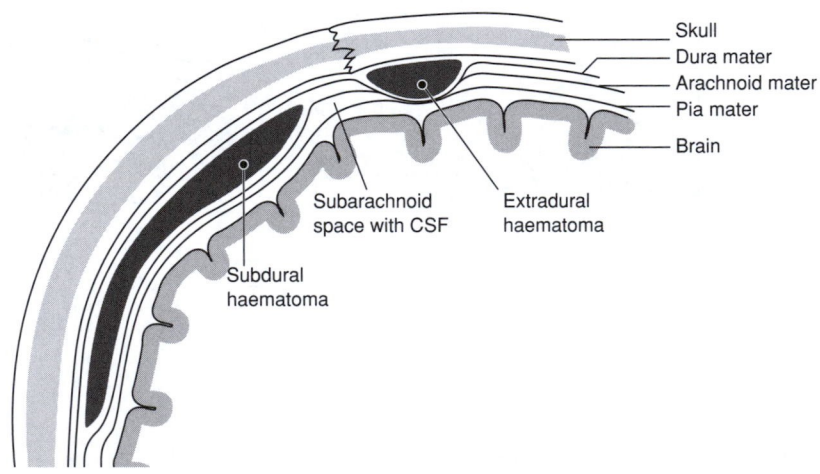

FIGURE 10.15 Subdural and extradural haematomas. CSF, cerebrospinal fluid.

bleeds into the cerebral cortex may occur (brain bruising, or **contusion**). The blood lost may build up if bleeding continues and puts pressure on the brain (compression). The process leading to RICP is often continuous, and the casualty deteriorates with loss of consciousness. Where the bleeding occurs inside the skull is important; the most common sites associated with head injuries being the **extradural haematoma** (blood in the extradural space, i.e. between the dura and the skull) or the **subdural haematoma** (blood in the subdural space, see p. 184 and Figure 10.15). When the meninges and the spaces between them were described, there was no mention of an **extradural space**. This is because the space does not normally exist; in fact, the space has to be created by the lesion, which must therefore be a high-pressure bleed to force the separation of the dura from the skull, i.e. it must be an arterial bleed (for example, in the **middle meningeal artery**). This kind of injury is rarer than the venous bleed that causes a subdural haematoma, (i.e. four subdural bleeds to every extradural bleed), and extradural bleeds are even rarer in the elderly, for the dura slowly fuses onto the skull with increasing age, making the creation of an extradural space almost impossible. The main difference, apart from the site and blood vessel involved, is speed of onset of symptoms. An extradural haematoma is *rapid*, i.e. life-threatening symptoms can occur within a few minutes, compared with the *slower* subdural haematoma, which causes problems over several hours or even days. This indicates two things:

1   The need for a scan or a 24-hour stay in hospital for head injuries to exclude an extradural haematoma; if a subdural haematoma develops at home after that, there is time to get the patient back to hospital.
2   The need for continuous observation, since the patient may deteriorate rapidly and die if vital symptoms of an extradural haematoma are missed.

The symptoms are those of RICP, and they fall into two categories:

1   **General symptoms**: those that indicate the presence of RICP but give no clue to the exact site of the pressure on the brain.
2   **Local** (or **focal**) **symptoms**: those that indicate both the presence and the site of pressure on the brain.

General symptoms are **headache** (which is worse on wakening), **nausea**, vomiting, slow pulse rate (bradycardia) and **raised blood pressure** (changes in the pulse and blood pressure may occur late as the patient deteriorates and should not be relied on), **altered state of consciousness** (see p. 177 and Figure 10.8), **blurred vision**, respiratory irregularities and **papilloedema** (see p. 225). The focal symptoms are **unilateral**, ipsilateral fixed dilated pupil followed later by **bilateral fixed dilated pupils**, nystagmus and **visual field defects** (see p. 218), **fits** (see p. 177), **aphasia** (loss of speech), **ataxia**, hemiparesis and/or **hemiplegia** (see p. 240), and **specific sensory losses**. These symptoms will develop at different speeds depending on many factors, as indicated here for extradural and subdural haematomas, including which blood vessel is bleeding, the location of the bleed on the brain and the brain's compensatory mechanism. This **compensatory mechanism** allows for a certain increase in SOL size without undue change in the ICP (see Figure 10.16).

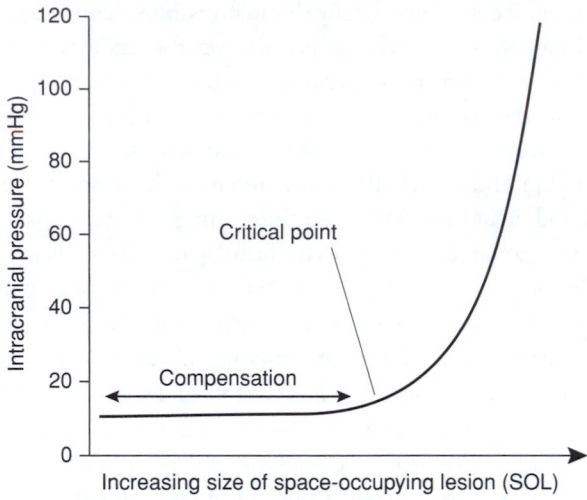

FIGURE 10.16   A sudden rise in the intracranial pressure occurs when the brain compensatory mechanism fails. This critical point must be watched for very carefully.

As the SOL grows, the pressure it exerts is *absorbed* at first by a *reduction* in both the volume of blood entering the skull and the volume of CSF produced. Remember, these two account for 20% of the ICP (see p. 184), and this percentage could drop to accommodate the growing SOL. This compensation only lasts for a while, after which the ICP will rise sharply (see Figure 10.16) since the SOL is now big enough to put pressure on the brain, which cannot reduce any of its 80% ICP value. This is the critical point, the change from compensation to decompensation, where the resultant RICP may kill the patient if this is not noticed urgently. Increasing RICP will displace the brain, forcing it downwards and/or sideways, referred to as **herniation** of the brain structures, with associated tearing of membranes and crushing of nerves. As the brain stem is forced downwards, it impacts on the **foramen magnum**, the large opening in the base of the skull through which the spinal cord emerges. This impaction blocks the flow of CSF through the opening from brain to cord and back, and it puts pressure on the vital centres of the brain stem: the cardiac and vasomotor centres (see Chapter 3), and the respiratory centre (see Chapter 4). This is a life-threatening situation, called **coning**, and is far better avoided by accurate observation. The treatment for RICP is generally a surgical opening made into the skull, called a **burr hole**, to let the haematoma out, and in the case of an extradural haematoma it may be necessary, in an emergency, to perform this *before* the patient is taken to theatre. This vital procedure, combined with accurate neurological observation, can save the patient's life.

Other causes of loss of consciousness

Many other causes of unconsciousness exist. A group of student nurses was asked to put together a list of causes, and between them they identified more than 15. The list was then passed to several trained nurses, who raised the total to 26. Finally, a number of doctors were asked for their contribution, and the list grew to nearly 40 causes. This illustrates just how vulnerable consciousness is to instabilities in both the internal environment of the brain and the external environment we live in, yet we take consciousness so much for granted. We do not notice it until we lose it. Here are a few important examples of causes of unconsciousness:

- lack of oxygen, either in the air or through strangulation, choking, drowning or airway obstruction;
- various poisons and toxins, such as the toxin that causes **tetanus** from the bacterium **Clostridium tetani**, which lives in soil and infects soil-contaminated wounds;
- central nervous system infections, such as **meningitis** (inflammation of the meninges) or **encephalitis** (inflammation of the brain substance);
- intoxication by alcohol or drug abuse or drug overdose;
- electric shock;
- loss of blood pressure, temporarily as in **fainting** (or **apoplexy**), or more profound as in severe shock;
- metabolic disorders such as **diabetes** (see Chapter 7), where both high and low blood sugar levels induce coma in response to instability in the blood insulin level.

Fainting is possibly the most common cause of unconsciousness; the one most people may suffer or encounter. The temporary drop in blood pressure causes a transient loss of blood supply to the brain, which then goes unconscious. It is usually temporary because it tends to treat itself. The original problem is caused by the brain being *vertically* above the heart, which then has the job of pumping blood *uphill*, against gravity, to the brain. This requires a good arterial blood pressure and therefore considerable heart pumping power, and if the left ventricle fails to deliver this blood, the brain suffers. However, it is somewhat self-treating because fainting causes the person to collapse and this puts the brain *horizontally in line* with the heart, and the pressure required to supply blood to the brain is then much reduced. In short, fainting does away with gravity. Now the left ventricle can happily supply blood to the brain at the new lower pressure, and the brain recovers. Of course, the fall can cause problems, and the casualty must remain flat until the ventricular pressure is high enough to supply the brain once more in the upright position. When asked, 'Under what circumstances could fainting be the cause of death?' one student answered 'If you faint on the edge of a cliff.' The real answer is: when the person faints while pinned in an upright position, i.e. unable to fall to the ground, such as standing in a tightly packed train on a long, hot journey. The drop in blood pressure results in the blood being unable to flow uphill to reach the brain, and since the person is unable to fall down, the brain is starved of blood for longer.

The anaesthetic drugs

Currently it is not possible to say exactly how many anaesthetic drugs create unconsciousness. The benzodiazepines, like diazepam, and the barbiturates, such as phenobarbitol, can induce unconsciousness in sufficient dosage. They work by binding to specific GABA receptors and enhance the inhibitory (or braking) effect of GABA, thus effectively shutting down brain activity. Other anaesthetics are less well understood, but they do appear to suppress excitation of the cerebral cortex without affecting nerve conduction. Lipid solubility is a common feature of these drugs and correlates well with their anaesthetic properties, i.e. the more lipid-soluble, the greater is their power of anaesthesia. Perhaps they get incorporated into cortical neuron cell membranes, which are themselves lipid-based. Distortion of these membranes by the drugs may disrupt ionic movement across the membrane and cause the neuron to fail temporarily.

Key points

- The cerebral cortex, particularly the prefrontal cortex, is the conscious brain.
- Awareness of the environment and control of activities are qualities of consciousness.
- The cortex is made up of nerve cells called neurons.
- Neurons have a cell body with dendrites and an axon that is often myelinated.
- Neuroglia (or glial cells) provide structural or chemical functions important for neuron activity.
- Grey matter is cell bodies packed together and white matter is axons packed together.
- Neurons connect to each other through synapses. These tiny gaps require a neurotransmitter, the most important of which for consciousness is glutamate.
- Another neurotransmitter is GABA (gamma-aminobutyric acid), which inhibits nerve impulses.
- The left and right hemispheres of the cortex are further divided into lobes given the same names as the skull bones: the frontal, parietal, temporal and occipital lobes.
- Association areas between the main functional areas of the cortex are essential for making sense of the sensory stimuli arriving at the cortex.
- The motor cortex is in the frontal lobe, the sensory cortex is in the parietal lobe. The cells are carefully arranged in a layout that matches the body plan.
- Sensations coming into the brain from the body must first pass to the thalamus, a sensory relay station that sends sensations on to the correct part of the cerebral cortex.
- Consciousness can be considered as a spectrum, from fully conscious at one end to coma at the other. The various points on this spectrum are the altered states of consciousness.
- Painful stimuli are achieved by applying pressure to the fingernails and toenails, which are dead tissue and therefore will not be damaged. The response to pain is motor, i.e. limb movements.
- Purposeful responses are signs of trying to stop painful stimuli; non-purposeful responses are limb movements without any attempt to stop painful stimuli.
- The Glasgow Coma Scale is the most widely adopted. This defines coma as an inability to open the eyes, to obey commands and to speak.
- The cause of epilepsy can be a small area of damaged or disturbed brain tissue, the epileptogenic focus.
- A grand mal fit involves collapse, tonic rigidity, clonic convulsions and then full recovery. Minor fits (petit mal or vacancies) are short periods of aimless staring with fumbling followed by complete recovery.

- Strokes, or cerebrovascular accidents (CVAs), are sudden, unpredictable disruptions to the blood supply to the brain, bleeding into the brain itself (intracerebral bleed) or sudden arterial obstruction (cerebral thrombosis or embolus).
- Unconsciousness in head injury is caused by shaking of the brain (concussion), damage or pressure on the brain. The difference between them means full recovery (associated with pressure), partial or no recovery (associated with brain damage).
- Some protection to the brain is afforded by the meninges, the pia mater next to the brain, the arachnoid mater, and beneath the skull, the dura mater, and by the cerebrospinal fluid, or CSF. The subdural space exists between the dura mater and the arachnoid mater below.
- The development of an extradural haematoma is rapid, within minutes, compared with the slower subdural haematoma, which takes several hours or days.
- The symptoms of raised intracranial pressure (RICP) are general (those that indicate RICP but no clue to the site of the pressure) or focal (those that indicate both RICP and the site of pressure). A slow pulse rate and raised blood pressure may occur late and should not be relied on.
- Coning, i.e. death by impacting the medulla through the foramen magnum, is avoidable with accurate observation.
- Fainting is a common cause of unconsciousness caused by a temporary drop in blood pressure with loss of blood supply to the brain. It is somewhat self-treating because collapse puts the brain level with the heart, and the pressure required to supply blood to the brain is much less. If a person faints while pinned in an upright position, i.e. unable to fall, it could be fatal.

References

Blows W. T. (2011) *The Biological Basis of Mental Health Nursing,* 2nd edition. Routledge, London.

Carlson N. R. (2010) *Physiology of Behaviour,* 10th edition. Allyn and Bacon, Boston.

Carter R. (1998) *Mapping the Mind.* Weidenfeld and Nicolson, London.

Hickey J. (2008) *The Clinical Practice of Neurological and Neurosurgical Nursing,* 6th edition. Lippincott Williams and Wilkins, Philadelphia, PA.

Juarez V. and Lyons M. (1995) Interrater reliability of the Glasgow Coma Scale. *Journal of Neuroscience Nursing,* **27**(5): 283–286.

McCance K. L., Huether S. E., Brashers V. L. and Rote N. S. (2010) *Pathophysiology: The Biological Basis for Disease in Adults and Children,* 6th edition. Mosby Elsevier, St Louis, Missouri.

Chapter 11 **Neurological observations (II)**

Pain

- Introduction
- The nature and causes of pain
- Pain pathways
- The observation of pain
- Pain management
- Key points
- References

Introduction

Pain is a topic that is naturally abhorrent to us, and one we would prefer to forget. But to health professionals, pain must be addressed because patient comfort is a major issue in all aspects of health care. However, observing pain in a patient is one of the most difficult assessments to make, but it is such an important assessment to get as accurate as possible. Of course, an important way of assessing a patient's pain is simply to ask them if they are in pain. The problem here is that this type of assessment is not really measurable, so there is little hard data upon which pain treatment can be based. And different people have different pain thresholds. Part of the problem is that medical and nursing staff could actually interpret a patient's pain while unconsciously colouring it with their own pain perceptions. This becomes evident when carers say things such as 'Come on, it can't hurt that much!' Pain observations are an attempt to overcome these problems. An interesting insight into pain was given by D'Costa (2011).

The nature and causes of pain

The three physiological causes of pain are **nociception** (pain causes by actual or potential tissue injury), **inflammatory pain** (caused by inflammatory processes) and **neuropathic pain** (caused by nerve damage) (Meijler 2006).

Nociception is a term used to describe pain caused by everyday injuries, such as stings, burns, bumps, and so on. There are several types of nociception. **Acute pain** has recently occurred and of relatively short duration. It alerts the individual that something is wrong and needs attention, and therefore it can protect the individual against further tissue injury. **Chronic pain** has a longer duration than acute, often lasting for weeks, months or even years. Some authors consider chronic pain as lasting for longer than three months (Wood 2002). **Intractable pain** is chronic pain with no detectable pathology causing it. It is very difficult to treat and is a major challenge to health care professionals. Apart from some theories, there is no known cause of intractable pain.

Localised pain is often caused by **inflammation** of the tissues involved (Figure 11.1). Inflammation is, in turn, caused by local trauma or irritation of the tissues, as seen in infections and mechanical injury. Inflammation is unpleasant to us, but the immune system could not function adequately without it. The increase in capillary wall permeability that occurs in inflammation causes increased amounts of water to leak into the tissues from blood plasma, along with proteins and large numbers of white blood cells, all entering the tissues. Extra protein in the tissue fluid attracts more water from the capillaries. This causes a local **oedema** (see p. 84). **Pain mediators** (i.e. chemicals causing pain) are released at the site; notably **histamine, prostaglandins** and **bradykinins** (Figure 11.2). These bind to receptor sites present on **nociceptors**, which are pain nerve endings. There are two types of nociceptors: **mechanoreceptors** and **polymodal receptors**. Mechanoreceptors are pain receptors

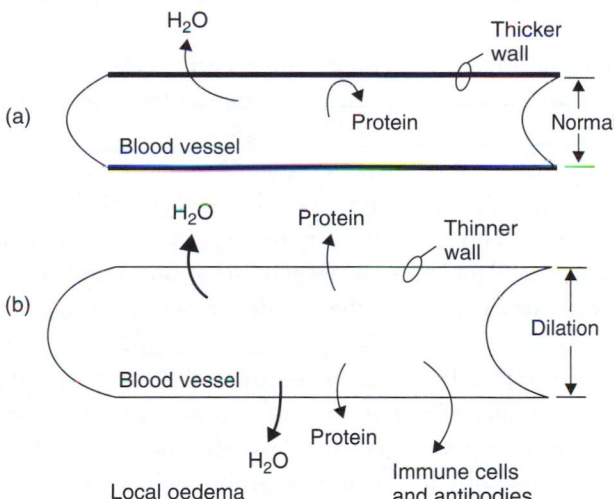

FIGURE 11.1 Inflammation. (a) The non-inflamed blood vessel is normal width and has a wall thick enough to prevent inappropriate leakage of blood contents into the surrounding tissues. (b) In inflamed tissues, blood vessels are dilated and the walls are stretched and thinner, and leakage of water, proteins and immune cells and antibodies can take place. Protein that has escaped into the tissues attracts further water out of the blood, causing local tissue oedema. This oedematous swelling puts pressure on nociceptors. Pain is generated by this swelling and locally released pain mediators (see also Figure 11.2).

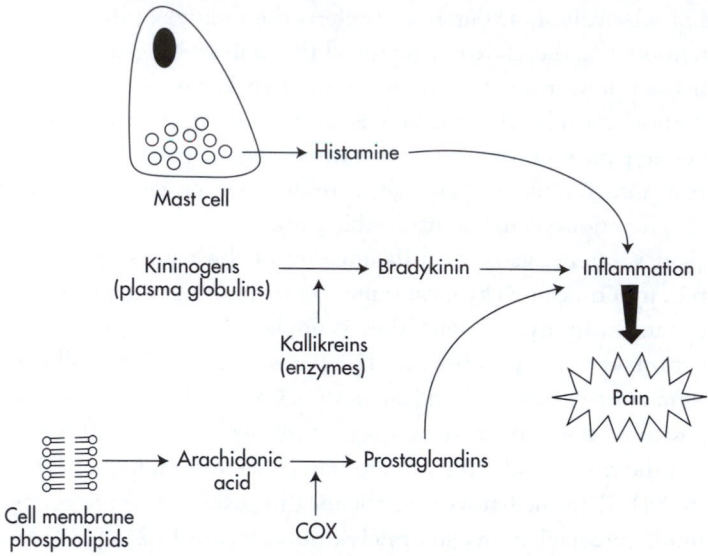

FIGURE 11.2 Pain mediators. Histamine is released from mast cells (found in most tissues), bradykinins are derived from the plasma globulins kininogens, and prostaglandins are formed from arachidonic acid.

that respond to mechanical injury, while polymodal receptors respond to pain caused by many types of tissue injury.

Conscious perception of pain relies on certain criteria being reached. First, sufficient chemical mediator must bind to the nociceptors to raise the level of stimulation to the **pain threshold** point or beyond. Threshold means the amount of chemical stimulation necessary to generate strong enough impulses from the nociceptors that are recognised as pain by the brain. With less chemical binding, i.e. below threshold level, impulses can still be generated from the nociceptor, but these are weaker, and are recognised by the brain as **irritation**, rather than pain. **Itching** is one form of irritation caused by mediators binding to nociceptors in concentrations below that needed to activate the pain threshold level (Figure 11.3).

Second, even if the pain threshold is exceeded, the nature, severity and duration of pain conceived by the brain are dependent on the intensity of neuronal firing from the nociceptor. If the nociceptor firing is weak (i.e. just above threshold level), the pain conceived by the brain will be significantly less than if the firing intensity increased. It is a simple relationship; the greater the intensity of impulses generated, the greater is the perceived pain.

Pain pathways

Pain impulses pass to the brain via the peripheral **sensory nervous system**. There are two major types of sensory nerve pathways which carry impulses destined to register as pain in the brain. These are **Aδ fibres** and **C fibres**. The A fibres (fast fibres) are divided into

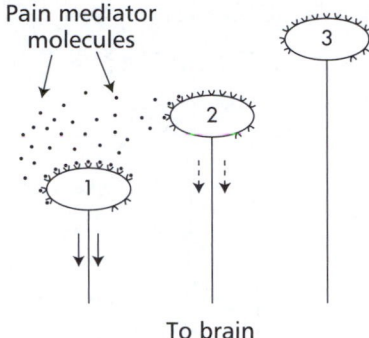

Pain mediator molecules

To brain

FIGURE 11.3 Pain mediator molecules bind to nociceptors (1, 2 and 3). Number 1 has bound a lot of molecules and sends rapid impulses to the brain, and pain is experienced. Number 2 has fewer molecules and sends a slower rate of impulses which the brain interprets as itching. Number 3 has no molecules and sends no impulses to the brain.

subtypes, **A\alpha**, **A\beta** and **A\delta**, of which the A\delta fibre carries pain. A\delta fibres are the fastest of the fast fibres, i.e. they convey impulses to the brain at speeds up to 30 metres per second, while C fibres are much slower than this (up to 2 metres per second). The speed difference is caused by the thickness of the fibres and the degree of **myelination** the fibre has. Myelin is the fatty covering along the axon of neurons that is involved in impulse conduction. The better the myelination (as in A fibres), the faster the impulse will travel. C fibres are unmyelinated and transmit impulses at the slowest speeds. They are important, however, since they carry about 80% of pain impulses to the brain. Nociceptors at the peripheral end of the A\delta fibres are found in the skin (see Chapter 9) and mucous membranes, where they are the first to warn the brain against sudden, sharp pain due to trauma. Compare that with nociceptors of C fibres, which are also in the skin but are found in most other body tissues as well.

The pathway from the periphery to the brain is a three-neuronal system, i.e. the impulse must pass through three **sensory neurons** to get from the nociceptor to the brain (Figure 11.4):

- *Neuron 1* passes from the nociceptor into the posterior part of the **spinal cord**. It is a specialised neuron having the cell body on a branch just outside the cord. This cell body is called the **posterior root ganglion (PRG)**. Placing the cell body near the cord protects it against everyday injuries. Death of this cell body would result in loss of the neuron and the skin would lose sensation.
- *Neuron 2* synapses with the first neuron in the cord, the axon first crossing the midline before passing up the cord to the part of the brain called the **thalamus**. The cross-over in the cord (called a **decussation**) means that impulses from the left of the body will continue up the right-hand side of the nervous system, and vice versa.
- *Neuron 3* synapses with neuron 2, the axon passing from the thalamus to the **sensory cortex** in the parietal lobe of the **cerebrum**.

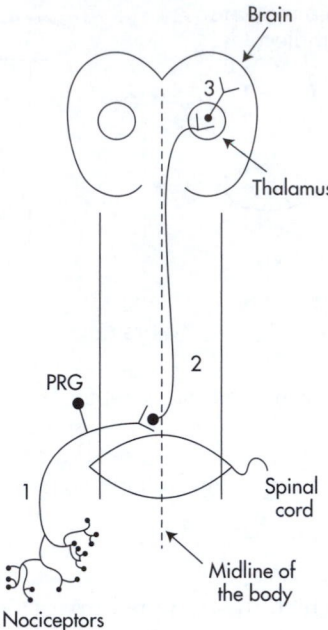

Figure 11.4 All sensations, including pain, use a three-neuronal system from periphery to the brain. Neuron 1 extends from the nociceptor in the periphery to the cord (PRG = posterior root ganglion, the cell body of neuron 1). Neuron 2 crosses the midline in the cord and extends to the thalamus. Neuron 3 relays the impulses from the thalamus to the cerebral cortex of the brain.

Synapses are connections between neurons. Synapses use chemicals called **neurotransmitters** to bridge a gap that the synapse creates. These gaps (called the **synaptic cleft**) and the neurotransmitters found there are important in the story of pain transmission. Beyond the nociceptor, therefore, the synapses conveniently divide the pain pathways into three main parts: (1) these are the pathway from the periphery to the spinal cord (via neuron 1); (2) the pathway to the thalamus (via neuron 2); and (3) the pathway to the sensory area of the cerebral cortex (via neuron 3) (Figure 11.4).

The spinal cord

Pain impulses are *not* recognised as a conscious sensation at spinal cord level. All impulses pass through the cord and its synapses purely automatically at subconscious level. The posterior spinal cord is the site of the first synapse, between neurons 1 and 2.

This connection permits the formation of a pain **reflex arc** (see Figure 13.10) and **cross-reflex** (see Figure 13.11). In the simple reflex arc, a connector (or association) neuron connects the sensory neuron at the back of the cord to the motor neuron at the front of the cord, i.e. the **lower motor neuron (LMN)**. This mechanism then allows pain impulses to trigger another impulse in the corresponding motor neuron in the cord, which then causes muscles to contract and withdraw the affected part away from the source of pain. This arc is also the location for a pain-blocking process called the '**gate-control theory**' (Figure 11.5).

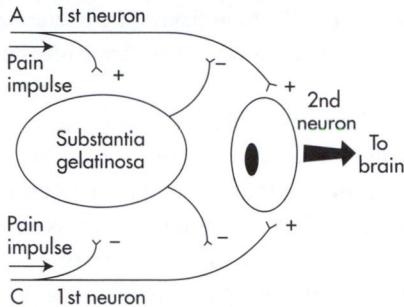

Figure 11.5   The gate control theory. The first sensory neurons (from the periphery to the spinal cord) are both A (fast) and C (slower) fibres. Both carry pain impulses and both stimulate (+) the second neuron in the cord. The A fibre also activates the substantia gelatinosa (SG) with stimulatory (+) synapses . The SG then blocks impulses along both the A and C fibres using its own negative (–) inhibitory synapses. This closes the gate to pain impulses reaching the second neuron. C stimulation shuts down the SG using negative (–) inhibitory synapses and therefore opens the gate to pain by switching off the SG (–) synapses, and allows impulses to reach the second neuron . Generally the 'gate' is neither fully open nor fully closed but varies between the two states and can be influenced by impulses from the brain.

The gate control theory of pain works like this. In the centre of the spinal cord is an area of nerve cell bodies called **grey matter**. Part of this grey matter is a collection of neuronal cell bodies known as the **substantia gellatinosa** (or 'jelly substance'). This can be activated (switched on) by Aδ fibre stimulation, but de-activated (switched off) by C fibre stimulation. Pain impulses arrive first via the faster A fibres of neuron 1, and these impulses pass on up to the brain via neuron 2. At the same time, A fibre impulses activate the substantia gellatinosa. The substantia gelatinosa then inhibits (= blocks) all further A, and also C fibre impulses, and the 'gate' is closed to pain (Figure 11.5). Slower pain impulses passing along C fibres arrive a little later. They cannot pass through this 'gate', but C fibre stimulation tends to switch off the substantia gellatinosa, thus opening the 'gate' to pain impulses, again along both the A and C fibres. In reality, the so-called 'gate' will not be either fully opened or fully closed, but will fluctuate between the two states depending on which has the greater stimulus at any given moment, A or C fibres. Anything that promotes A fibre stimulus will help to block pain at spinal cord level, and this may be how mechanisms like **transcutaneous electrical nerve stimulation (TENS)** or **acupuncture** may work. Also, what should not be overlooked is the fact that the 'gate control' mechanism, and the reflex arc, are significantly influenced by the higher intellectual centres of the brain. Impulses descending from the **brain stem**, the **hypothalamus** and especially from the cerebral cortex all modify the events at cord level. The brain does this because factors such as emotions, culture, personal beliefs and learning are all involved in the total pain experience. In Chapter 10, pain was used as a means of assessing conscious levels (see p. 176), but it may not always be possible to determine how much of, let's say, a limb response to pain is cortical (i.e. conscious) and how much is spinal (automatic), and this is one of the problems of choosing pain as a stimulus in assessing consciousness (see Chapter 10). Descending neurons from the brain create synapses in the cord that use a variety of neurotransmitters such as **enkephalins, endorphins** and **dynorphins** (see p. 202) to block further pain transmission up the cord (Clancy and McVicar 1998).

The thalamus works at a subconscious level for most sensory stimuli except pain, which registers as conscious at thalamic level. Pain impulses begin to become part of our consciousness as they pass through our brain. As impulses travel up neuron 2 and enter the brain, they first pass through the **brain stem**. Here pain impulses are recognised as something different from other sensory impulses, but the true obnoxious nature of the stimulus is not known at this point. On arrival at the thalamus, pain impulses are, for the first time, consciously recognised as unpleasant. As a sensory relay station, the thalamus is normally dealing with thousands of sensations every minute, all of which are still at subconscious level except pain. The thalamus must pass sensory impulses onto the conscious part of the brain, and those sensory stimuli from the body must pass to the **sensory cortex** of the cerebrum (in the **parietal lobe**), via neuron 3. With pain impulses this still happens, but the thalamus also communicates with the **motor cortex** of the cerebrum (in the **frontal lobe**) and thus influences movement in response to the pain (called a **thalamic response** to pain) (Figure 11.6). So, both synapses in the three-neuronal system, i.e. in the cord and in the thalamus, have motor connections facilitating responses to the pain impulses.

Finally, the nociceptive impulses arrive at the sensory cortex of the parietal lobe, part of the cerebrum, via neuron 3. This is the conscious brain, where the individual will become fully aware of the pain as a noxious and unpleasant sensation. But by then, both the pain-blocking mechanisms and the muscle responses to pain at spinal and thalamic level would have activated and reduced the pain intensity. The cells of the sensory cortex are laid out in a plan representative of the body layout (Figure 10.5, p. 172). Having been 'relayed' from the thalamus, the pain impulses will arrive at that part of the cortex that represents the area of the body from where the pain has originated. Thus, pain impulses arising from the abdomen,

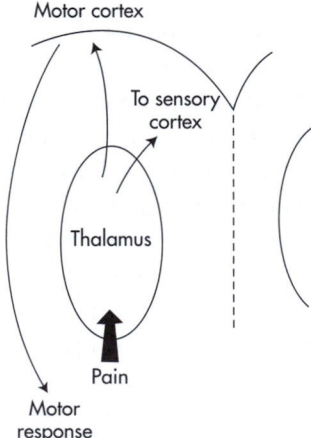

FIGURE 11.6 Pain impulses are not only passed from the thalamus to the sensory cortex, but also, by including the motor cortex, the thalamus can initiate a motor response to pain.

for example, will arrive in that part of the cortex that specialises in the abdomen. Remember, there is also a cross-over of the sensory neuron 2 in the cord, so pain impulses from the left of the body will arrive in the right cortex, and vice versa. The conscious nature of the cortex allows the individual to make decisions and to act on the pain, e.g. to rest, to take pain-killing drugs or to see a doctor. This is very different to the responses found at cord or thalamic levels, which are less sophisticated, and are only there to save life and prevent further injury.

What is also interesting is that the pain sensation is only fully conscious to us when it reaches the cerebrum of the brain, but still we recognise the pain as arising from the body part affected. As an example, consider pain impulses arising from a leg. These impulses are not conscious (and therefore not recognised as pain) until they reach the brain. Yet as soon as we are aware of them in the cortex we actually 'feel' the pain in the leg, not the brain. This is because, as said before, the cerebral cortex receiving the impulses is laid out in a body plan. So, in our example, there is a part of the cortex where the brain cells are representatives of the leg. When these brain cells receive pain impulses, they make the person aware of pain in the leg, *not* in the brain. The brain *itself* does *not* feel pain! This has been demonstrated many times by surgeons who have operated on the brains of *conscious* patients. The scalp and other tissues require local anaesthesia, but the brain itself does not require any anaesthesia as it cannot 'feel' pain. When the surgeon stimulates the cortex, the patient feels sensations in that part of the body represented by the cerebral cortical cells stimulated. In our previous example, if the surgeon stimulated that part of the cortex representing the leg, the patient would feel sensation in the leg. So, this means that the brain makes you aware of pain arising from all other parts of the body except itself. This should make sense because the cerebral cortex could not be both the *initiator* (i.e. the nociceptor) and the *receiver* of pain impulses at the same time!

The observation of pain

The question arises 'How can you quantify and measure pain?' It not difficult to identify when a person is in pain; they can usually tell you and they may show the signs of pain (Figure 11.7). But how *much* pain are they suffering (i.e. is it quantifiable?), and is it getting

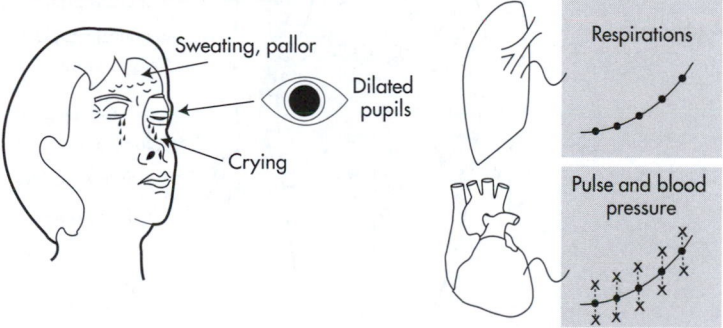

FIGURE 11.7   The signs of pain. The pulse, blood pressure and respiration rates rise. The pupils dilate and the person may show sweating, pallor and they may cry.

better or worse? How *much* pain is similar to asking 'How blue is the sky?' You can see it is blue, but measuring its 'blueness' accurately is very difficult. Pain is very much an individual (or subjective) concept: what is mild pain to one person would be severe to another. It raises questions such as how much does conscious or subconscious exaggeration of the pain, or other factors, enter the equation?

Pain assessment requires judgement concerning the following factors:

- Pain site; i.e. where is the pain? Remember that not all pain occurs at the site of the pathology (or the cause of the pain). **Referred pain** occurs some distance away from the site of the cause (Figure 11.8). This is because pain impulses travel along nerve pathways and sometimes gives the brain a false impression of where the pain is originating from.
- Pain intensity, which is very subjective and will vary between individuals and at different times in the same individual.
- The nature of the pain, i.e. is it sharp like a knife, is it a dull ache or is it burning?
- Is the pain associated with specific activities, such as eating, vomiting or urinating, or with a specific movement or position?
- Duration of the pain, i.e. is it sudden or acute, or is it chronic?

In an attempt to be as objective as possible about such a subjective phenomenon, **pain assessment tools** (**pain charts** or **pain scales**) have been devised. Pain assessment tools fall into three categories:

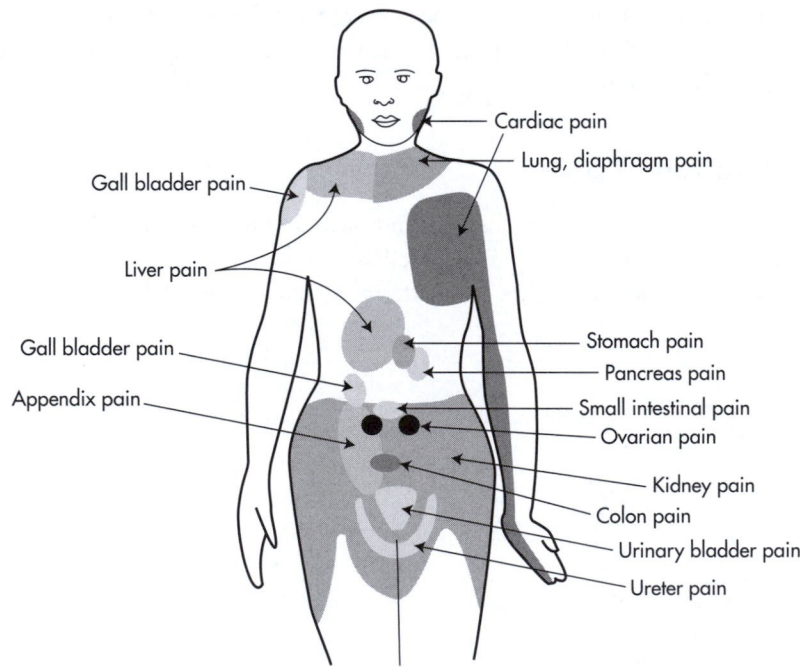

FIGURE 11.8   The areas where referred pain is experienced and the organs the pain is derived from.

Source: redrawn from LeMone and Burke (2007)

1 **Verbal descriptor scales** use words that may be appropriate to describe pain ranked in order of severity, e.g. *none (no pain)*; *slight pain*; *moderate pain*; *severe pain*; *agonising pain*. Patients indicate the word most applicable to their pain, and a numerical ranking alongside the words will aid in charting the response (Figure 11.9). The word list may provide rather limited choice when applied to some patients' pain, but it is easy to score and analyse.

2 **Visual analogue scales** consist of a line representing a pain continuum, with descriptive word 'anchors' at both ends. An example is the continuum that stretches from '*no pain*' at one end of the line to '*pain as bad as it could be*' at the other end. Patients must indicate where along this line their pain ranks. Additional word descriptions may be added along the line to aid the patient in their choice (Figure 11.10). They are relatively easy to use and do not rely heavily on the choice of wording. However, they may not be suitable to all patients, particularly the elderly and confused, or those with educational disabilities.

3 **Pain behaviour tools** are based on the understanding that patients in pain demonstrate certain behaviour patterns. These behaviour patterns are most likely to consist of *verbal responses to pain* (e.g. crying or swearing); *pain-related body language* (e.g. holding affected area or rubbing); *specific facial expressions*; *certain behaviour changes* (e.g. seeking analgesia or medical attention); *changes in conscious level* and *pain-related physiological responses* (e.g. mild pain causes a rise in blood pressure; severe pain causes a drop in blood pressure). These scales can be used on patients with communication problems but they are more time-consuming and complex than the previous tools, and they exclude the patient's own subjective assessment (Manchester Triage Group 1997).

Description	Score
No pain	0
Slight pain	1
Mild pain	2
	3
Moderate pain	4
	5
Severe pain	6
More severe pain	7
Very severe pain	8
	9
Worst possible pain	10

FIGURE 11.9 Verbal descriptor scale for pain.

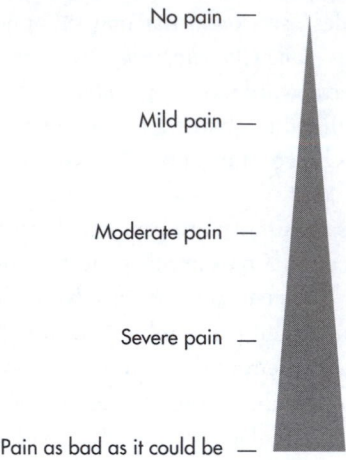

FIGURE 11.10   Visual analogue scale for pain.

Numerous variations of these tools will be seen in clinical practice where they have been combined or modified to suit specific patient needs.

There is now new research that is attempting to quantify the amount of pain an individual suffers. At the present time, the work involves the brain's response to thermal (heat) pain in controlled environments, but it may be possible in the future to extend it to other forms of pain and other circumstances. The technique involves brain scans taken on subjects while experiencing thermal pain and while not in pain, and sophisticated computer programs that were more than 80% accurate in predicting pain from the brain scan changes identified. This technique is expected to expand into other types of pain and may become the standard method for determining pain levels in patients (Brown *et al.* 2011).

Pain management

Drugs have been the mainstay of pain control for a long time, and continue to be so. **Analgesia** (an = without, algesia = increased sensitivity to pain; thus 'without sensitivity to pain') is the absence of pain *without* causing loss of consciousness (as caused by general anaesthesia) or loss of touch sensation (as caused by local anaesthesia). Two major groups of analgesic drugs exist: the **opioids** and the **non-steroidal anti-inflammatory drugs (NSAI drugs)**. Basically, they work in very different ways, not only in their mechanism of action but also in the location of action within the nervous system. NSAI drugs act in the tissues where pain originates from, i.e. they work *peripherally*, while opioids work in the brain stem and spinal cord, i.e. they work *centrally*.

Non-steroidal anti-inflammatory (NSAI) drugs

Linoleic acid is a natural fat-based component of the diet. In the body, linoleic acid is converted to another substance called **arachidonic acid**, and this becomes an important part of **phospholipids**, a large component of our cell membranes. But arachidonic acid is not only part of our cell membranes, it can be recovered from cell membranes if the need arises, since arachidonic acid is the basic substance (or **substrate**) from which other substances can be made (see Figure 11.2, p. 192).

One large group of these other substances are **prostanoids**, a major class of chemicals that includes **prostacyclins**, **prostaglandins** and **thromboxanes**. Prostacyclins, prostaglandins and thromboxanes act similarly to hormones, mostly locally but sometimes systemically. Unlike many hormones, which are produced on a daily basis, these substances will only be produced if required. However, when they are produced, they cause changes in the tissues, similar to hormones, but generally close to where they are produced. Prostacyclins, for example, cause several tissue changes, including local **vasodilation** (i.e. dilation of local blood vessels). Thromboxane A_2 does the opposite by causing **vasoconstriction**. Prostaglandins are a large group of substances that have many effects, both locally and more widespread, including some like the prostaglandin E (PGE) and prostaglandin F (PGF) groups, which cause pain. These prostaglandins are very important pain mediators that increase the sensitivity of nociceptors, making them respond more to other pain mediators, i.e. lowering the threshold to pain (see p. 192).

To produce all these chemicals from arachidonic acid requires the enzyme **cyclo-oxygenase** (**COX**), which occurs in two forms: COX-1 and COX-2. COX-1 is found in most cells most of the time (i.e. it is *constitutive*; part of the constituents of the cells), while COX-2 is found in inflammatory cells when activated during inflammation (i.e. it is *induced*; produced only when required). NSAI drugs work primarily by blocking (or inhibiting) COX-1 in peripheral tissues where the pain is generated. The best-known drug in this group is **aspirin (acetylsalicylic acid)**, which causes irreversible blockage of COX-1, thus preventing the formation of the prostaglandin pain mediators. **Indometacin** (a derivative of **indole acetic acid**) also inhibits COX-1, **diclofenac** (derived from **phenylacetic acid**) and **naproxen** (derived from **propionic acid**) inhibit COX-1 and COX-2 equally, while **nabumetone** (derived from **naphthylacetic acid**) blocks COX-2 specifically (naproxen and nabumetone are used mainly for musculo-skeletal pain). Such selectivity for COX-2 means that nabumetone improves gastric tolerance when given by mouth, gastric intolerance being a problem noted for the COX-1 inhibitors.

Paracetamol, a well-known and popular analgesic drug, is only a weak inhibitor of both COX-1 and COX-2, so its mode of analgesic action is still somewhat unclear. What is known is that some metabolites of arachidonic acid caused by the action of COX are **hydroperoxides**, and these in turn then further stimulate COX to produce more cytokines. Paracetamol blocks this feedback pathway, therefore inhibiting COX indirectly by stopping the activity of hydroperoxides. In this respect, paracetamol is particularly active in the brain, where it has an analgesic and an antipyretic effect, but no anti-inflammatory effect (Waller *et al.* 2009).

As the group name NSAI suggests, most of these drugs are also **anti-inflammatory** (except for paracetamol, as we have just seen), and reduction of inflammation may be of importance in pain relief. The NSAI drugs are often marketed as tablets that have a combination of several drugs in one, and sometimes with **caffeine** added as this is said to enhance their analgesic property.

Aspirin and other NSAI drugs are a very good means of controlling mild pain, but for severe pain, however, there is often a need for an additional stronger analgesia: the opioids.

The opioid drugs

Opium, a natural product of the opium poppy plant, is a powerful analgesic and psychoactive drug. Its use in pain management, and also for sedation and even recreation, has been important for many years. It was used extensively in the nineteenth century as 'tincture of opium' (known then as **laudanum**), which contained **morphine**, an opium derivative. Laudanum is no longer used, but morphine is still used along with other opium derivatives, and these are a major means of solving the pain problem.

Unlike the NSAI drugs, the opioid drugs work *centrally* within the central nervous system (CNS, i.e. the brain and cord). They bind to special receptors within the brain and cord to provide a degree of analgesia at spinal cord level (called **spinous analgesia**) or brain stem level (called **supra-spinous analgesia**). There are three main kinds of receptors on the surface of cells in the CNS that bind opioid drugs: the **mu (μ)**, **kappa (κ)** and **delta (δ)** receptors. These receptors are referred to as **metabotropic**, i.e. their activation changes the metabolism of the cell (see Blows 2011, pp. 58–59). The mu receptor is found mostly in the brain stem, and is the one mostly associated with supra-spinous analgesia, respiratory depression, euphoria and dependence. This is the receptor to which morphine and drugs like morphine mostly bind. The kappa receptor is found in the upper spinal cord and provides spinous analgesia by blocking substance P (see below). The relative importance of the delta receptor in pain control is not fully known, although its analgesic effects are less than those of the mu receptor.

Opioid receptors bind naturally produced substances called **ligands**, i.e. ligands are products of the nervous system that bind to specific receptors. All nervous system receptors have their own particular ligand. In the case of the opioid receptors mu, kappa and delta, there are a number of *natural* ligands called **endorphins**, **enkephalins**, **dynorphins** and **endomorphins**. In addition, some less well-known small peptide ligands also exist, such as **dermorphins** and **morphiceptins**.

Endorphins are the largest peptide molecules of the group. They come in various forms called **alpha (α) -endorphin, beta (β) -endorphin** and **gamma (γ) -endorphin**. They tend to be produced in the brain in response to severe pain and provide some degree of analgesia for around four hours or so.

Enkephalins are smaller peptide molecules. There are two types: **met-enkephalin** (where met = **methionine**) and **leu-enkephalin** (where leu = **leucine**). They are present in the ratio of about 4 met to 1 leu. They are produced in response to milder pain and provide analgesia for around 2 minutes or so. **Substance P** was identified as a facilitator for the passages of pain impulses across the synapse between neurons 1 and 2 of the pain pathways (see p. 194). Substance P is therefore a pain mediator at spinal cord level. By binding to kappa receptors in the spinal cord, enkephalin inhibits the release and therefore the function of substance P, thus reducing pain impulses at spinal cord level (see p. 194).

Dynorphins are of two known types: **dynorphin A** and **dynorphin B**. These are small peptide molecules. Endomorphins are also small peptide molecules that fall into two categories: **endomorphin-1** and **endomorphin-2**.

We take advantage of the receptors that naturally bind these ligands by delivering drugs that also bind to them: the **opioid drugs**. The principal members of this drug group include:

- **Morphine**, which remains the major drug for pain relief in this group. It is the analgesic against which all others are compared. It is a potent analgesic for the management of severe pain, but it does cause respiratory depression (see p. 63), nausea, vomiting and constipation as side effects. Morphine also causes a state of euphoria (the reason for morphine addiction when taken in the absence of pain), and some degree of mental detachment (Blows 2011), which is useful in reducing the psychological response to pain.

  Morphine has variable absorption when taken by mouth, and undergoes considerable **first-pass metabolism** in the liver, making injection more efficient as a route of administration. First-pass metabolism is the alteration of the drug in the liver after absorption from the bowel. These changes do not apply to the injected drug since only the drug delivered by the oral route is taken first to the liver by the hepatic portal vein. The metabolism of morphine in the liver results in a metabolite called **morphine-6 glucuronide**, which is a greater analgesic than morphine itself. **Morphine-3 glucuronide** is also produced but it has no analgesic effect. Morphine glucuronides are excreted through the urine, but also through the biliary system to the bowel where the morphine component is largely reabsorbed. The duration of activity for morphine is about 3–4 hours.

- **Diamorphine (heroin)** is a powerful analgesic that is converted to morphine in the body, although diamorphine itself is more active as an analgesic than morphine. Diamorphine has greater powers than morphine in crossing the blood–brain barrier, and therefore enters the brain faster, especially when given intravenously (IV). This makes it attractive as a drug of illicit use. Diamorphine is active in the body for about 2 hours.

- **Pethidine** provides rapid but short-lasting analgesia. It is less potent than morphine, even in higher doses, but it is less constipating. Severe pain on a long-term basis is better managed with drugs other than pethidine. Pethidine is metabolised in the liver to **norpethidine**, a metabolite with hallucinogenic and convulsant properties.

- **Codeine** is made from morphine (codeine is **3-methylmorphine**), but is better absorbed when given by mouth than morphine, although it has only about 20% of the analgesic effect. Codeine is effective for treating mild to moderate pain but is not advisable for long-term use due to its side effect of causing constipation. It causes little or no euphoric effects and is therefore rarely addictive, and can be purchased without prescription.

- Other opioid analgesics include **fentanyl**, a drug with similar but shorter-lasting actions to morphine, and available in transdermal skin patches for the prevention of 'breakthrough' pain (i.e. transient periods of pain not prevented by other drugs). **Hydromorphone** has a similar efficacy to morphine but with fewer side effects, especially nausea and vomiting.

The dosage of opioid analgesics has to be accurately calculated to combine a complete pain-free state without excessive drug administration, which would lead to unwanted side effects. Finding the right dosage level is called **titration**.

Opioid drug titration is defined as *calculating the least amount of the drug required in circulation to achieve full analgesia*. Opioid titration relies on feedback from the patient on their pain status, and this is where a pain assessment tool is of value. If they are still in pain, then they require more analgesia. Each additional dose is less than the previous doses, and these 'top-up doses' are given until a pain-free state is achieved. Consideration must be made of the serious side effects of opioids. A serious side effect that must be avoided is **respiratory depression**, i.e. the reduction in breathing caused by opioid drugs binding to receptors on the respiratory centre in the brain stem. Respiratory depression is particularly dangerous in the elderly (due to their reduced lung capacity) and in those with pre-existing respiratory disease. The other concern, that of drug addiction, does not apply to this situation. Giving opioids to treat pain does not cause addiction. Opioid addiction occurs only when the drugs are administered to individuals who are already pain-free from the start.

Analgesia can and should be given, so long as it is needed, in any setting from hospital to the patient's home or hospice care. In those patients where further treatment options are not possible, the term **palliative care** is used. Palliative care indicates the management of symptoms, such as being pain or nausea-free, so that the patient will live out their remaining life in comfort and will not suffer at the time of their death. Under these circumstances it is not necessary to be concerned about drug addiction risks, but care must be taken to prevent respiratory depression or accidental drug overdose.

The analgesic ladder and adjuvant therapy

The **World Health Organization (WHO)** (1986) introduced the concept of a stepped approach to pain management in cancer, known as the 'analgesic ladder' (Figure 11.11, Vargas-Schaffer 2010).

- *Step 1*: The baseline treatment to start with is a *non-opioid* drug, e.g. a **non-steroidal anti-inflammatory drug**, with or without **adjuvant therapy** (see below). Such non-opioids include aspirin (except in children), paracetamol or ibuprofen.
- *Step 2*: If pain persists or increases, an **opioid drug** suitable for moderate pain is introduced, with or without the NSAI drug, and with or without the adjuvant therapy. Such

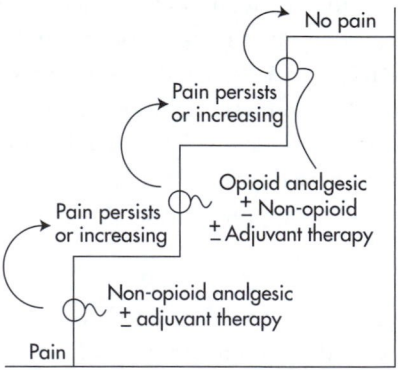

FIGURE 11.11 The analgesic ladder. If pain persists or increases, the next level of analgesia must be attained.

Source: Redrawn from Souhami and Tobias (2007).

opioid drugs include codeine, dihydrocodeine, pentazocine, dipipanone (not suitable for palliative care) or oxycodone.

- *Step 3*: If pain continues to persist or increase, a stronger opioid drug is introduced, one reserved for severe pain, such as morphine, diamorphine, pethidine, methadone or fentanyl (see p. 203). The addition of the NSAI drug and adjuvant therapy remains an option as well. This is pursued until the patient is pain-free.

In all cases, drugs must be given:

- in a dose sufficient to induce a pain-free state;
- regularly, not on demand;
- with a warning about potential side effects;
- in conjunction with adjuvant therapy as required.

Adjuvant therapy is non-drug treatment for pain, and consists of a wide range of possibilities, from simple massage techniques to surgery. The following is a summary of adjuvant therapies available:

- Local **radiotherapy**, which can be good for relief of symptoms including pain.
- **Epidural infusion** of local anaesthetic, perhaps given slowly via an infusion pump. Opioid drugs can be prescribed for delivery by this route when they cannot be tolerated by mouth. Infusions are into the **epidural space** (a space outside the **dura mater**; the outer of the three covering of the central nervous system) within the spinal canal, and may be continuous or intermittent. Effectiveness is usually only for a few weeks, after which tolerance becomes a problem, but it is very good for acute pain control without paralysis or disturbance of the autonomic nervous system.
- **Transcutaneous electrical nerve stimulation** (**TENS**) uses an electrical apparatus for delivery of a small charge across the skin surface, the purpose of which is relief of pain. It is effective, being used frequently in midwifery during labour, but its uses extend to other causes of pain. The analgesia comes on about 20 minutes or so after starting and continues for a significant period after use has stopped. There are no significant side effects. Limitations of use are few, i.e. it should not be used near the eye or over the heart if the patient has had a heart complication, not used on the head or neck in epileptic patients, and used with caution in pregnancy. It can interfere with the function of pacemakers and electrocardiographs (ECG) or electroencephalograms (EEG). How it works is not known but it may induce the closure of the spinal gate to pain (see gate theory of pain, p. 195).
- Massage and **aromatherapy**.
- **Acupuncture**, the Chinese art of inserting needles to relieve pain and other conditions. Like TENS, the way acupuncture works is unknown but it may prevent the flow of pain impulses through the gate control mechanism. It may release hormones from the endocrine system, stimulate the immune system, release antibodies and increase the body's resistance to inflammation (L. Zhang-Lheureux, personal communication).
- **Psychological support**, i.e. staying with the patient, comforting, distracting their attention away from the pain (e.g. reading to them). Distraction, like television or favourite games, is particularly useful with children in pain.

- **Nerve block** is carried out by injecting parts of the sensory nerves (e.g. the **dorsal root**) or sympathetic nerves with phenol or alcohol, thus blocking pain sensations. The destruction of the nerve by the chemical is irreversible, so the procedure is not carried out until other avenues have been tried.
- **Surgery** is a last resort because it is also irreversible. The aim is to permanently divide the pain pathways and therefore stop the passage of pain impulses.

Patient-controlled analgesia (PCA)

The ability for patients to take control of their own analgesia has become increasingly important and useful for patients and staff alike. Self-administration of even the more potent opioids in hospitals and hospices has provided the patients with greater and more consistent pain relief, and provided the staff with more time for other matters. The analgesia is delivered by means of a PCA pump (or **syringe driver**) attached to an intravenous (IV) or subcutaneous line (Figure 11.12). This line consists of a cannula in a vein (IV) or under the skin (subcutaneous), usually in the arm, to which a delivery tube is attached. On the other end is the syringe driver, or PCA pump. The pump houses a syringe containing the analgesia, and by operating a switch, the pump pushes a controlled dose of a drug from the syringe, along the line into the patient. The line is usually separate from any other IV line, but could be combined with an IV fluid delivery system if this was desirable. Once operated by the patient, the pumps usually provides a 'lock-out' period, perhaps about 5 minutes or so, during which the patient cannot operate it again. After the 'lock-out' period the pump is again ready for use. Patients can therefore keep pain under control according to their own needs. This saves the patient the need to alert staff whenever pain is a problem, and removes the difficulties for staff to try and assess the pain level that the patient is in (see p. 197). The drug and dose are prescribed by the doctor and prepared by the pharmacy, so the nurse has only to set up the pump and change the syringe when empty, according to the prescription chart.

A typical drug regime for PCA may consist of intravenous morphine, or subcutaneous diamorphine. Many units offering this treatment may prefer to use diamorphine as the drug of choice because its higher rate of solubility than morphine allows adequate dosages to be delivered in smaller fluid volumes.

Key points

- Acute pain tends to be recently occurred and of short duration. Chronic pain has a longer duration of weeks, months or even years. Intractable pain is chronic pain unrelated to any detectable pathology.
- Localised pain is often caused by inflammation of the tissues involved.
- Pain mediators are released at the site, e.g. histamine, prostaglandins and bradykinins.

Pain pathways

- Nociceptors are pain nerve endings occurring in two types: mechanoreceptors and polymodalreceptors.

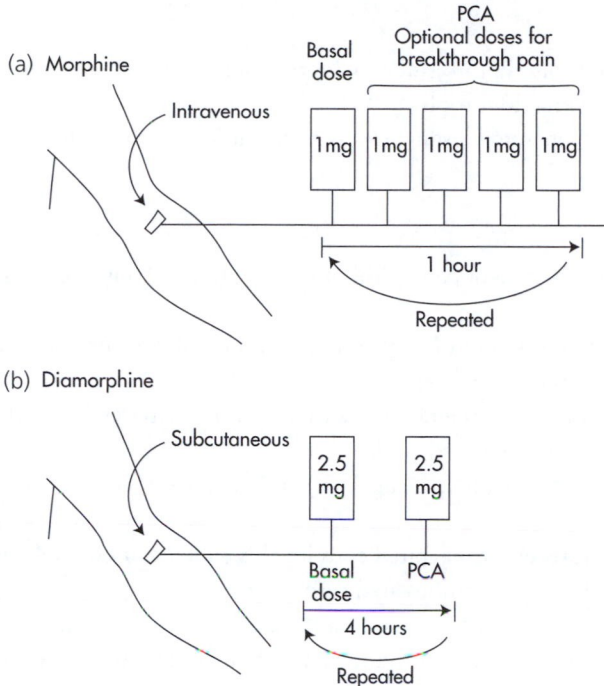

FIGURE 11.12 A diagrammatic representation of patient-controlled analgesia (PCA). Patients with severe chronic pain may be prescribed morphine or diamorphine. Morphine is usually given by continuous intravenous (IV) infusion, while diamorphine is the better drug to give by continuous subcutaneous infusion because larger doses of diamorphine can be concentrated in smaller volumes. Subcutaneous infusion is slower (0.1–0.3 ml per hour) than IV, and subcutaneous infusions are usually driven by a syringe pump. (a) Morphine: a basal rate of IV infusion of 1 mg per hour is a standard dose, with a bolus dose of 1 mg every 15 minutes that can be given by the patient themselves by pressing a button on the delivery apparatus if 'breakthrough' pain occurs. The total dose in 1 hour would be 5 mg. The delivery apparatus would be set to have a 'lock-out' period of 15 minutes, meaning the patient could not press the button twice in that time. (b) Diamorphine: a basal rate of subcutaneous infusion of 2.5 mg per 4 hours is a standard dose, with a 2.5 mg bolus dose available for the patient to self-administer to treat break-through pain (via pressing the button). The 'lock-out' time (and therefore the maximum 4-hourly dose) should be determined by the doctor. Irrespective of which drug or route is used, the patient should be reassessed for pain every 8 hours to determine if the basal infusion rate (and dose) needs adjustment (either up or down) to reduce the need for bolus doses.

- Two types of sensory nerve pathways carry pain impulses to the brain: fast Aδ fibres and slower C fibres.
- The Aδ and C fibres are the first neurons of a three-neuronal system from the periphery to the brain.
- The 'gate-control theory' describes a pain-blocking process in the spinal cord.
- The thalamic response to pain is to influence movement to help overcome the pain.

Pain assessment

- Pain assessment tools fall into three categories: verbal descriptor scales; visual analogue scales; and pain behaviour tools.
- Referred pain occurs some distance away from the site of the cause.

Analgesia

- Analgesia is the absence of pain without causing loss of consciousness or loss of touch sensation.
- There are two major groups of analgesic drugs: the opioids and the non-steroidal anti-inflammatory drugs (NSAI drugs).
- NSAI drugs act in the peripheral tissues where pain originates from, while opioids work centrally in the brain stem and cord.
- Opioid drugs bind to the mu (μ), kappa (κ) and delta (δ) receptors within the brain and cord.
- A drug acting on receptors at spinal cord level is called spinous analgesia, and at brain stem level is called supra-spinous analgesia.
- The opioid receptors mu, kappa and delta are there to bind the naturally produced endogenous opioids called endorphins, enkephalins, dynorphins, endomorphins, dermorphins and morphiceptins.
- Morphine is the major opioid drug for pain relief, against which all others are compared. It is a potent analgesic for the management of severe pain, but it does cause respiratory depression, nausea, vomiting and constipation as side effects.
- Finding the right dosage level of analgesia is called titration.
- Opioid drug titration is defined as calculating the least amount of the drug required in circulation to achieve full analgesia.
- A serious side effect that must be avoided is respiratory depression.
- Respiratory depression is particularly dangerous in the elderly (due to reduced lung capacity) and in those with pre-existing respiratory disease.
- Opioid titration relies on feedback from the patient on their pain status.
- The World Health Organization (WHO) introduced the concept of a stepped approach to pain management known as the 'analgesic ladder'.
- Adjuvant therapy is non-drug treatment for pain, and consists of a wide range of treatments from simple things like massage, TENS, acupuncture, and aromatherapy, to nerve block and surgery.
- Patient-controlled analgesia (PCA) is delivered by means of a PCA pump (or syringe driver) attached to an intravenous (IV) or subcutaneous line.

References

Blows W. T. (2011) *The Biological Basis of Mental Health Nursing*, 2nd edition. Routledge, London.

Brown J. E., Chatterjee N., Younger J. and Mackey S. (2011) Towards a physiology-based measure of pain: patterns of human brain activity distinguish painful from non-painful thermal stimulation. *PLoS ONE*, 6 (9):e24124 DOI: 10.1371/journal.pone.0024124.

Clancy J. and McVicar A. (1998) Homeostasis: the key concept to physiological control (neurophysiology of pain). *British Journal of Theatre Nursing*, 7(10): 19–27.

D'Costa K. (2011) The ways we talk about pain. *Scientific American*. http://blogs.scientificamerican.com/anthropology-in-practice/2011/09/27/the-ways-we-talk-about-pain/?WT_mc_id=SA_CAT_MB_20110928 (accessed 28 September 2011).

LeMone P. and Burke K. (2007) *Medical-Surgical Nursing: Critical Thinking in Client Care*, 4th edition. Pearson Education Inc., Prentice Hall, NJ.

Manchester Triage Group (1997) Pain assessment as part of the triage process, in Mackway-Jones K. (ed.) *Emergency Triage*. BMJ Publishing Group, London.

Meijler W. J. (2006) Nociception and sensitisation. *Nederlands Tijdschrift Voor Tandheelkunde*, 113(11): 433–436.

Souhami R. and Tobias J. (2007) *Cancer and Its Management*, 5th edition. Blackwell Science, Oxford.

Vargas-Schaffer G. (2010) Is the WHO analgesic ladder still valid? Twenty-four years of experience. *Canadian Family Physician, Médecin de famille canadien*, 56(6): 514–517, e202–e205.

Waller D. G., Renwick A. G. and Hillier K. (2009) *Medical Pharmacology and Therapeutics*, 3rd edition. W. B. Saunders, London.

World Health Organization (1986) http://www.who.int/cancer/palliative/painladder/en/ (accessed July 2011).

Wood S. (2002) Special focus: pain. *Nursing Times*, 98(38): 41–44.

Chapter 12 **Neurological observations (III)**
Eyes

- Introduction
- The basic neurology of the human eye
- Visual disturbance
- Basic eye observations
- Advanced visual neurobiology
- Advanced eye observations
- Key points
- References

Introduction

It has been said that the eyes are the window on the soul. However, for medical purposes, it would be more accurate to say that the eyes are the window on the brain. This is because observation of the eyes gives so many clues about pathological changes taking place within the brain. This should not be surprising since the light-sensitive retina at the back of the eye is the only part of the nervous system visible from the outside world.

The basic neurology of the human eye

This is a simplified account of the complex nervous system that consists of both motor and sensory nerves and their control areas within the brain that serve the eye.

The sensory system (vision)

The sensory nerve component is the visual pathway extending from the retina posteriorly into the brain. Light passes through the **pupil** at the front of the eye onto the **retina** at the back (Figure 12.1). The majority of light falls on that part of the retina that lies directly opposite the pupil: the **macula**, the central part of which is the **fovea**. The fovea has the greatest concentration of daylight-sensitive cells, the **cones**. The straight line from the pupil to the retina is known as the **visual axis**. Cones produce nerve impulses in response to daylight and colour, unlike the other type of light-sensitive cells, the **rods**, which create impulses in response to low light levels and black and white stimuli. Just off-centre to the macula, i.e. a little divergent from the visual axis, is the **optic disc** (Figure 12.2), the area where the retina attaches to the **optic nerve** (Figure 12.1). This nerve is the sensory pathway of vision from the eye: the second cranial nerve (cranial nerve II), which passes posteriorly through the rear of the orbit into the brain.

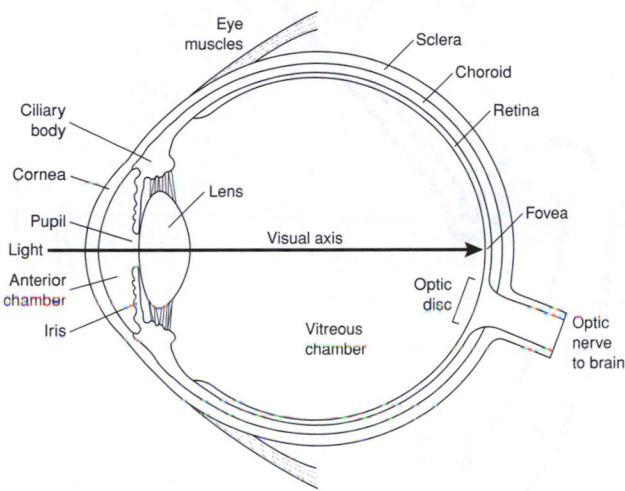

FIGURE 12.1 Section through the eye.

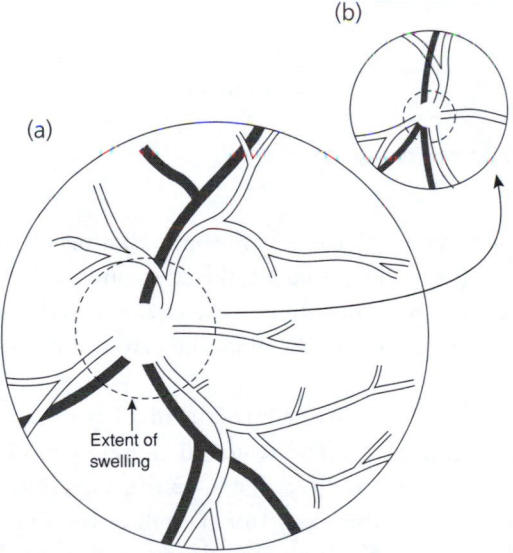

FIGURE 12.2 View of the retina through an ophthalmoscope. (a) papilloedema, with the extent of the optic disc swelling indicated; (b) a normal optic disc.

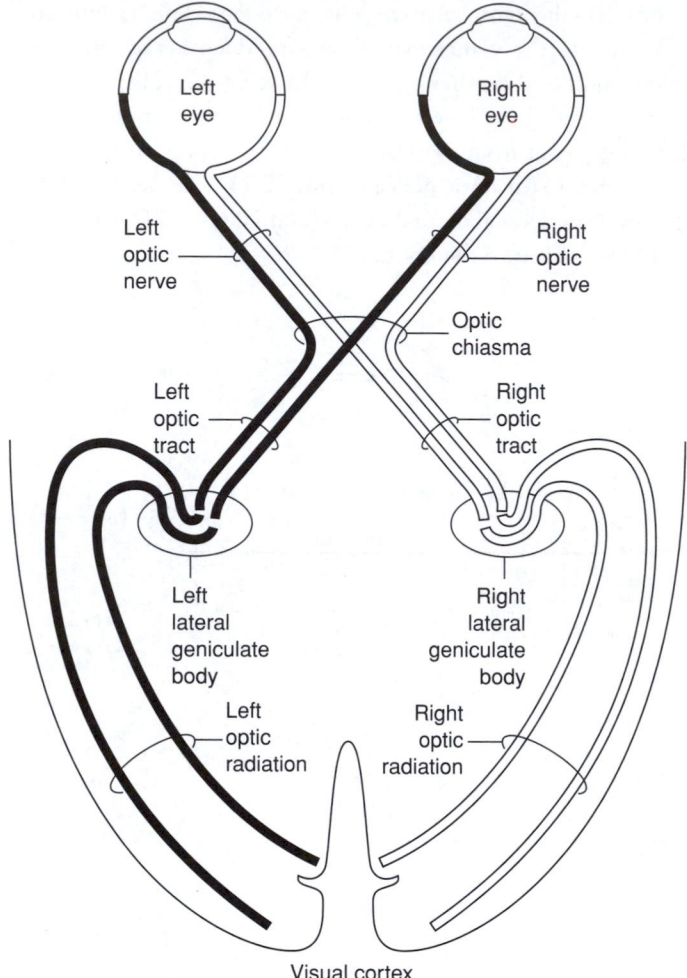

FIGURE 12.3 Superior view of the optic pathways.

The left and right optic nerves converge at the **optic chiasma** (Figure 12.3). By the definition of the word 'nerve' (i.e. pathways *outside* the brain and cord), the visual pathways are called the optic nerves *only* from the retina to the chiasma. Pathways from the chiasma to the visual cortex are *within* the brain, therefore they are not nerves, they are *pathways* or *tracts*.

The optic chiasma is the point where 50% of the fibres cross to the opposite side (crossover = **decussation**) (Figure 12.3). The **temporal** (outer) half of each retina generates impulses that remain ipsilateral, i.e. they remain on the same side as they originated from without crossing over, whereas the **nasal** (inner) half of each retina generates impulses that decussate, i.e. they cross to the opposite side in the chiasma. The result is that each half of the brain, both left and right, receives visual impulses from the temporal retina of the same side but impulses from the nasal retina of the opposite side. But despite this, the brain interprets these signals as a normal complete visual image. From the chiasma backwards to the thalamus the pathways are *inside* the brain and are therefore called the **optic tracts** (Figure 12.3). After the thalamus, the main pathways continue posteriorly as the **optic radiations**, and these terminate at the back of the brain in the **visual cortex** within part of the **cerebrum** called the **occipital lobe** (Figure 12.3). Here, the visual stimulus becomes conscious, i.e. we actually see with the rear of the brain, *not* the eye. The retina converts light to nerve impulses that pass through these pathways subconsciously until they reach the visual cortex, at which point we become aware of them. Of course, all these pathways are crucial in the delivery of the impulses to the visual cortex, which is why **blindness** can occur from a disorder at any point along this pathway. The area of vision we see before us constitutes the **visual fields**, the centre of which falls on the visual axis and is the point of our gaze. Nothing that exists outside the periphery of the visual fields can be seen without turning our eyes and head (i.e. adjustments to form new centres for our gaze).

The motor system (movements inside and outside the eye)

The motor supply to the eye operates the three muscular aspects of vision: (1) muscle movements of the *whole* eye within the **orbit** (the eye socket); (2) the movement of the **iris** governing pupil size; and (3) the movement of the **lens** for the purpose of accommodation (focusing on objects at differing distances from the eye).

1   Movement of the whole eye is achieved by the six *striated* muscles *outside* each eye but *within* the orbits. These muscles are controlled by several cranial nerves: **cranial nerve III**, the **oculomotor nerve**, part of which innervates four of the orbital muscles on both sides; **cranial nerve IV**, the **trochlear nerve,** which innervates one orbital muscle on each side (the **superior oblique**); and **cranial nerve VI**, the **abducens nerve**, which innervates one other orbital muscle on each side (the **lateral rectus**) (Figure 12.4). Cranial nerves are so called because they come directly from the brain (i.e. *not* via the cord), with cranial nerves III, IV and VI arising in nuclei within the **brain stem**: III and IV in the **midbrain**, and VI in the **pons**. They operate a **reciprocal innervation** of the muscles, i.e. contracting one muscle while relaxing the muscle that moves in the opposite direction. This allows the eyes to both move in one direction at a time, i.e. the eye muscles are **yoked**, which means that their movements are tied together. Although this brain stem function is automatic, it can also occur at a conscious level from the cerebrum (see Chapter 10). In addition, the oculomotor nerve also operates striated muscle that elevates the upper lid.

2   Pupil size is a function of *smooth* muscle activity *inside* the eye. Pupils respond to light stimuli automatically; the smooth muscle is operated by the **autonomic nervous system** (**ANS**), which has both **sympathetic** and **parasympathetic** components. **Pupil constriction** is caused by the *parasympathetic* component of the oculomotor nerve, which innervates the iris **sphincter** muscles in response to bright light. In low light the *sympathetic* component controls the iris **radial dilator** muscles and opens the pupil, i.e. **pupil dilation**. The sympathetic supply to the smooth muscle of the iris

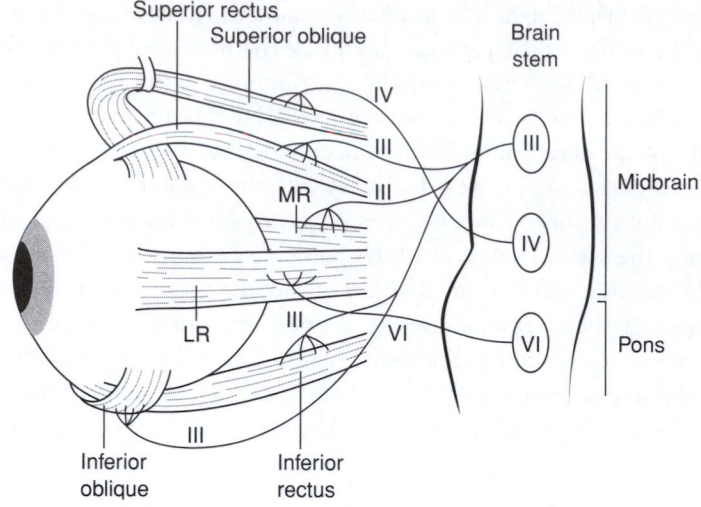

FIGURE 12.4 The external (skeletal) eye muscles and their innervation from the brain stem nuclei of the cranial nerves III, IV and VI. LR, lateral rectus muscle; MR, medial rectus muscle.

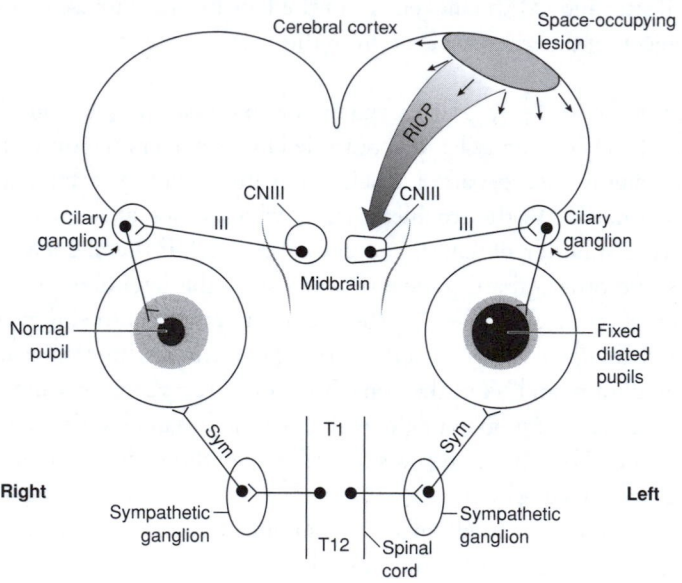

FIGURE 12.5 Pupil size innervation in normal conditions (right) and in head injury (left). The parasympathetic supply that constricts the pupil comes via the third cranial nerve (III) from the cranial nerve III nuclei (CNIII) in the midbrain. They reach the pupil via the ciliary ganglion. The sympathetic (sym) supply to the eye that dilates the pupil comes from the thoracic spinal cord; the sympathetic emerges from the cord between vertebrae T1 and T12 via the sympathetic ganglion. Raised intracranial pressure (RICP) comes from a space-occupying lesion and compresses the nucleus on the same side, causing an ipsilateral fixed dilated pupil.

214

comes from the upper thoracic spinal cord (T1 to T3, i.e. first to third thoracic vertebral level), part of the **sympathetic outflow** (Figure 12.5). Thus, the sympathetic component is a *spinal* outflow (cord and spinal nerves) while the parasympathetic component is a *cranial* outflow (medulla and cranial nerve III); a point of importance when considering pupil observations as part of head injury care.

3   The *parasympathetic* component of the oculomotor nerve (cranial nerve III) also controls **accommodation**. This is the process of stretching or relaxing the suspensory smooth muscles that control the shape of the lens for the purpose of focusing on objects that are different distances from the eye. The **near point** is the closest an object can get to the eye and remain in focus, and the eye should be able to focus on an object from this point to infinity.

Visual disturbance

Opacity of the lens, called a **cataract**, will prevent light from entering the posterior chamber of the eye. The lens is normally made from clear cells to allow light through, but they are unable to receive a direct blood supply since blood entering the lens would mean that we would see the world through a volume of blood, giving us a permanent red view of the world. This would obviously be disadvantageous for us as well as unpleasant, so these cells must acquire their nutrients and oxygen via a pass-along system. In this system, the cells at the edges collect what is needed from the blood and pass it, cell by cell, to all the others in the lens. Waste products flow in the opposite direction. Failure of this transport mechanism, as can occur in old age or exposure to prolonged radiation from the sun, leads to the milky opacity seen in cataracts. This is an observable sign that the cells are not getting adequate nutrients or oxygen and are dying. Cataracts are still a common cause of blindness, especially in developing countries, despite the fact that the relatively simple surgery of cataract removal can restore sight quickly.

Glaucoma is becoming better understood, not just as a disturbance of vision with acute eye pain caused by raised **intraocular pressure (IOP)**, but by the fact that beneath these symptoms hides a neurodegenerative disorder affecting retinal cells and their axons (Vasudevan *et al.* 2011). With raised IOP, the fluid inside the front of the eye builds up in volume and then stretches the front of the eye, and this is a major risk factor in causing the retinal degeneration. Patients complain not only of severe pain but of seeing distorted images surrounded by a halo. The urgent treatment is to administer drops to constrict the pupil (see p. 218) to improve drainage of the front chamber of the eye. Long-term treatment may require surgery to remove a segment of the iris (called a partial **iridectomy**), creating a keyhole-shaped pupil, which may be observed in patients with a history of the disease. Other long-term treatments are being developed to reduce the neurodegenerative effects of this disease (Vasudevan *et al.* 2011).

Damage or death of cells in the retina, as may occur from looking directly at the sun, or detachment of the retina from the inner wall of the eye can all impair vision. Anything that interrupts the function of the optic nerve, such as pressure from a tumour or injury, will block impulses from the retina from reaching the brain. Inside the brain, similar tumour growths, bleeding (as in strokes) or trauma from head injuries can disrupt the pathways from the chiasma to the thalamus or on to the visual cortex of the occipital lobe. The visual cortex itself can be affected by intracranial bleeds, infarcts or direct injury causing trauma to the cells that interpret what we see. It seems odd that loss of vision can be the result of a blow to the back of the head. Some blind patients report only a partial visual loss, which could be a reduction in the ability to see light across the entire visual field, or it may be a narrowing of the field itself. Defects of the visual fields can be detected on examination or reported by the patient. **Tunnel vision** is one such defect, where the peripheral aspects of the fields are gradually or suddenly lost; the patient only sees what is on or close to the visual axis.

Basic eye observations

Pupil size and reaction to light

The normal average pupil size is about 3.5 mm, with a range from 2 to 6 mm diameter (Clark *et al.* 2006). A light shone into one eye should cause a fast constriction of the pupils in *both* eyes, a **direct reaction** in the pupil to which the light was applied and a **consensual reaction** in the opposite pupil. The opposite pupil reacts because some branches of the neuronal connections in the brain stem decussate, whereas others remain ipsilateral (Figure 12.6). The pupil size is partly governed by a **pupillary reflex**, an autonomic motor response to the sensory stimulus of light intensity falling on the retina. As noted above (p. 213), the reflex action to bright light has a sensory input from the retina, the optic nerve (cranial nerve II); a motor output to the pupillary muscles of the iris, the parasympathetic oculomotor nerve (cranial nerve III); and brain stem relay areas (Figure 12.6). Pupil size is also partly governed by optical needs, the pupil will constrict as part of the mechanism for regulating depth of focus, and under these circumstances the constriction is independent of light intensity.

Abnormal pupils

Abnormal pupils are an important nursing observation and require careful interpretation and sometimes urgent intervention. Blindness in one eye due to causes involving the front of the eye, the retina or the optic nerve will mean the loss of the sensory component of the light pupillary reflex. Light shone in the blind eye will not affect either pupil size, but light will cause pupillary constriction in *both* eyes if it is shone in the good eye (provided the oculomotor nerve is functioning). Problems *inside* the brain that cause blindness are beyond the pupillary reflex and the pupils should therefore still react to light.

In **pinpoint pupils** (i.e. **miotic pupils**) (Figure 12.7), pupil size is at its minimum, i.e. the pupils are just visible at 1 mm or less in diameter, and are unlikely to constrict further to light. **Opioid drugs,** such as heroin, in large doses can cause this, and pinpoint pupils are a sign used to observe for opioid abuse. Alternatively, it may be caused by anything that obstructs the sympathetic supply to the eye, thus allowing the parasympathetic supply full control, e.g. spinal lesions with cervical nerve damage, causing **Horner's pupil**

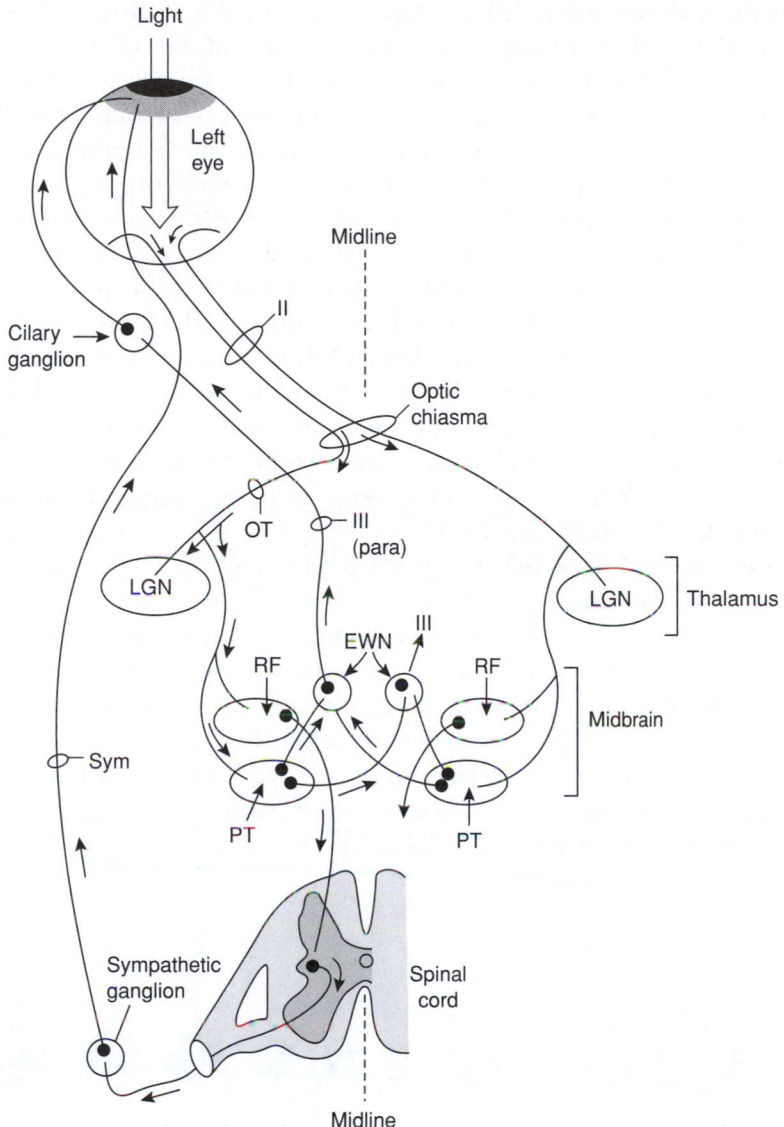

FIGURE 12.6 Detail of the pathways involved in establishing pupil size in response to light. Light enters the eye and impulses return to the brain from the retina via the optic nerve (II, cranial nerve II). Medial retinal impulses cross the midline at the optic chiasma; lateral retinal impulses do not cross. Impulses then pass to the lateral geniculate nucleus (LGN) via the optic tracts (OT). Some impulses are redirected to the reticular formation (RF) and the pretectum (PT). From the pretectum the impulses pass to the Edinger–Westphal nucleus (EWN), which is part of the cranial nerve III (III, oculomotor nerve) nucleus. This nerve provides parasympathetic (para) innervation to the pupil via the ciliary ganglion to cause constriction in bright light. From the reticular formation pathways descend the spinal cord to the sympathetic output of the thoracic cord. From here the pupil is supplied with sympathetic (Sym) fibres that dilate the pupil in dull light. Only the left side is shown.

(or **Horner's syndrome**, see p. 225 and Figure 12.7) (Patel and Ilsen 2003; Mojon and Stehberger 2005). Pinpoint pupils may also be a feature of direct trauma to the orbit (eye socket), which is identified by other signs of orbital injury, such as bruising filling the orbit and causing swelling around the eye. Small pupils (i.e. smaller than 3 mm) are naturally going to occur in bright light, and should be capable of further constriction if the light gets brighter. Abnormal small pupils could be the result of any of the conditions identified under pinpoint pupils, but to a lesser degree. In addition, if the small pupils are bilateral and respond to light, they could also be found in comas caused by a number of abnormal metabolic conditions (e.g. diabetic ketoacidosis or coma due to imbalance of blood electrolytes), or they could be due to bilateral injury to the thalamus or hypothalamus (referred to as **bilateral diencephalic damage**). Small irregular pupils that do *not* react to light but do constrict on accommodation of close objects are called **Argyll Robertson** pupils, and have long been associated with **syphilis** (a sexually transmitted infection often involving the brain), but can also be a feature of other brain stem disorders. Small or pinpoint pupils can result from the use of miotic drugs, such as pilocarpine or physostigmine, as a treatment for glaucoma (see p. 215).

Normal average-sized pupils that, however, are *not* reacting to light indicate a failure of both components of the autonomic nervous system and may be a feature of midbrain injury from **infarction** (a sudden loss of blood supply leading to an area of dead or dying tissue) or **herniation** (part of the brain forced out of position, usually downwards).

Dilation of the pupils (or **mydriasis**, 6–8 mm diameter) occurs normally in low-light conditions, but the pupils will constrict again on exposure to light (Figure 12.7). Pupil dilation can also be caused by high-dosage **amphetamines** (nervous system stimulants) or by the use of a **mydriatic** or **cycloplegic** drug for eye examination purposes. These drugs (e.g. **tropicamide**, **cyclopentolate** and **homatropine**) dilate the pupil by blocking the parasympathetic

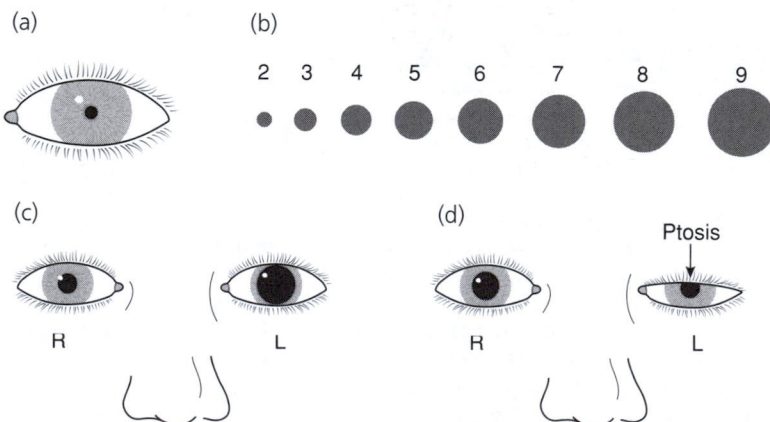

FIGURE 12.7 Pupil sizes. (a) pinpoint pupils; (b) various sizes from 2 to 9 mm; (c) unilateral fixed dilated pupil on the left seen in oculomotor nerve compression or damage due to raised intracranial pressure; (d) Horner's syndrome, with right dilated pupil and left ptosis.

and thus increasing the sympathetic balance to the eye. Large pupils may also be due to direct orbital injuries (as with small pupils) if the trauma causes pressure on the third cranial nerve with concurrent loss of pupillary constriction.

Chapter 10 identified the abnormal changes in pupil size and reaction to light as a focal sign of raised intracranial pressure (RICP), but they could be due to other intracranial disorders. In head injury, these changes are initially a dilated pupil that is *unilateral* (on one side), *ipsilateral* (the same side as the injury) and *fixed* (no response to light). Later (and this could be anything from minutes to hours), the fixed dilated pupil becomes *bilateral* (both sides). The time taken for the progression from unilateral to bilateral is dependent on the rate of increase in the space-occupying lesion (SOL) that is causing the increased pressure, e.g. extradural haematoma, which progresses much faster than subdural haematoma in head injuries (see Chapter 10). The observation made is twofold; first, identification of the size of the pupil on both sides so that equality of the left pupil with the right pupil can be assessed, and, second, the pupil's reaction to light. Pupils that are widely dilated (9 mm or more in diameter) and fixed (not reacting to light) are a very serious observation suggesting intracranial bleeding after head injury, or some other SOL, such as a brain tumour or cerebral oedema, and must be reported and acted upon urgently. RICP from the developing SOL causes failure of the brain stem areas controlling pupil constriction or compression of the oculomotor nerve. This is often unilateral at first, becoming bilateral as the RICP increases, causing compression down onto the brain stem. Continued compression of the brain as the SOL gets larger will result in **coning**, a herniation of parts of the brain, especially the medulla (the lowest part of the brain stem). The herniation is usually downwards into the foramen magnum at the base of the skull. As the cardiac and respiratory centres are in the medulla, they will be compressed and both the heart and the lungs will stop functioning, with little chance of resuscitation. Fixed, bilateral dilated pupils are also seen in the terminal stages of many conditions, including **cerebral ischaemia** (loss of blood supply to the brain) and severe **cerebral anoxia** (loss of oxygen); and indeed it is also the state seen after death has occurred.

Advanced visual neurobiology

Sensory pathways

The optic tracts link the chiasma with parts of the thalamus (see p. 173) known as the **lateral geniculate nucleus (LGN)**. About 10% of the visual stimulus passing along this optic tract connects with part of the **midbrain**, the **superior colliculus** (Figure 12.8). This area responds to retinal impulses by operating the muscles that are keeping the eye and head in a position to retain the viewed image on the fovea. It is therefore responsible for maintaining the eye's *gaze* on a subject, especially if that subject is moving. The superior colliculus is linked to the three cranial nerves operating the orbital muscles that move the eye (see p. 213). These muscles are attached to the external surface of the eyeball. Gaze is a vital requirement for hunting and survival, and in lower vertebrates the superior colliculus is the main area to which *all* the retinal output goes. The fact that only

10% of the pathway goes there in humans suggests that it may be less important for us, although 10% of *human* retinal output is roughly the equivalent to the *entire* retinal output of a cat (Bear *et al.* 1996).

Another area of the midbrain that receives light-induced impulses is the **pretectum**, the relay nucleus that has partial control over pupil size and some eye movements in response to light intensity. The pretectum is an intermediary link between the incoming sensory impulses from the retina and the outgoing motor impulses of the parasympathetic third cranial nerve (see below). Another area that receives light-induced impulses from the optic tracts is the **hypothalamus** via the **retinohypothalamic tract** (Figure 12.8). Through this

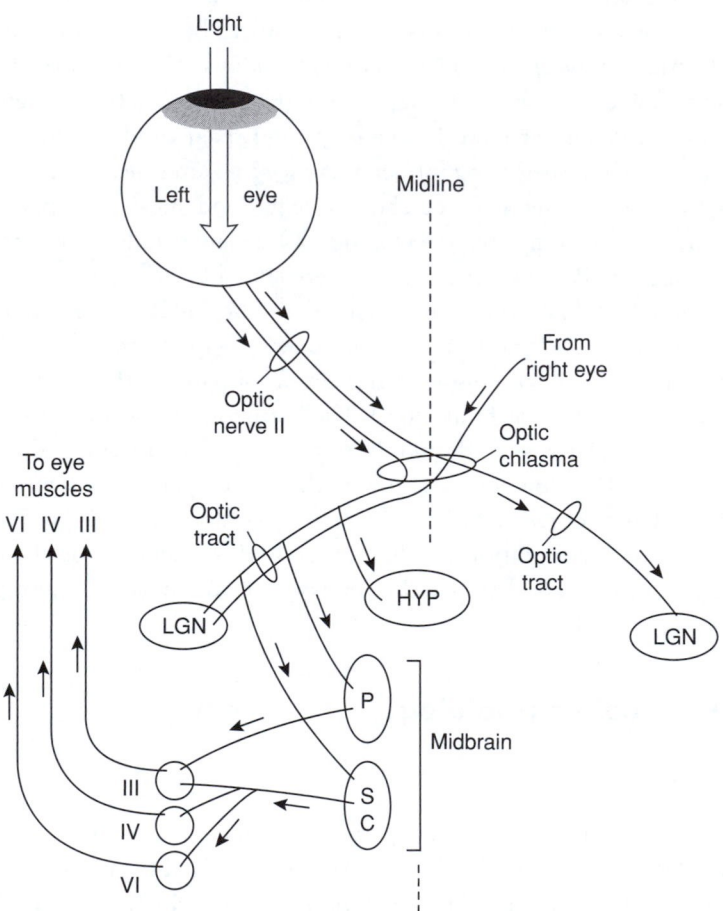

FIGURE 12.8 Pathways in the brain that respond to light intensity. Nerve impulses passing down the optic nerve not only go to the lateral geniculate nucleus (LGN, on the visual pathway), but some pass to the hypothalamus (HYP), via the retinohypothalamic tract. The hypothalamus governs the sleep–wake cycle in response to light intensity. Some light also pass to the pretectum (P), which helps to control pupil size, and some go to the superior colliculus (SC), which aids in eye movements via the cranial nerves III, IV and VI. Only the left side is shown.

pathway, the **sleep–wake cycle** is controlled by the light intensity falling on the retina and transmitted as impulses to the hypothalamus via the retinohypothalamic tracts. This cycle determines when the brain will sleep (in response to low light) and when it will awake (in response to greater light).

The retina causes impulses to travel along the optic nerve (sensory) to the pretectum, then onto the **Edinger–Westphal nucleus**, which is part of the **third cranial nerve nucleus** in the midbrain (Figures 12.6 and 12.8). The Edinger–Westphal nucleus is the pupillary control centre and origin of the *parasympathetic* component of the oculomotor nerve. From here, the oculomotor nerve passes to the orbit, where a **synapse** occurs with the cell body of the second neurons, called the **ciliary ganglion**, before the nerve entering the iris. Second, neurons of the oculomotor nerve also pass from the ciliary ganglion into the **ciliary body** inside the eye, where they control suspensory *smooth* muscles that pull on the lens. The first neurons of the *sympathetic* outflow pass down the upper thoracic spinal nerves into the **sympathetic trunk** on each side of the spine and then pass up the trunk to synapse with the **superior cervical ganglion**, the cell body of the second neurons. From here the second neurons pass up towards the head and follow the arterial pathway into the eyes.

Motor system and eye movements

Eye movements are essential to allow the subject of visual interest to remain on the fovea when it is stationary (**gaze holding**) or moving (**gaze shifting**) and also to respond quickly to new visual stimuli entering the visual fields. A rapid eye movement (or sudden attention change) in order to bring a new or peripheral object onto the fovea is called a **saccade**. Saccades are the fastest specialised form of *gaze shift* and can be vertical, horizontal or a combination of these. Vertical saccades are controlled by an area at the highest point of the midbrain, close to the thalamus, from where connections pass to the oculomotor and trochlear nuclei. Horizontal saccades are commanded from lower in the brain stem, close to the pons (Figure 12.9).

Bilateral lesions in either of these command areas, as may be possible in brain stem ischaemia or bleeds, can result in a loss of the corresponding saccade. Other gaze shifts include **smooth pursuit** (retaining the image of a moving object on the fovea) and **vergence** (the eyes move in opposing directions to retain the image simultaneously on both foveae). These are conscious motor activities and are therefore controlled by specific areas of the cerebral cortex (Figure 12.10). Since they are in response to visual sensory stimuli, neuronal connections occur between the sensory visual cortex in the occipital lobe and the various ophthalmic motor centres of the parietal and frontal lobes. From these centres motor pathways descend through the basal ganglia and via the superior colliculus, the gaze control centre, with output to the cranial nerve nuclei in the brain stem that govern eye muscle movement. In general, nuclei in the midbrain (cranial nerves III and IV) control vertical gaze, whereas the nucleus in the pons (cranial nerve VI) controls horizontal gaze.

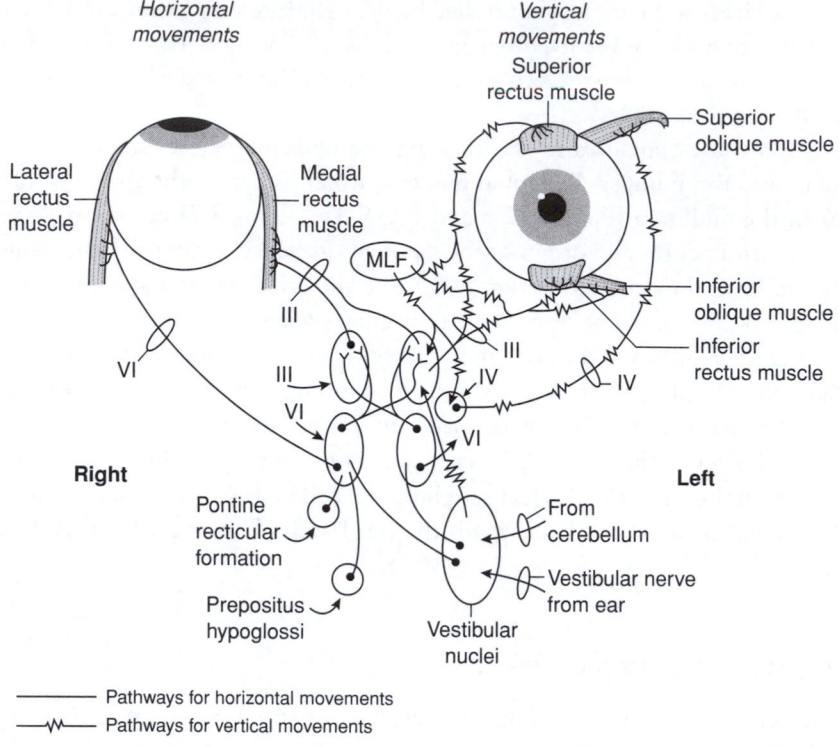

FIGURE 12.9 Control of eye movements. The right side shows control of horizontal movements. Input to the cranial nerve VI nucleus is from the pontine reticular formation, the vestibular nuclei and the prepositus hypoglossi. The cranial nerve VI nucleus connects to the cranial nerve III nucleus on both sides. The left side shows control of vertical movements. Input to the cranial nerve III nucleus is from the cerebellum and vestibular nerve via the vestibular nuclei and from the medial longitudinal fasciculus (MLF), which also has direct output to the superior and inferior rectus muscles.

Advanced eye observations

Abnormal eye movements

Health care professionals may note abnormalities of both gaze holding and gaze shift in conscious patients (but to a much lesser extent in an unconscious patient, who is unable to co-operate). Abnormal gaze holding can be seen in unilateral paralysis of each of the cranial nerves that control eye muscles, and these present with the characteristic symptom of the two eyes no longer functioning together (Figure 12.11). **Diagonal diplopia** (diplopia = double vision) is seen in unilateral **cranial nerve III palsy** (paralysis of one oculomotor nerve), where the eye *on the affected side* looks 'down and out' with ptosis (see p. 225) and pupil dilation, while the other eye appears normal. Unilateral **cranial nerve IV palsy** results in a **vertical diplopia**, as the eye on the affected side becomes unable to

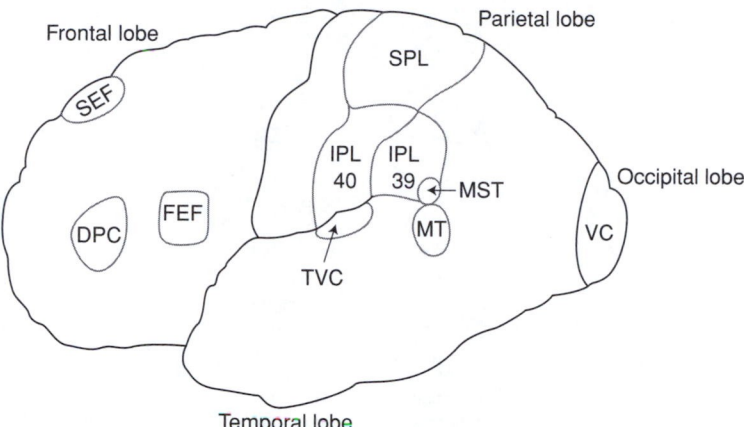

FIGURE 12.10   Areas of the cerebral cortex involved in eye movement control. DPC, dorsolateral prefrontal cortex (area 46); FEF, frontal eye fields (parts of areas 4, 6, 8, 9); IPL inferior parietal lobe (areas 39, 40); MST, medial superior temporal visual area (parts of areas 19, 37, 39); MT, mid-temporal visual areas (parts of areas 19, 37); SEF, supplementary eye fields (part of area 6); SPL, superior parietal lobe (areas 5, 7); TVC, temporal vestibular cortex (parts of areas 41, 42); VC, visual cortex (area 17).

look down when adducted (brought towards the nose). Unilateral **cranial nerve VI palsy** causes **horizontal diplopia,** as the affected eye cannot be abducted (moved outwards) (Figure 12.11).

Abnormal **gaze shift** may be seen when the patient is asked to follow the examiner's finger through a range of up, down, left and right movements. **Nystagmus** describes the involuntary rhythmic oscillations of the eyeball, a rapid back and forth movement that the patient has no control over (Figure 12.12) (Nebbioso *et al.* 2009). Nystagmus may occur in the horizontal, vertical, mixed or rotary directions. Two types of nystagmus have been identified: the more common *jerky* form, in which movements in one direction are faster (rapid saccade) than in the other direction, and the *pendular* form, in which the movements in both directions are equal in speed. Nystagmus can be artificially induced in normal individuals by putting cold water into an ear, a procedure called a **cold caloric** test. It causes **vestibular** (= balance or equilibrium) stimulation by chilling the fluid within the **lateral semi-circular canal,** part of the **labyrinth** (= cavity) of the inner ear, and thus creating convection currents in this fluid. This tests the function of the pathway passing from the semi-circular canals of the inner ear (the vestibular branch of cranial nerve VIII) to the brain stem and **cerebellum,** then on to the cranial nerve nuclei controlling eye movements (see p. 213). The cerebellum controls balance (in response to semi-circular canal activity) and both the speed and the co-ordination of eye saccades. **Labyrinthine vestibular nystagmus,** a rotary jerky form, may be caused by diseases of the inner ear. Other jerky forms can be caused by brain stem or cerebellar diseases, or as the result of barbiturate overdose. Pendular nystagmus is usually a feature of **intraocular disease,** i.e. disorders of the retina or fluid pressures inside the eye.

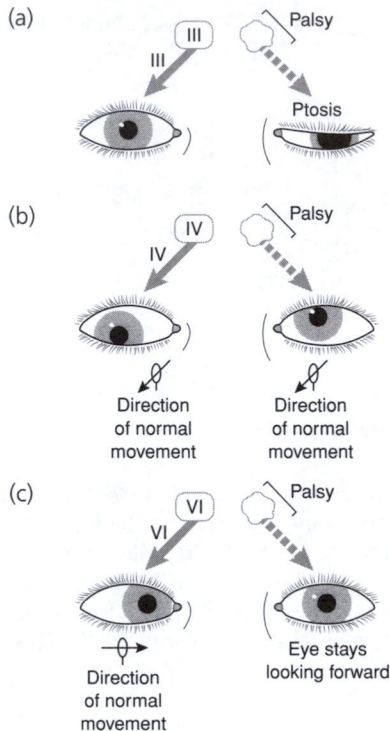

FIGURE 12.11 Disturbance of eye positions in various cranial nerve palsies. (a) Cranial nerve III palsy causes the 'down and out' appearance of the affected eye with dilated pupil and ptosis of the lid. (b) Cranial nerve IV palsy causes the affected eye to have limited ability to look down when it is adducted (moved towards the nose). (c) Cranial nerve VI palsy causes the inability to abduct (move towards the ear) the affected eye when both eyes are commanded to look in that direction.

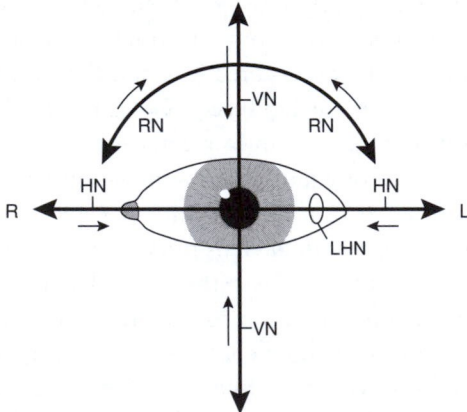

FIGURE 12.12 The range of movements in nystagmus. Nystagmus has a slow movement phase (short, thin arrow) and a rapid return phase (long, thick arrow). The rapid phase is the direction given for the nystagmus (HN), rotary nystagmus (RN) or a mix of these in either left, right, up or down directions.

Papilloedema

Papilloedema is swelling of the optic disc due to oedema. Using an **ophthalmoscope**, the retina is viewed (known as a **funduscopic examination** since the **fundus**, or deepest part of the eye where the retina lies, will be seen), and the retinal blood vessels can been identified (Figure 12.2). These vessels spread out to all parts of the retina from a single point, the optic disc, just off centre from the macula. The blood vessels are the **retinal arteries and veins**, the blood supply to this light-sensitive layer, and they follow the optic nerve pathway between the brain and the eye. The veins are some 30% larger than the arteries, but, like everywhere else, the retinal arteries carry blood at greater pressure than the veins. Papilloedema is usually caused by raised intracranial pressure (RICP, see Chapter 10). This is because the meninges surrounding the brain are continuous along the optic nerve to the optic disc, and any RICP will exist along the optic nerve and onto the disc itself. When pressure is applied to the blood vessels from RICP, the veins will tend to be occluded before the arteries (i.e. at an early stage of RICP). This means that blood passing along the vessels enters the retina easier via the arteries than it can leave via the veins. RICP together with some venous congestion causes excess tissue fluid to accumulate, called oedema, at the point around the vessel entry, the optic disc. This obscures the normally obvious disc margins; they become distorted and swollen, with the disc becoming a reddish colour, i.e. visual proof of the existence of RICP. This becomes a very important visual check for RICP (remember the statement at the start of this chapter about the retina being the only part of the nervous system visible from the outside world). It is not only carried out as part of the neurological examination of the patient but is usually also done to exclude the existence of RICP before a **lumbar puncture** (**LP**). A lumbar puncture is the introduction of a needle into the spinal canal below the level of **lumbar vertebra 2** (**L2**) in order to obtain a sample of **cerebrospinal fluid** (**CSF**). If RICP was present during a lumbar puncture, the sudden decompression of the cord by removing CSF could cause coning (see p. 186).

Ptosis

The elevation of the upper eyelid is a function of the oculomotor nerve (see p. 213) and incomplete opening of the upper lid is a condition called **ptosis** (or **lid lag**). It can be seen by observing the narrowed **palpebral fissure**, i.e. the gap between the upper and lower lids, when the patient is asked to open the eyes. Ptosis may be unilateral or bilateral, and may be the result of oculomotor nerve or brain stem injury or compression, as in RICP. It could be part of several neurological disorders, e.g. **Horner's syndrome**, where ptosis, constricted pupils and dry facial skin indicate the presence of a spinal cord lesion (syndrome = a collection of symptoms that tend to be present together) (Figure 12.7). Some drugs, e.g. the **benzodiazepines**, such as **diazepam**, may cause ptosis when given in sufficient dosage to induce sedation before minor surgical procedures.

Key points

* The optic nerve (cranial nerve II) is the sensory nerve of vision from the eye. It passes posteriorly into the brain.
* The left and right optic nerves converge at the optic chiasma.

- The optic tracts link the chiasma with the lateral geniculate nucleus (LGN), part of the thalamus.
- Ten per cent of the visual stimulus passing along this optic tract connects with the superior colliculus, part of the midbrain. This area operates the muscles that keep the eye fixed on an image, maintaining the gaze.
- The pretectum in the midbrain receives retinal impulses and has partial control over pupil size and some eye movements in response to light intensity.
- Posteriorly to the LGN, the optic radiations pass to the visual cortex, part of the occipital lobe of the cerebrum.
- Cranial nerve III (oculomotor) innervates four of the orbital muscles, cranial nerve IV (trochlear) innervates the superior oblique muscle, and cranial nerve VI (abducens) innervates the lateral rectus muscle.
- The third cranial nerve nucleus in the medulla contains the Edinger–Westphal area, the pupillary constriction centre and origin of the parasympathetic component of the oculomotor nerve.
- The sympathetic supply to the iris comes from the upper thoracic spinal cord (T1 to T3), part of the sympathetic outflow, and causes pupillary dilation.
- The pupil size is partly due to a pupillary reflex, an autonomic motor response to the sensory stimulus of light intensity falling on the retina, and partly due to optical adjustments required for depth of focus.
- Miotic pupils are pinpoint, and mydriatic pupils are dilated. Miotic and mydriatic drugs can be used to close and open the pupils respectively.
- Unilateral, followed by bilateral, widely dilated and fixed pupils may be due to intracranial bleeding after a head injury and must be reported urgently.
- A rapid eye movement or sudden attention change is called a saccade.
- Nystagmus is the rapid involuntary rhythmic back and forth movement (fast saccades) of the eyeball and may be due to vestibular (balance) disorder, intraocular diseases or barbiturate overdose.
- Diplopia is double vision.
- Papilloedema is swelling of the optic disc and is visual proof of the existence of RICP.
- Incomplete opening of the upper lid is a condition called ptosis (or lid lag).

References

Bear M., Connors B. and Paradiso M. (1996) *Neuroscience: Exploring the Brain*. Williams and Wilkins, Baltimore, MD.

Clark A., Clarke T. N. S., Gregson B., Hooker P. N. A. and Chambers I. R. (2006) Variability in pupil size estimation. *Emergency Medicine Journal*, **23**(6): 440–441.

Mojon D. S. and Stehberger B. (2005) Diagnosis of Horner syndrome by pupil dilation lag. *Klinische Monatsblätter für Augenheilkunde*, **222**(3): 211–213.

Nebbioso M., D'Innocenzo D., Rapone S., Di Benedetto G. and Grenga R. (2009) Nystagmus in ophthalmology. *La Clinica Terapeutica*, **160**(2): 145–149.

Patel S. and Ilsen P. F. (2003) Acquired Horner's syndrome: clinical review. *Optometry*, **74**(4): 245–256.

Vasudevan S. K., Gupta V. and Crowston J. G. (2011) Neuroprotection in glaucoma. *Indian Journal of Ophthalmology*, **59**(Suppl. 1): S102–S113.

Chapter 13 **Neurological observations (IV)**
Movement

- Introduction
- The neurology of human movement
- Movement observations
- Movement losses
- Movement excesses
- The immobile patient
- Key points
- References

Introduction

The ability to move is fundamental to our existence and survival. It therefore becomes life-threatening when movement is disturbed by disease or injury, requiring a great deal of nursing care. We are not born with full movement; indeed the human newborn is extremely limited in what movement it can make. Most movements achieved by adult age are learnt throughout childhood, often after bitter trial and error. This learning process does not involve gaining extra neurons; we are born with about 100 billion neurons and gradually lose them through life. Learning is still somewhat of a mystery, but it seems that it involves gaining both neuronal connections, called synapses, and specific chemical receptors at those synapses. And learning is also facilitated by sensory feedback at every stage. The normal child will gain the usual movement abilities, such as walking and talking, but specific movement skills, like playing the piano, require additional learning involving considerable practice. Despite how much we take it for granted, movement, it seems, does not come easy. This is partly due to the complexity of the motor system, which has far more to do than just control muscles.

The neurology of human movement

This simplified version of motor activity introduces the concepts of muscle movement in relation to balance and posture, muscle tone, co-ordination and smoothing out of muscle activity, special skills like synergy (see p. 236) and the importance of sensory feedback. We do have conscious control over the obvious movements; we can decide when to walk, to grasp an object, and so on. There are, however, many thousands of subconscious (or automatic) muscle changes and neuronal activities going on continuously, many of which make the conscious movements possible.

Conscious muscle control begins with the **primary motor cortex** within the frontal lobe of the cerebrum. Cells here are the start of the **pyramidal system**, which initiates the contraction of the skeletal muscle that moves the body (Figure 13.1). The pyramidal system is so named because it forms a pyramid shape as it passes down through the brain. Consciousness suggests that each movement is purposefully thought about, but in reality we move *without* thinking. Most movements are pre-programmed and require little if any thought. Pre-programming of movement is the essence of the learning process. This is seen in the pianist who plays a Beethoven sonata effortlessly, the finger movements being pre-programmed by years of practice. The conscious aspect involves the ability to initiate the movement in response to sensory stimuli, to be aware of the movement as it happens and to modify the motor response according to sensory feedback. The muscle co-ordination, extent and smoothness of contraction, repetition of muscle action (as in running) and other features of movement are controlled at a subconscious level by the **extra-pyramidal system** (extra = outside, i.e. a system outside the pyramidal system functioning at an automatic level; see p. 231).

The pyramidal tract system

The cells of the primary motor cortex are not randomly arranged; rather, they are positioned in a manner that reflects the basic body plan (Figure 13.2). Larger surface areas housing greater cell numbers occur on the cortex representing those parts where fine intricate muscle movement is required, notably the hands. Pathways descending from the motor cortex, the **pyramidal tracts**, pass through the brain to the brain stem and onward into the cord (Figure 13.1). At the level of the medulla about 75% of these fibres decussate (i.e. cross to the other side) and become contralateral (i.e. from the *opposite* side), whereas the other 25% remain **ipsilateral** (i.e. from the same side). Since both cerebral hemispheres have a motor cortex, there are four pyramidal pathways descending the cord from the brain; two contralateral that have crossed (one from each side) and two ipsilateral that have not crossed (one on each side). Neurons occupying these pyramidal tracts are called **upper motor neurons (UMNs)**, i.e. they extend from the brain to the cord within the **central nervous system (CNS)**. The descending tracts pass down the spinal cord in specific positions within the **white matter** (Figure 13.3). The fibres enter the anterior **grey matter** of the cord, where they synapse with other neurons at all the spinal levels, i.e. from high in the cervical (neck) region to low in the sacral (pelvic) region.

Lower motor neurons (LMNs) are those that begin with the cells in the anterior grey matter of the cord, and the fibres pass via the **anterior root** into the **spinal nerve** to the voluntary skeletal muscles of the body. The LMN is therefore part of the **peripheral nervous system (PNS)**, being a component of the spinal nerves. Therefore, the pyramidal system is two-neuronal, consisting of a UMN and an LMN, from motor cortex to muscle (Figure 13.1).

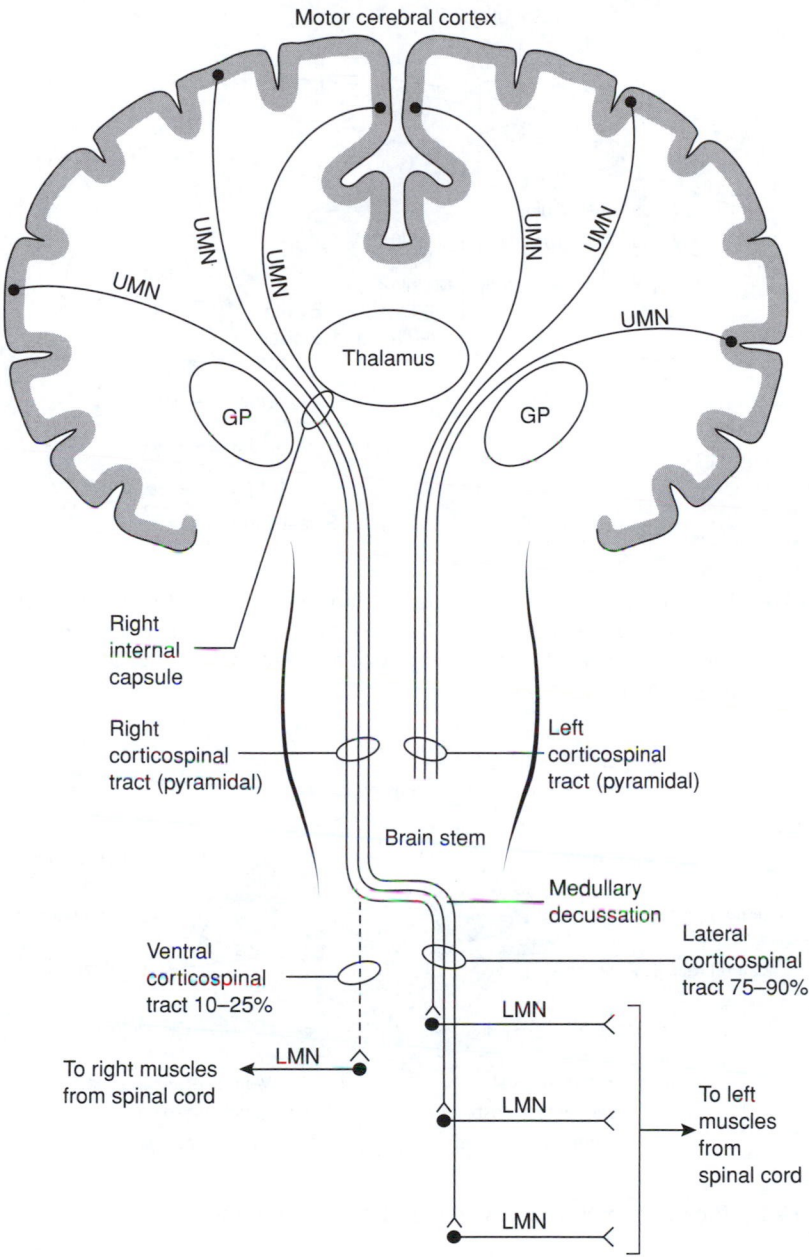

Motor cerebral cortex

UMN

UMN

UMN

UMN

UMN

UMN

Thalamus

GP

GP

Right internal capsule

Right corticospinal tract (pyramidal)

Left corticospinal tract (pyramidal)

Brain stem

Medullary decussation

Ventral corticospinal tract 10–25%

Lateral corticospinal tract 75–90%

LMN

To right muscles from spinal cord

LMN

LMN

To left muscles from spinal cord

LMN

FIGURE 13.1 The pyramidal tracts. The corticospinal (known as pyramidal) tracts begin with widely distributed neuronal cell bodies within the motor cortex (three shown) on both sides. The collected pathway passes between the globus pallidus (GP) and the thalamus at the internal capsule. The fibres (70–90%) cross (decussate) to the opposite side (contralateral) in the medulla to form the lateral corticospinal tract; 10–25% remain on the same side (ipsilateral) to form the ventral corticospinal tract. LMN, lower motor neuron; UMN, upper motor neuron.

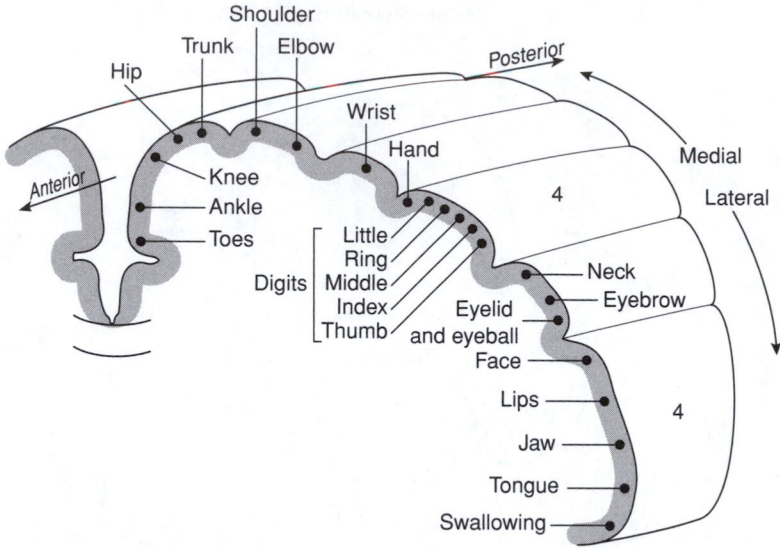

FIGURE 13.2 The left main motor cortex (area 4) showing the layout of the cells according to function (i.e. the muscle sites they control). Notice the large area controlling finger and hand movements compared with the area for feet and toes, which indicates great manual dexterity.

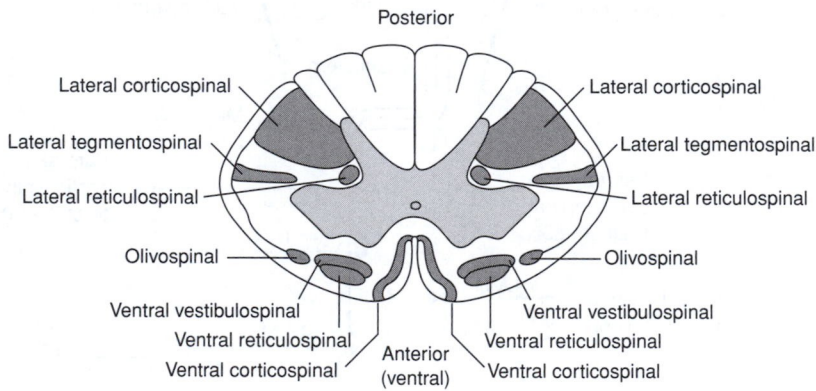

FIGURE 13.3 The motor pathways within the white matter of the cord.

The pyramidal system also operates through some of the **cranial nerves** that control muscles of the head, face and neck. The **corticobulbar tracts** (Figure 13.4) begin as neuronal cell bodies in the head and neck areas (lateral areas) of the motor cortex (hence *cortico*). These UMN fibres pass down to nuclei in the pons and medulla of the brain stem (note: the pons, part of the brain stem, is called *bulbar*, i.e. shaped like a bulb). From a nucleus in the pons, LMN fibres become components of the **trigeminal nerve** (cranial V) and pass to

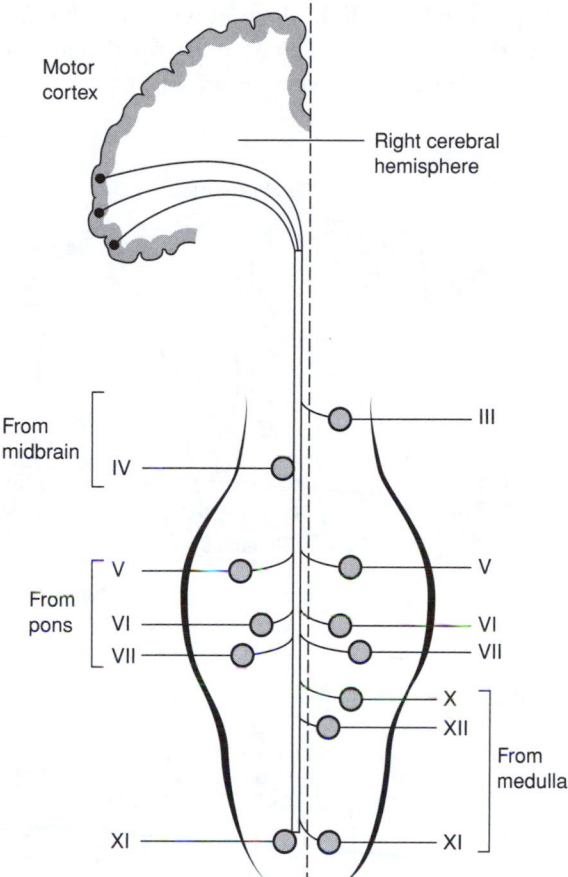

FIGURE 13.4 The corticobulbar tracts to the cranial nerves. This schematic diagram shows motor pathways coming from the head and neck area of the right motor cortex (see Figure 13.2) and passing into the brain stem. The cranial nerve nuclei are indicated, showing their brain stem locations, the corticobulbar input (unilateral or bilateral), which cross the midline. The left hemisphere (not shown) has a mirror image input.

the muscles of the lower jaw (e.g. for eating). Also from the pons, LMN fibres form part of the **facial nerve** (cranial VII) and pass to muscles of the face (e.g. for facial expression). Separate *medullary* nuclei give rise to LMN fibres within the **glossopharyngeal nerve** (cranial IX, to pharyngeal muscles), the **vagus nerve** (cranial X, to muscles of the pharynx, larynx, oesophagus and soft palate) and the **spinal accessory nerve** (cranial XI, to the neck muscles).

The extra-pyramidal system

This system operates skeletal muscle at the subconscious level, i.e. it controls the automatic aspects of voluntary movement. The main areas of the brain involved are parts of the brain stem (nuclei of the pons and medulla), which in turn are influenced by the basal ganglia, some sensory parts of the cerebral cortex, and parts of the thalamus and cerebellum, including all their pathways and feedback circuits (Figure 13.5).

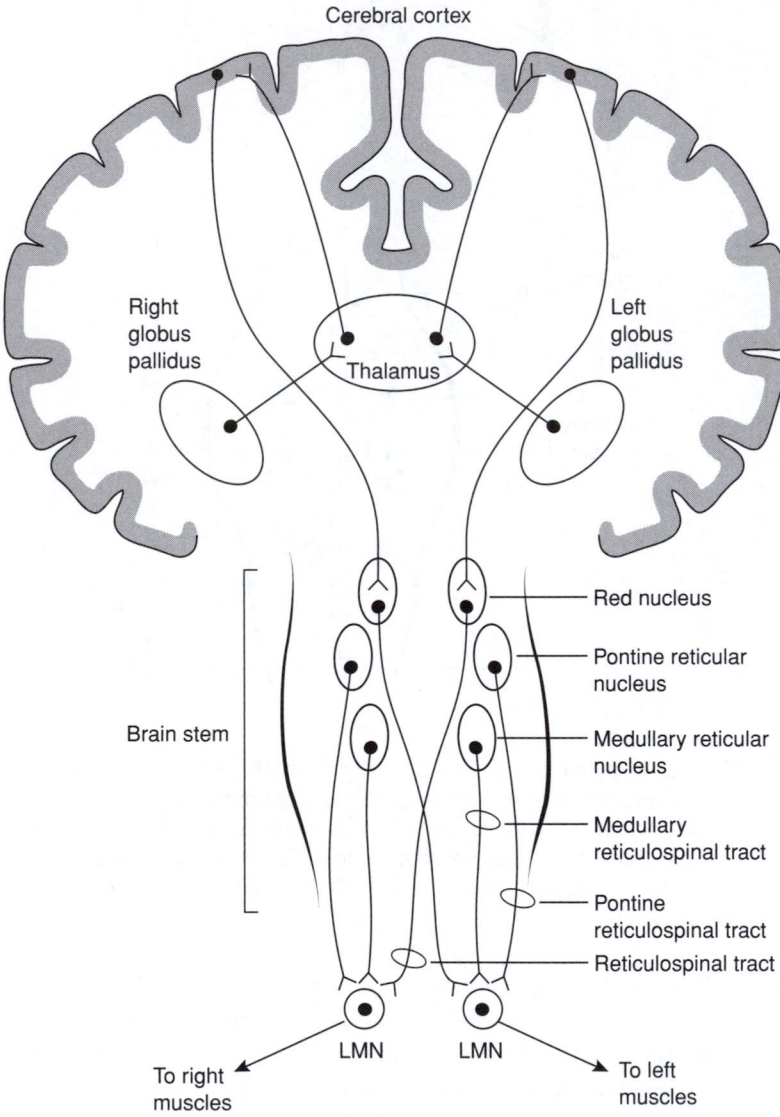

FIGURE 13.5 Some extra-pyramidal tracts. Pathways of the extra-pyramidal system extend from the cerebral cortex to the red nucleus, and from the red nucleus to the contralateral LMN (lower motor neuron) in the cord (a pathway called the rubrospinal tract), from the globus pallidus to the thalamus with feedback pathways to the cortex, from the pontine nucleus to the ipsilateral LMN (called the pontine reticulospinal tract) and from the medullary reticulospinal nucleus to the LMN (called the medullary reticulospinal tract).

Some pathways involved are:

- *Primary* cells within the cerebral cortex that have fibres that end in the red nucleus within the midbrain, the **corticorubral tract**. In the red nucleus, *secondary* cells give rise to fibres that pass down the cord, forming the **rubrospinal tract**.
- Several nuclei towards the base of the brain are collectively called the basal ganglia (Figure 13.6). One of these nuclei, the **globus pallidus**, has *primary* cells providing fibres that terminate in some areas of the thalamus. From the thalamus, *secondary* cell fibres feed back to the motor cortex of the cerebrum (part of the basal ganglia motor loop, see p. 234 and Figures 13.5 and 13.8).
- Areas of the pons and medulla, known as the **reticular formation**, have *secondary* cells with fibres extending down the cord, creating the **reticulospinal tract**.

The basal ganglia and thalamus

The five nuclei of the basal ganglia (Figure 13.6) are responsible for a major influence, both **facilitatory** and **inhibitory**, on movement (Anderson 2001). Facilitatory promotes move-

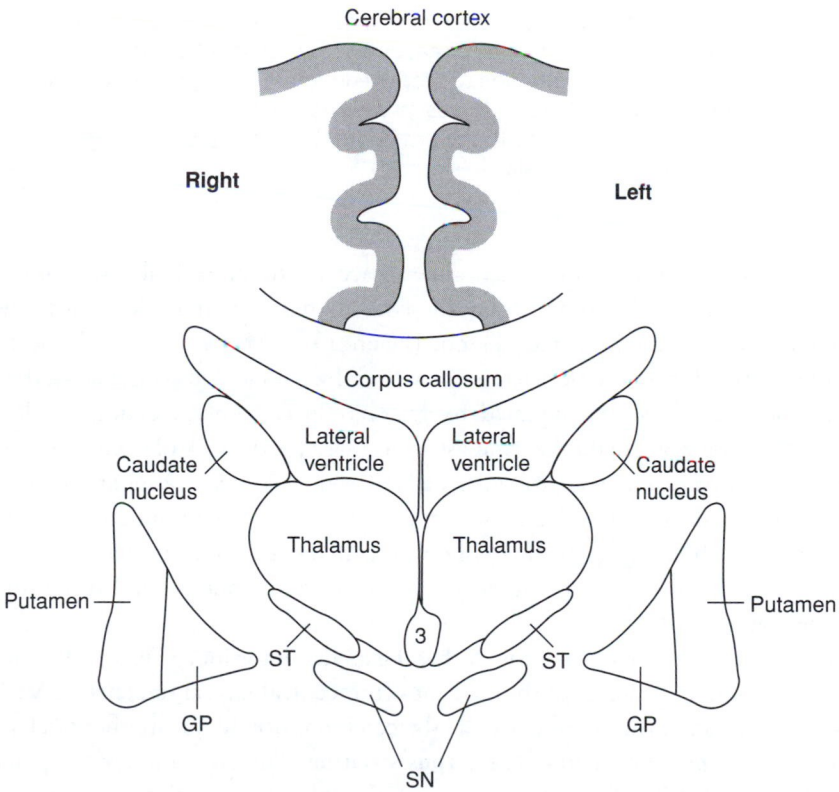

FIGURE 13.6 Areas that make up the basal ganglia. GP, globus pallidus; SN, substantia nigra; ST, subthalamus; 3, third ventricle.

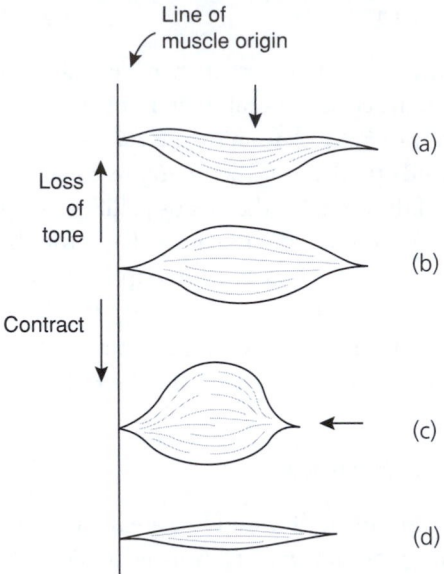

FIGURE 13.7 Muscle tone. (a) loss of muscle tone: the muscle is soft, loose and floppy, sinking in response to gravity (i.e. after long immobilisation); (b) normal muscle tone: the muscle is firm and retains its shape ready for contraction; (c) contraction of the muscle, where the insertion (opposite end to the origin) moves towards the origin (which does not move); (d) muscle wasting, where muscle bulk is lost. Excessive muscle tone appears as the opposite of (a), i.e. the muscle is tight and stiff and cannot contract normally.

ment and inhibitory prevents movement, like an accelerator and a brake in a car providing fine control of the vehicle. In particular, these nuclei have a major role in slow, sustained movements and in maintaining **muscle tone** (Figure 13.7). Muscle tone can be described as a state of readiness for contraction; a tension within the muscle that is essential if the muscle is to function instantly when stimulated. Exercise has the effect of increasing muscle tone, as identified by those who attend the gymnasium regularly, and a lack of exercise causes a loss of tone. This is one reason why prolonged bed rest is no longer a treatment for patients, for this results in muscle tone loss, i.e. loose, floppy muscles that do not function properly. But this effect is not the only factor, since the basal ganglia provide *inhibition* (or *reduction*) of excessive muscle tone, and this is notably a major role of the nucleus called the **substantia nigra** (see Figure 13.6).

A major influence on movement is the **basal ganglia motor loop** (Figure 13.8), in which the globus pallidus *inhibits* part of the thalamus (the **ventral lateral nucleus**, or **VLN**) during rest. Activation of the motor cortex of the cerebrum *switches on* another nucleus of the basal ganglia, the **putamen**, part of the **corpus striatum**. This activation of the putamen in turn *inhibits* the globus pallidus, thus removing the inhibition on the thalamus. Free now to act, the thalamus has considerable influence on an area close to the motor cortex, the **supplementary motor area** (**SMA**), which in turn focuses the activity of the main motor

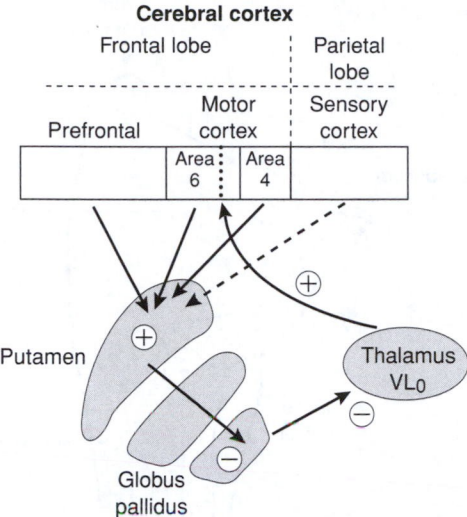

FIGURE 13.8 Basal ganglia motor loop. Input to the putamen comes from the frontal cortex, with less input from the parietal sensory cortex. This activates (+) neurons running from the putamen to the globus pallidus, which, in turn, then deactivate (−) neurons linking the globus pallidus with the ventral lateral nucleus of the thalamus (known as VL_0). These globus pallidus neurons prevent (i.e. inhibit, shown as −) any feedback from the VL_0 to the cerebral cortex. However, deactivation from the putamen has removed this inhibition, and the VL_0 then has freedom to feedback to the cortex (+), more precisely the supplemental motor area (SMA) of area 6 of the motor cortex.

cortex. Thus the loop is complete when motor cortex activity switches on the mechanism that focuses that activity.

The cerebellum

The **cerebellum** (Figure 13.9) contributes several aspects of movement, not least of which are **balance** and **posture**. The equilibrium of the body requires the **centre of gravity** (in the mid-lumbar spinal area) to remain within the base, i.e. the floor area occupied by the two feet. Should the centre of gravity drift outside the base, the individual will fall to one side. To prevent this, many minute muscular adjustments are constantly made to keep the body upright inside the base, correcting any defects in posture at the same time. These muscular contractions are co-ordinated by the cerebellum at an unconscious level, but they require *sensory* feedback to tell the cerebellum what the second-by-second state of the body's balance is. This sensory feedback on balance (known as **vestibular** stimuli) comes from the semi-circular canals of the inner ear, via the **vestibulocochlear nerve** (cranial nerve VIII). Additional sensory information on balance comes from receptors in the joints and muscles; this is sensory feedback called **proprioception** and arrives in the brain stem via the

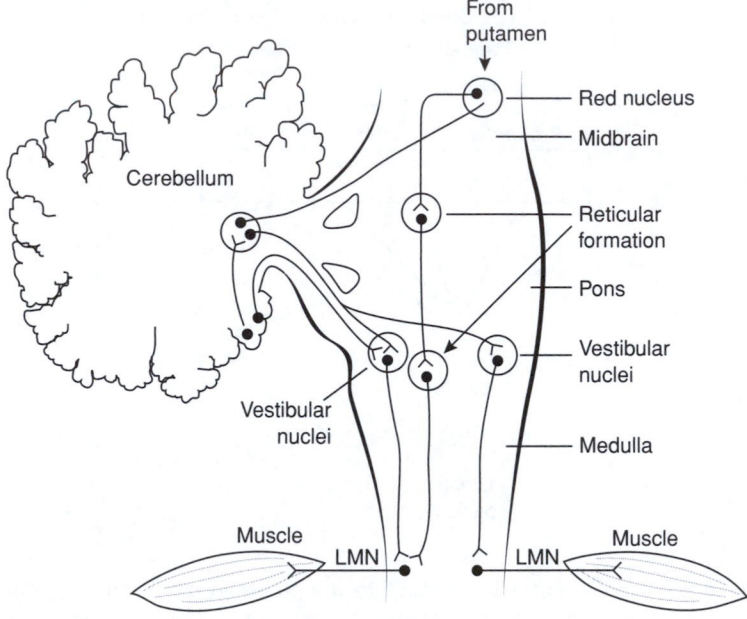

Figure 13.9 The pathways from the cerebellum that control balance by adjusting the body's skeletal muscles (see also Figure 8.3). LMN, lower motor neuron.

spinal cord. The cerebellum, like the cerebrum, is divided into a left and right **hemisphere**, both of which communicate with the rest of the brain entirely via the brain stem. This is through connections called the **cerebellar peduncles** (ped = foot; the 'cerebellar feet'), and three such peduncles exist: the **superior**, **middle** and **inferior**. The vestibular stimuli from both ears arrive at one of the three cerebellar lobes that occur within each hemisphere, the **flocculonodular lobe**, the area ultimately responsible for balance. Proprioception stimuli arrive at another cerebellar lobe, the **anterior lobe**, where posture can be maintained. The cerebellum's **posterior lobe** receives impulses from the high centres of the cerebrum via the brain stem. These cerebral connections allow the cerebellum to step in and control the fine co-ordination of voluntary movement at an unconscious level. For example, the cerebellum smooths out muscle activity that otherwise would be jerky and erratic, especially fast movements, and it determines the extent and timing of muscle fibre contractions. In this respect it also has some influence *increasing* muscle tone, providing a balance to the muscle tone function of the basal ganglia (see p. 234). It also learns and perfects the skills of **synergy**. Synergistic skills involve the ability to co-ordinate muscle activity in relation to a moving object, using visual information from the visual cortex of the cerebrum to plot the direction and speed of the moving object. It works out the muscle response required to allow the chosen part (e.g. hand or foot) to intercept with that object, such as returning a ball over the net in tennis. It means predicting ahead, since it takes time to move a limb to a new position, during which the object itself has moved. Children are born without these skills, and both synergistic skills and balance are learnt and practised from an early age. They are then pre-programmed (like many other motor skills) and function with very little or no conscious thought. A Wimbledon tennis champion must spend many hours teaching the cerebellum that particular synergistic skill. Since visual information is crucial for this function, the cerebellum has some influence and control over eyeball movements, vital in tracking moving objects.

Reflexes

Various **reflexes** exist to provide stability during movement and fast responses to adverse stimuli and are a safeguard against falling and injury (Pomfrett 2005). A reflex consists of a sensory input to the brain or cord, an integration or control centre, and a motor output to the relevant muscle group, i.e. the components of a **reflex arc** (Figure 13.10). Painful sensory impulses pass into the posterior spinal cord and cross to the front on the same side via a **connector** (or **association**) neuron to the cell body of an LMN. The impulses from this LMN pass out of the cord to the muscle, which then contracts to pull the limb away from the source of the pain. **Deep tendon** (or **stretch extensor**) reflexes include the **patellar reflex**, when the patellar tendon is tapped below the patellar bone with a clinical hammer. The **knee jerk** that follows is caused first by stretching the sensory **muscle spindle** within the thigh muscle with the hammer tap, thus sending impulses into the cord. This then activates the LMN at the same level as the sensory input, and motor impulses are sent back to the same muscle, making it contract slightly (to correct the original stretch). The **flexor** (or **withdrawal**) **response** is created by the application of painful stimuli to a limb, causing pain stimuli to pass into the cord. Again an LMN fires in response to contract the flexor muscles

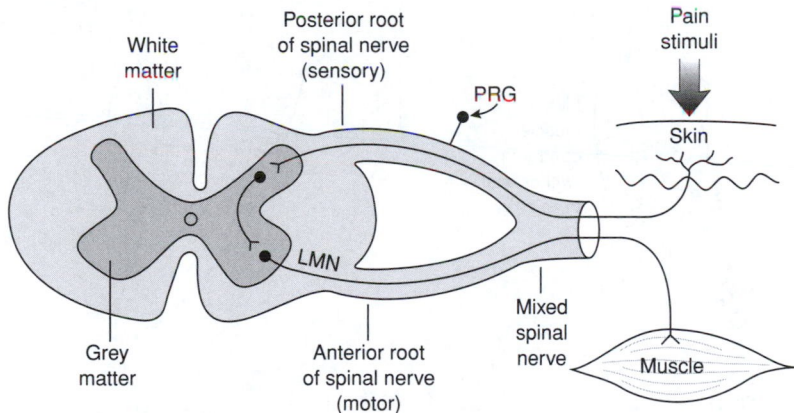

FIGURE 13.10 The reflex arc. A special sensory neuron takes painful impulses from the periphery to the cord. Impulses pass to the brain, but at the same time interneurons cross the cord from the posterior sensory to the anterior motor areas of the grey matter, and the lower motor neuron conveys an impulse to the muscles to move the part from harm. LMN, lower motor neuron; PRG, posterior root ganglion.

of that same limb while relaxing the extensor muscles. At the same time, the impulse crosses the midline in the cord and causes the opposite response in the other limb, which then extends (called the **crossed extensor response**) (Figure 13.11).

The muscles

The **end organ** of any motor system is the **muscle**, a specialist tissue with the sole function of contraction. Muscles are of three types: **skeletal muscle**, which is attached to the bones and serves to allow *voluntary* movement; **smooth muscle**, which forms the walls of internal *tubes*, such as blood vessels and the digestive tract, and is *involuntary*; and **cardiac muscle** in the heart wall, which contracts *involuntarily*. Muscle is the only tissue in the body that can itself move; anything else that moves, like bones or blood, is moved by a muscle. Muscles *pull*, but cannot *push*; but smooth muscle constructed in a ring or around a tube wall can

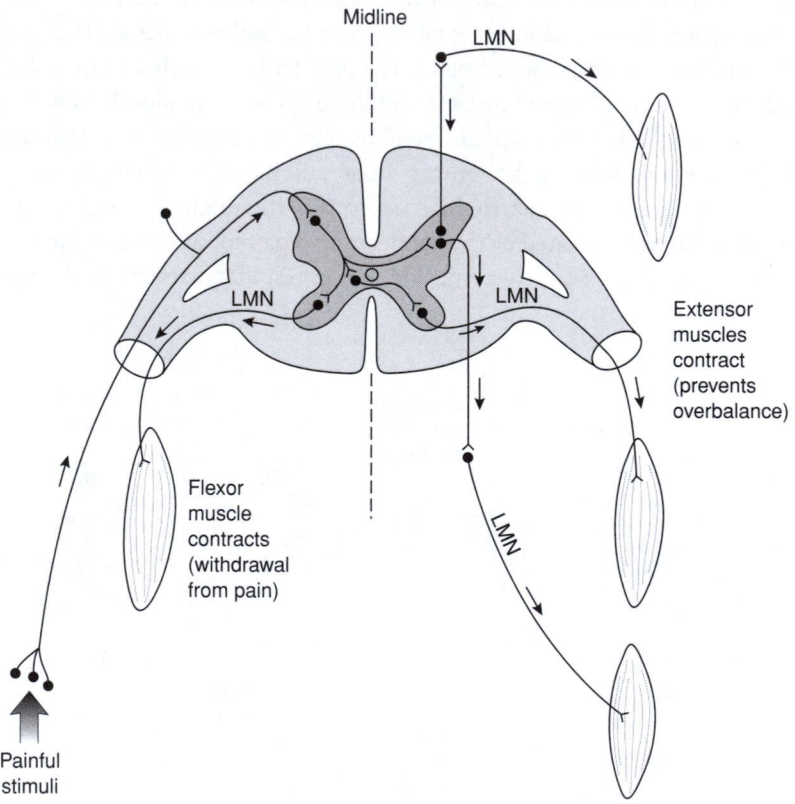

FIGURE 13.11   The cross-reflex. Painful stimuli affecting one side of the body cause flexion of the muscles on that side via the reflex arc (Figure 13.10) in order to withdraw from the pain. At the same time impulses cross to the other side and stimulate extensor muscles at several levels above and below the level affected to prevent overbalancing.

constrict to close the ring or tube lumen, e.g. a **sphincter** or the wall of the bronchus. In the limbs, skeletal muscles are set in opposing positions around joints, **antagonistic pairs**, so called because these muscles have opposing functions: one muscle to *bend* the joint (the **flexor**), and one muscle to *straighten* the joint (the **extensor**) (Figure 13.12). Contracting the flexor muscle stretches the extensor muscle, and vice versa. Muscle contraction involves moving the **insertion** (the *travelling* and mostly lower end of the muscle) towards the **origin** (the *fixed* and mostly upper end of the muscle). The nerve innervation of the various types of muscle is different: the skeletal muscle is *controlled* by the pyramidal and extra-pyramidal tract systems, the smooth muscle is *controlled* by the **autonomic nervous system** (**ANS**) and the cardiac muscle is *regulated* by the ANS. Between the nerve and the *voluntary skeletal muscle* is the **neuromuscular junction**, a gap where a neurotransmitter called **acetylcholine** is active in passing the impulse from the neuron to the muscle cells.

Movement observations

Disorders of movement can be classified according to the system that is causing the problem, i.e. pyramidal or extra-pyramidal tract disorders, basal ganglia or cerebellar disorders, or diseases of the muscles themselves. Nurses can contribute significantly to the understanding of the patient's problem, identifying the patient's needs and necessary medical interventions by observing abnormalities of movement.

Observations of movement are best achieved in conscious patients, either by watching as patients attempt movement or by requesting patients to undergo specific movements for the purpose of observation. Walking is a good opportunity to observe a patient's ability to move, whereby different forms of **gait**, i.e. the manner an individual walks, may be seen and balance can be assessed. Loss of consciousness removes all such *purposeful* movements

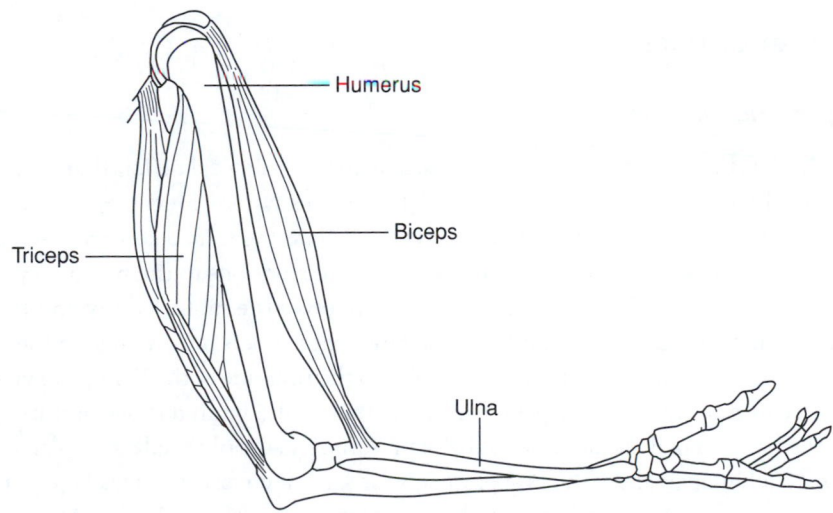

FIGURE 13.12 Antagonistic muscle pairs. In this example the flexor is the biceps and the extensor is the triceps muscles of the upper arm.

and would probably mean that any movements observed are likely to be spontaneous and probably reflex-type activities.

Neurological assessment of the motor systems is usually carried out by specialist doctors or nurses who work in neuromedical or neurosurgical units. However, all nurses should be able to identify gross abnormalities of movement in many care settings: in particular the accident and emergency or trauma unit, establishments caring for elderly people, and outpatients' departments. The basic questions to establish are:

- Can the patient walk properly, or are there noticeable difficulties with mobility, for example, dragging one foot or being unable to balance?
- Can the patient talk properly, or are there noticeable problems with speech, e.g. slurring of words? Remember, there is a major motor component to speech.
- Does the patient show any abnormal movements, such as shaking or inability to sit still?

We are all familiar with the normal and expected range and types of movement, which is why abnormalities of movement tend to become quite obvious as patients make efforts to get around and communicate.

Movement problems can be classified into **losses** and **excesses**. Losses include a reduced level of movement, called **hypokinesia** (kinetics = movement, hypo = lower than normal level), the inability to *initiate* a movement, for example, being unable to start to walk, called **akinesia** (the letter *a* before a word means 'without'), and a total loss of movement, referred to as a **paralysis**. **Paresis** is a weakness of muscle movement and is a condition similar to, but less severe than, paralysis. Excesses include **dyskinesia** (abnormal movements), **hyperkinesia** (an increase in involuntary movement, such as tremor, which is an uncontrolled shaking of limbs) and **akathisia** (motor restlessness that prevents the individual from sitting down).

Movement losses

Paralysis and weakness

A total loss of the ability to move is paralysis, a major neurological deficit that may be local (e.g. in one limb) or involve wider aspects of the nervous system. **Hemiplegia**, a paralysis of either the left or right side of the body, affects those suffering from a **cerebrovascular accident (CVA, or stroke)** to various degrees. CVAs are disruptions to the blood supply of the brain resulting in brain damage. This very often involves the motor cortex and the major pathways from this area, the pyramidal tracts. Since these tracts mostly cross in the medulla (Figure 13.1), a *left* hemiplegia indicates a stroke on the *right* side of the brain, and vice versa. The degree of movement loss depends on the extent of the brain damage and its location within the brain. Small bleeds close to the brain surface may only result in *weakness* on one side, called a **hemiparesis**, with good prospects for some recovery, whereas larger or deeper bleeds may cause profound paralysis with some permanent deficit. A CVA is an example of a UMN lesion leading to **spastic paralysis** in the longer term, where spastic means the stiffening and contracture of the muscles of the affected limbs if inadequate preventative measures are taken. The arm is held in a bent (= **flexed**) position and the spastic hemiparesis creates a characteristic gait where the leg *circles* stiffly outwards then inwards with a pointed toe while walking.

Unlike hemiplegia, **paraplegia** results in the loss of function of the lower limbs, and mobility usually requires a wheelchair. Paraplegia is often associated with spinal injuries where the cord is damaged, severing the pyramidal motor tracts at a point in the **thoracic** or **lumbar** regions. Such trauma cuts off any opportunity for the brain to control the muscles below the level of the injury. Of course, it could also affect the sensory neurons as well, causing sensation losses in the lower limbs. A similar injury higher in the spine, the **cervical** (neck) region, may include a loss of movement below this level, i.e. a **tetraplegia**, involving all four limbs and the trunk. Another cause of lower limb paralysis is **poliomyelitis**, an infectious disease that damages the cell body of the LMNs or their axons passing from the cord. LMN lesions result in a **flaccid paralysis**, where muscles of the paralysed limbs become loose and floppy (loss of muscle tone) with complete loss of reflexes, and **foot drop** (a failure of the muscles that retain the foot at the normal right angle to the leg).

The loss of the ability to perform *purposeful* movements is **apraxia** (a = without, praxia = performing movements), i.e. movements are possible but meaningless. The problem is *not* caused by simple paralysis or weakness, nor is it due to a lack of comprehension or motivation. It may be the result of a lesion in the parietal association cortex (see p. 172) along with disturbance to sensory interpretation and integration. Different forms of apraxia may occur and this depends on which side of the brain is affected (see p. 170). **Dyspraxia** (dys = difficulty; praxia = performing movements) is a difficulty in carrying out skilled movements with no evidence of disorder of the primary motor pathways. This is *not* the same as paralysis, which usually *does* involve the primary motor pathways. Apraxia and dyspraxia are functional developmental disorders of differing severity: apraxia is a total loss of purposeful movements and dyspraxia is a difficulty in carrying out skilled purposeful movements. Both disorders disturb the development of different systems, e.g. **verbal dyspraxia** (speech difficulty and delay), or **motor dyspraxia** (difficulty with body movement co-ordination, including balance and walking). A child with **motor dyspraxia** may be called a *clumsy child*.

Another motor problem is **multiple sclerosis** (**MS**), an **autoimmune disease** of the neuronal myelin sheath, which breaks down and is replaced by scar tissue (a **demyelination** disease). Autoimmune diseases occur when the body's immune system identifies part of the body as foreign (or *alien*) tissue and begins to destroy it. The reason is not fully known but viral infections of the affected tissues are suspected. MS can affect any neuron, motor or sensory, and it causes a wide range of symptoms of varying degrees that can pass from **remissions** (periods of no or few symptoms) to **relapses** (periods of worse symptoms). Those signs affecting movement include spastic limb weakness with exaggerated reflexes (UMN pyramidal signs) and an ataxia (a cerebellar sign, see p. 245).

Motor neuron disease (**MND**) is another progressive degeneration of motor neurons, this time the pyramidal (corticospinal) tract fibres, some cranial nerve nuclei and some LMNs within the cord. It causes severe movement losses involving motor control of the swallow reflex, and death occurs within a few years. The usual age of onset is 40–60 years. Now a number of genes have been identified in the causation of motor neuron disease that runs in families, and the following is some information on the main ones (Corcia *et al.* 2008):

- The gene *SOD1* (**superoxide dismutase-1**; found 1993) on chromosome 21q codes for the enzyme superoxide dismutase 1, which is a cellular defence against free radicals, which damage cells. Over 150 gene mutations are known in this gene, one of the most common being a codon change from alanine to valine.
- The gene *ANG* (**angiogenin**; found 2006) is a autosomal dominant gene on chromosome 14q which codes for a protein that is both an enzyme and a blood vessel growth factor (**angiogenesis** is the growth of new blood vessels). Patients with this gene mutation have predominant bulbar symptoms.
- The gene *TARDBP* (**TAR DNA-binding protein**) on chromosome 1p codes for the protein **TDP-43** (**TAR DNA-binding protein 43**). Normally this protein has important functions in gene transcription and translation.
- The gene *C9orf72* (**chromosome 9 open reading frame 72**; found 2011) on chromosome 9p. This is a DNA sequence repeat. The gene normally has up to 20 repeats, while sufferers have hundreds of repeats. It affects about one-third of all familial MND sufferers.
- The gene *FUS* (**fused in sarcoma**; found 2009) on chromosome 16p. It codes for a protein that has multiple functions within the nucleus of motor neurons, but mutations cause this protein to accummulate outside the nucleus.

Unfortunately there is no treatment available for MND. Three different aspects characterise this disease: (1) **progressive muscular atrophy (PMA)**; (2) **progressive bulbar palsy (PBP)**; and (3) **amyotrophic lateral sclerosis (ALS**, also known as Lou Gehrig's disease). Most of the discovered genes are linked to the causation of ALS.

Patients with this disorder will first develop one of these three aspects first, either (1) muscular atrophy; or (2) bulbar symptoms of the mouth, throat or face, including difficulty swallowing; or (3) muscle weakness with twitching and some paralysis. These symptoms will remain dominant as other symptoms occur. Most patients will eventually show signs of all three to varying degrees. Those in whom PMA is dominant have the least severe form and can have a survival rate of up to 15 years or more. PBP causes deterioration of parts of the brain stem, and it has the worst symptoms and the shortest life expectancy. It causes deterioration of swallowing, with choking on food, and muscle paralysis of the tongue and throat, including speech loss. ALS is a progressive combination of **amyotrophy**, i.e. muscle wasting caused by a loss of LMNs, and **lateral sclerosis**, a loss of UMNs in the corticospinal tracts of the spinal cord. The main features are muscular weakness and **atrophy** (= wasting of muscles), with **fasciculation** (= twitching of muscles) in two or more limbs. The intellect and sensory systems are completely unaffected and remain intact throughout.

Muscular diseases also cause weakness and paralysis. **Myasthenia gravis** is a disorder of the neuromuscular junction. Acetylcholine (see p. 239) cannot bind to the receptors properly and muscle cells are unable to sustain repeated contraction during exercise so that they fatigue quickly. The receptors are blocked by antibodies, plus there is a reduced amount of acetylcholine available at the synapse. The **thymus gland**, part of the lymphatic and immune systems in the chest, may be the site of production of the antibodies concerned, and removal of this gland, plus drugs to improve acetylcholine function, are options for treatment.

The various **muscular dystrophies** form a group of disabling diseases involving the muscle itself. Several of these disorders are genetically inherited, such as **Duchenne muscular dystrophy (DMD)**. This disease is the most common in the group and affects mostly boys because the gene involved (the *DMD* gene) is on the X chromosome. Normally the gene codes for the protein **dystrophin** found in muscles. The role of dytrophin is to strengthen and protect muscle proteins as they contract and relax. In DMD, muscles become weakened and damaged due to repeated muscle contraction, leading to deterioration in walking and other movement, with complete mobility loss by the time of adolescence. It can affect cardiac muscle, and life expectancy may only be 20–29 years.

Myopathies (myo = muscle, path = disease) is the term used to describe a failure of muscle development with weakness, muscle pain and cramps early in life, again often due to genetic inheritance. The weakness may be severe and cause major mobility difficulties that can be progressive throughout life.

Increased muscle tone (rigidity)

Disturbances to basal ganglia function, as in **Parkinson's disease (PD)**, can cause an increase in muscle tone, known as **hypertonia**; muscles become rigid and fail to allow full body movement. In Parkinson's disease, the limbs are severely limited in function; the legs in particular create a shuffling gait and sufferers cannot lift their feet properly. The body takes on a forward stance and often moves faster than the feet can; patients may therefore lose their balance and fall. Nurses observing these patients should be aware of the potential for injury. The muscle tone increase is due to the failure of the basal ganglia's role of inhibiting excess muscle tone; an excess that is therefore passed onto the muscle. James Parkinson, a Shoreditch apothecary surgeon, described the condition as *paralysis agitans* (i.e. agitated paralysis), which neatly describes the two main features: rigidity and tremor. Parkinson's disease is progressive due to the relentless destruction of the substantia nigra, with a corresponding gradual loss of the neurotransmitter dopamine in the pathway from the substantia nigra to the corpus striatum, the **nigrostriatal pathway**. The reason for the loss of cells in the substantia nigra is unknown and untreatable, and will eventually lead to the patient's death. It would appear that the symptoms do not occur until the dopamine loss reaches 80%, indicating the **asymptomatic** (= without symptoms) onset of this disease, which is very gradual over a number of years. On average, the age that symptoms become obvious is about 60 years or more, but the process leading to those symptoms must have started earlier in life. There is no cure, but treatment is aimed at the replacement of the dopamine in this part of the brain, effectively reducing the symptoms, particularly the rigidity, and therefore improving the quality of life.

Other forms of rigidity are **decortication**, an *abnormal flexion response*, and **decerebration**, an *abnormal extensor response* of the limbs (Figure 13.13). The symptoms of these disorders and their causes are shown in Table 13.1. Decerebrate symptoms can be severe enough to include stiff clenching of the jaw, neck extension and arching of the back.

Explanation of the terms is as follows:

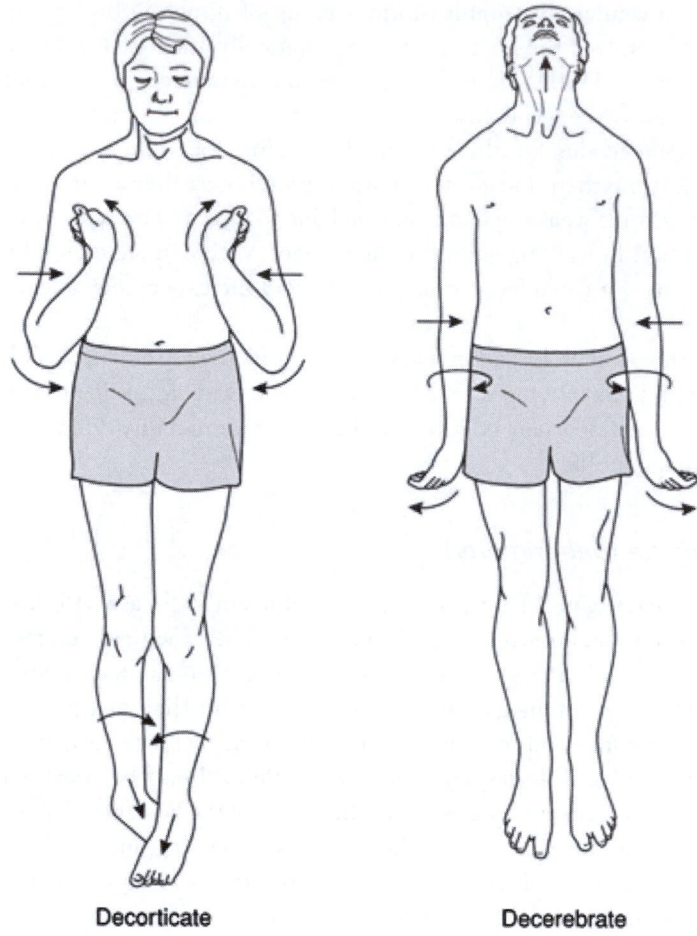

Decorticate   **Decerebrate**

FIGURE 13.13 Decorticate and decerebrate symptoms. In decorticate symptoms the elbows, wrists and fingers are flexed with adduction of the arms, the legs are inwardly rotated and the feet are plantar flexed. In decerebrate symptoms the head is extended with the jaws clenched shut, the arms are adducted with stiffly extended elbows, the forearms are hyperpronated and the wrists and fingers are flexed, the legs are stiffly extended and the feet are plantar flexed.

TABLE 13.1 The symptoms and causes of decortication and decerebration

Rigidity	Arms	Legs	Cause
Decortication	Hyperflexion of each of the joints with adduction of the limb	Extension of legs with internal rotation and plantar flexion of foot	A high cerebral lesion interrupting the corticospinal (pyramidal) tracts
Decerebration	Elbow extension, wrist flexion with limb adduction and pronated forearms	Stiff extension of legs with plantar flexion of foot	A hypothalamic or thalamic lesion involving the brain stem

- **Adduction** is movement of a limb *towards* the midline of the body, i.e. held against the side of the body.
- **Internal rotation** is a twisting of the limb *inwards*.
- **Pronation** is a *palm downwards* position of the forearm and hand (Figure 13.13).
- **Extension** is straightening of a limb.
- **Flexion** (or **hyperflexion**) is bending (or excessive bending) of joints.
- **Plantar flexion** is a downward movement of the foot; the toes point away from the body at an angle of as much as 45° from the normal right-angle position of the foot.

Ataxia

Ataxia is a difficult and abnormal gait, or walking, with specific forms of ataxia indicating particular neuromuscular disorders (Bastian 1997). The gait of spastic hemiparesis seen in CVA and the shuffling gait of Parkinson's disease have both been described (see p. 240 and p. 243). **Cerebellar ataxia** is caused by a disorder of the cerebellum or its tracts. It produces an unsteady staggering gait with difficulty on turning and balance loss when the feet come together, so the feet are held apart. **Sensory ataxia** is an unsteady gait, again with feet wide apart. During walking, each leg is lifted high, followed by the foot being *slapped* on the floor. Since the patient is unable to feel the floor because of absent sensory feedback, it becomes necessary for the patient to watch the ground to ensure his foot is safely in contact before putting any weight on it. This is due to a destruction of the somatic sensory pathways of the spinal cord, as in **tabes dorsalis**, a spinal cord complication of the infectious disease **syphilis**. **Scissor gait** is caused by a bilateral spastic weakness of the leg muscles. The legs are moved slowly forwards over short steps; the thighs tend to cross over each other in turn.

Movement excesses

Tremor

The uncontrollable and involuntary shaking seen in the limbs of sufferers of Parkinson's disease comes in two forms: a **coarse** tremor noticed in the whole limb and a **fine** tremor found in the hands and fingers. This fine tremor has been called **pill-rolling**, since this is the action taken during the manual production of pills before mechanisation and quality control. Parkinson's tremor disappears as the limbs are put into conscious motion, but returns at rest. Tremor is a very noticeable symptom and is very destructive of the patient's confidence, motor activities and natural behaviour patterns (Tarsy *et al.* 2010).

Tremor may also be the result of multiple sclerosis, strokes, brain injury, various neurodegenerative disorders, and even excess consumption of some drugs (e.g. amphetamines and caffeine), alcohol abuse and withdrawal, hypoglycaemia (low blood glucose levels), sleep deprivation, thyroid hormone excess, anxiety, and stress. Some nutritional deficiencies (e.g. of magnesium and niacin) also show tremor as a symptom.

Athetosis, chorea and ballism

Huntington's disease is a genetically inherited disorder caused by a gene mutation on the fourth chromosome (Bentley 1999). It results in a progressive degeneration of several areas of the brain, in particular, the **corpus striatum** (composed of the caudate nucleus and putamen) of the basal ganglia, with cell losses in the frontal and parietal lobes of the cerebral cortex. Unwanted involuntary movements are a characteristic of this disease, and these are **athetosis** (slow writhing movements of the limbs, face and tongue) and **chorea** (fast twitching of whole limbs and body). If these two movements occur together, the words are combined, i.e. **choreoathetosis**. The major distinctions between them are the speed (*sudden* chorea movements compared with the *slow* athetosis movements) and the nature of the movement (in chorea, *jerky* and *twitching* movements that are not repeated; in athetosis, *writhing* movements). Observers will note that the patient appears to be unable to sit still. Chorea can sometimes occur in children (Sydenham's chorea), often as a result **of rheumatic fever**, caused mostly by an immune response to the bacterium *Streptococcus*. The child or adolescent shows sudden, irregular and uncontrolled movements of no real purpose, but, unlike Huntington's disease, this is not a permanent problem (Gasser and Kieburtz 2000).

Uncontrolled violent movements of a whole limb, involving flinging the arm suddenly in any direction, is called **ballism**. The appearance of this phenomenon may be sudden and frightening. **Monoballism** is the term used if a single limb only is involved, and **hemiballism** indicates that both limbs on one side are affected. The violent nature of this movement is due to the involvement of the **subthalamic nucleus** in the lesion.

The immobile patient

Mobility is a precious asset that we usually take for granted. Immobility reduces independence to varying degrees, and this can easily remove some or all of the patient's ability to sustain the very basic needs of life. In many cases, these needs must be provided by the family or nurse. But practical care alone is not enough, observations of the immobile patient are critical to understanding the patient's needs, for identifying the early stages of the complications of immobility, and for maintaining the patient's progress towards mobility. In this observations checklist, the complications directly caused by immobility are shown in *italics*:

Observations checklist

Observing the skin is vital for:

- Assessing for any *dehydration*, i.e. when the skin is dry and can be pulled into folds that remain when released. Dehydration is a severe lack of fluids in the tissues, both the **intracellular** fluids (intra = inside, cellular = the cells) and the **extracellular** (extra = outside, also know as **tissue fluid**, see Chapter 5).
- Preventing **decubitus ulcers** (**pressure sores**), caused both by constricted blood supply to the tissues when compressed by body weight and by friction eroding the surface of the

skin when the patient is moved around the bed. Assessment of a patient's risk of skin breakdown is often made using the **Waterlow scale** (Baxter 2008) or the **Norton scale** (Lewko *et al.* 2005) (see Chapter 9).

- Assessing for *poor personal hygiene* and maintaining cleanliness.

Observing the mouth is vital for:

- Preventing dehydration, which would result in a *dry mouth with poor saliva production*.
- Preventing *infections*, which would cause red, swollen gums and halitosis (foul-smelling breath), pain and difficulty with eating, and the risk of complications, such as throat, chest, ear and brain infections.

Observing the urine is vital for:

- Assessing the output to maintain fluid balance and reduce the risk of *renal disorders* (see Chapter 7).
- Preventing *urinary tract infections* (see Chapter 7).

Observing the bowel function is vital for:

- Assessing the output, to prevent *constipation or diarrhoea* (see Chapter 8).

Observing the level of consciousness is vital for:

- Preventing *confusion or coma* (see Chapter 10).

Observing respiration is vital for:

- Maintaining adequate ventilation and oxygenation (see Chapter 4).
- Preventing *chest infections* (see Chapter 4).

Observing body temperature is vital for:

- Assessing the patient's ability to control body temperature (see Chapter 1).
- Preventing or detecting any underlying *infections*.

Observing the ability to communicate is vital for:

- Assessing mental function, especially mood, which may be *depressed*;
- Assessing of problems such as *pain*, and maintaining a pain-free state (see Chapter 11).

Observing the ability to eat and drink is vital for:

- Assessing the patient's nutritional status (see Chapter 6).
- Preventing *hunger, dehydration* and *malnutrition*.

Observing the sleep cycle pattern is vital for:

- Assessing that the patient has enough rest.

Observing the pattern of mobility possible in each limb and joint is vital for:

- Assessing what mobility the patient can achieve and maximising this to prevent *joint stiffness* and *muscle atrophy* (muscle atrophy = wasting of the muscles, or loss of muscle bulk) (see p. 104).

- Assessing what mobility assistance the patient will need in terms of professional help (such as physiotherapy) and mobility aids (such as a wheelchair) to prevent excessive periods of immobility.

With modern technology available, and given what is known about the complications of bed rest, mobility should be achieved or maximised as quickly and efficiently as possible. Immobility must *not* mean a lifetime, or even long periods, confined to bed.

Key points

The neurobiology of human movement

- Pre-programming of movement is the essence of the learning process and allows movement to occur at a subconscious level.
- The motor cortex cells are arranged in a manner that reflects the basic body plan.
- The pyramidal tracts descend from the motor cortex.
- The pyramidal system is two-neuronal, consisting of an upper motor neuron (UMN) from brain to cord and a lower motor neuron (LMN) from cord to muscle.
- The extra-pyramidal system controls voluntary movement at a subconscious level.
- The basal ganglia have a role in controlling slow, sustained movements and in maintaining muscle tone.
- Muscle tone is a state of tension of the muscle essential for contraction.
- The cerebellum is important for balance, posture, smoothing out muscle movements and synergistic skills, i.e. the ability to match muscle activity to a moving object.
- Reflexes provide stability during movement and fast responses to adverse stimuli. A reflex arc has a sensory input to the cord, a control centre and a motor output to the muscle.
- Muscles are of three types: skeletal muscle attached to bones, allowing voluntary movement; smooth muscle forming walls of internal tubes, allowing involuntary movement; and cardiac muscle in the heart wall.
- The various types of muscle have different nerve innervation: skeletal muscle is controlled by the pyramidal and extra-pyramidal systems, smooth muscle is controlled by the autonomic nervous system, and cardiac muscle is regulated by the autonomic nervous system.

Disorders involving movement

1 Paralysis is a loss of movement: hemiplegia is paralysis of either the left or right half of the body, paraplegia is paralysis of the lower half of the body and tetraplegia is paralysis of the body from the neck down.
2 Cerebrovascular accident (CVA) or stroke is a bleed into the brain or an obstruction of the blood supply to the brain.

3 Poliomyelitis is an infectious disease that damages the cell body of the lower motor neuron.

4 Multiple sclerosis is an autoimmune disease of the myelin sheath, which breaks down and is replaced by scar tissue.

5 Myasthenia gravis is the inability of acetylcholine to bind at the neuromuscular junction, which causes the muscles to be unable to sustain repeated contraction.

6 Muscular dystrophies are often genetically inherited. Duchenne muscular dystrophy affects mostly boys. Fat accumulates in the main muscles during childhood, leading to deterioration of walking with complete mobility loss by the time of adolescence.

7 Parkinson's disease is a degeneration of the basal ganglia, causing an increase in muscle tone resulting in rigidity and tremor.

8 Decortication is an abnormal flexion response caused by a high cerebral lesion interrupting the corticospinal (pyramidal) tracts. Decerebration is an abnormal extensor response caused by a hypothalamic or thalamic lesion involving the brain stem.

9 Ataxia is difficult or abnormal gait (method of walking).

10 Motor neuron disease is a progressive degeneration of neurons of the pyramidal and bulbar tracts.

11 Huntington's disease is a genetically inherited disorder resulting in a progressive degeneration of the corpus striatum with cell losses in the frontal and parietal lobes.

12 Unwanted involuntary movements are called chorea (sudden and jerky movements) and athetosis (slow writhing movements).

References

Anderson M. E. (2001) Basal ganglia and the regulation of movement. *Current Opinion in Neurobiology*, 1–7. DOI: 10: 1038/npg.els.0000020.

Bastian A. J. (1997) Mechanisms of ataxia. *Physical Therapy*, **77**(6): 672–675.

Baxter S. (2008) Assessing pressure ulcer risk in long-term care using the Waterlow scale. *Nursing Older People*, **20**(7): 34–38.

Bentley P. (1999) Dementia demystified. *Nursing Times* **95**(45): 47–49.

Corcia P., Praline J., Vourch P. and Andres C. (2008) Genetics of motor neuron disorders. *Revue Neurologique*, **164**(2): 115–130.

Gasser T. and Kieburtz K. (2000) Huntington's disease and Sydenham's chorea. *Movement Disorders* **125**(19): 2214–2217.

Lewko J., Demianiuk M., Krot E., Krajewska-Kułak E., Sierakowska M., Nyklewicz W., and Jankowiak B. (2005) Assessment of risk for pressure ulcers using the Norton scale in nursing practice. *Roczniki Akademii Medycznej w Bialymstoku Annales Academiae Medicae Bialostocensis*, **50**(Suppl. 1): 148–151.

Pomfrett C. J. D. (2005) Neural reflexes. *Anaesthesia and Intensive Care Medicine*, **6**(5): 145–150.

Tarsy D., Hurtig H. I. and Dashe J. F. (2010) Overview of tremor. *Science*, 1–16.

Chapter 14 **Drug side effects, interactions and allergies**

- Introduction
- Pharmacokinetics and pharmacodynamics
- Drug side effects
- Drug interactions
- Drug allergies
- Key points
- References

Introduction

Drugs are now, and have been for many years, the main treatment used in combating the causes and symptoms of disease. However, drugs often cause unwanted side (or toxic) effects, including allergies, and may also interact with each other when taken simultaneously. Such problems can cause misery, severe health problems and sometimes even death of the individual (Gottlieb 2001). In the past, serious side effects have resulted in patients being reluctant to take their medication and others being admitted to hospital (Gutierrez 2010). Some drugs have been rapidly withdrawn from medical use because the side effects were unacceptable. Clearly side effects, interactions and allergies are a serious problem, and this chapter addresses the known biology behind some of the most important and most common drug side effects, drug interactions and allergies.

Pharmacokinetics and pharmacodynamics

Pharmacology is the study of drugs, but this is an umbrella term incorporating several more specific sciences, the main ones being pharmacokinetics and pharmacodynamics.

Pharmacokinetics ('drug movement') is the study of the way drugs move through the body, from the point of entry to the point of exit. There are four stages:

1 absorption (the point of entry);
2 distribution;

3 metabolism; and
4 elimination (the point of exit).

Drug side effects, and particularly drug interactions, can occur at any of these stages.

Pharmacodynamics is the study of how drugs work, or how they do what they are expected to do. There are many different drugs, and to study their functions requires detail at the cellular level. Many drugs work through receptors on cell surfaces. Again, drug side effects and drug interactions can occur during the pharmacodynamic process.

A commonly used way to distinguish pharmacokinetics from pharmacodynamics is to say the former is the way the body handles the drug, and the latter is the way the drug handles the body.

Drug side effects

Drug side effects (or sometimes called 'toxic effects') can be defined as those effects that the drug has on the body that are seen as unpleasant, unwanted and harmful to the patient taking them, and are mostly unrelated to the expected function of the drug. However, there are examples of drug side effects that are, or can be, beneficial or therapeutic to the patient. In either case they usually occur through a different mechanism separate from that for which the drug was given (i.e. separate to the pharmacodynamic activity).

Side effects are known to involve almost every body system, but some systems are more affected than others. The most likely effect would be with the system responsible for the drug's entry into the body, i.e. the first point of contact. For example, the digestive system is more affected mainly because most of our drugs are administered by mouth, so it is the first system to be in contact with the medication and the first system to process the drug. Similarly, topically administered drugs (i.e. drugs in creams rubbed in through the skin) and subcutaneous injections (injected just under the skin surface) can cause skin reactions.

Gastrointestinal (GI) side effects

It is amazing how many drugs can be given by mouth, considering what oral medication is subjected to. Oral drugs have to survive chemical attack from digestive enzymes and wide changes in pH, from acid to alkaline. Gastrointestinal (GI) side effects, such as nausea and vomiting, diarrhoea, or constipation, are probably the most common side effects listed for most drugs. Thankfully most of the GI side effects are mild and not life-threatening, although they can be unpleasant. Not only can drugs given by mouth upset the digestive tract, intravenous injections can also cause these GI side effects quite quickly by affecting the brain centres that control digestion.

Nausea and vomiting

Nausea (the feeling of sickness) and vomiting are very common side effects of drugs because oral drugs may irritate the mucosal lining of the stomach, and because both oral and injected drugs may stimulate and activate the chemoreceptor trigger zone (CTZ) in the brain stem (Figure 8.2, p. 138). Absorbed drugs (or their metabolites) stimulate and activate the CTZ via the blood circulation. Local mucosal irritation sends sensory stimuli to the brain stem via the vagus nerve (cranial nerve X, Figure 8.4, p. 140). Chapter 8 discusses vomiting and the major drugs that cause nausea and vomiting

Diarrhoea and constipation

The problems of constipation and diarrhoea are discussed in Chapter 8, and morphine, a drug well known for its constipating side effect, is highlighted (see p. 136).

Indigestion (dyspepsia)

Dyspepsia is a collection of stomach-related symptoms, including a feeling of bloating and being overfull from excess gas, 'heartburn' (the burning pain caused by gastric acid refluxing into the lower oesophagus), and upper abdominal pain and distension. Acidic drugs, notably the non-steroidal anti-inflammatory (NSAI) drugs, may induce dyspepsia, and sometimes even gastric bleeding, by two different mechanisms. First, the acidic drug molecules can cause direct irritation of the gastric mucosa of the inner lining. Some aspirin products are **enteric-coated**, which is a protective coating over the tablet to reduce this gastric irritation. The coating dissolves once the tablet gets further down the digestive tract. Second, the drug inhibits the enzyme **cyclo-oxygenase (COX)**, which occurs in two forms, COX1 and COX2 (see p. 201). By blocking these enzymes, there is a loss of production of certain prostaglandins (locally produced chemicals) that normally protect the gastric mucosa against stomach acidity. With this protection lost, the stomach lining becomes inflamed and irritated by its own hydrochloric acid (HCl) production. NSAI drugs that are COX2-specific are more gastric-protective with fewer GI side effects (see p. 201) (Makins and Ballinger 2003).

Anorexia

Anorexia is loss of appetite, and this would accompany any patient suffering from the drug side effects of nausea and vomiting, and possibly also those with chronic constipation. Drugs that cause these problems will also be listed as a cause of anorexia. The consequence of prolonged anorexia is weight loss and nutrient deficiencies, notably a loss of energy food intake.

The opioid drugs, such as morphine and diamorphine (heroin), are well known to cause appetite loss. They bind to opioid receptors in the brain. These receptors are called **mu (µ) kappa (κ)** and **delta (δ)** (see also p. 202, and drowsiness, p. 260). Morphine activity on the mu receptor in particular suppresses brain function because the receptor is inhibitory (i.e. they reduce brain function). Various parts of the brain are involved in appetite control (Blows 2011), and activation of mu receptors by opioid drugs will lead to suppression of these appetite systems.

Central nervous system (CNS) side effects

Drug side effects involving the central nervous system occur in many different types and severity, dependent on which part of the brain is involved. Drugs entering the brain must first cross the blood–brain barrier. This cellular barrier controls what crosses into the brain from the blood circulation, and this also applies to everything, including drugs. Some drugs can cross without needing help, but others do need help (in the form of transport proteins), while some are unable to cross at all. It is remarkable how so many drugs do cross into the brain unaided and contribute to both beneficial and adverse effects on the brain.

Antimuscarinic side effects

Acetylcholine (ACh), a brain neurotransmitter, binds to two acetylcholine receptor types: the nicotinic and muscarinic receptors. They are named after two alkaloids (nicotine and muscarine, from plants and mushrooms respectively) that bind to them in laboratory conditions, although the natural binding agent (i.e. the ligand) in the brain is acetylcholine. Acetylcholine is the neurotransmitter found in the autonomic nervous system (ANS), i.e. the sympathetic and parasympathetic systems. Both these parts of the ANS are two-neuron systems (i.e. they involve two neurons) passing between the central nervous system (brain and cord) and the target organ. The first synapses, occurring between the two neurons in both systems, are the pre-ganglionic synapses, and these use acetylcholine. The terminal synapse in the target organ for the parasympathetic system also uses acetylcholine. The terminal synapse in the target organ for the sympathetic system uses noradrenaline (see Figure 14.1).

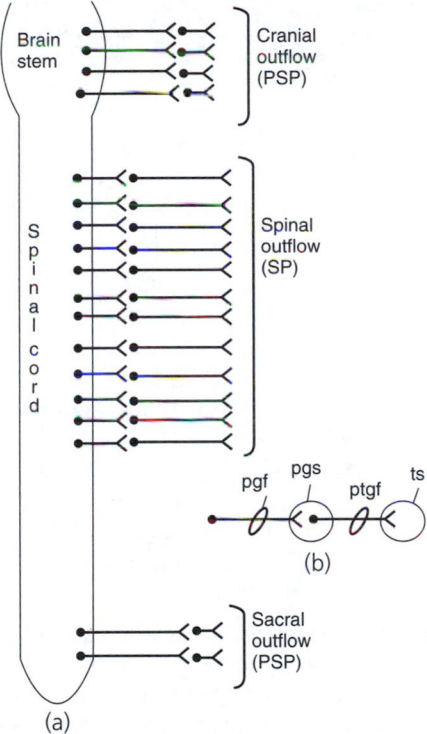

FIGURE 14.1   The two parts of the autonomic nervous system (ANS). (a) The parasympathetic (PSP) cranial outflow comes from the brain stem (via cranial nerves III, VII, IX and X) and the sacral outflow comes from the lower end of the spinal cord. The sympathetic (SP) outflow comes from the thoracic section of the spinal cord. (b) Both systems involve two neurons from the source to the terminal organ: the pre-ganglionic fibre (pgf) or neuron and a post-ganglionic fibre (ptgf) or neuron. The pre-ganglionic synapse (pgs) in both systems use acetylcholine (ACh), and the terminal synapse (ts) at the target organ uses acetylcholine in the parasympathetic system, and noradrenaline in the sympathetic system.

Antimuscarinic drugs (also called muscarinic antagonists) block the muscarinic receptors, and therefore block activity of the parasympathetic system. They are sometimes used to treat a range of conditions such as Parkinson's disease and motion sickness, and even used in optical diagnostics (see blurred vision, p. 255). However, antimuscarinic side effects are caused when other drugs, i.e. those drugs *not* used for their affect on the acetylcholine in these systems, then bind to the muscarinic receptor and prevent acetylcholine from binding. Typical antimuscarinic side effects include **dilated pupils**, **urine retention**, **constipation**, **dry mouth**, **dry eyes**, **blurred vision** and **palpitations** (Figure 14.2).

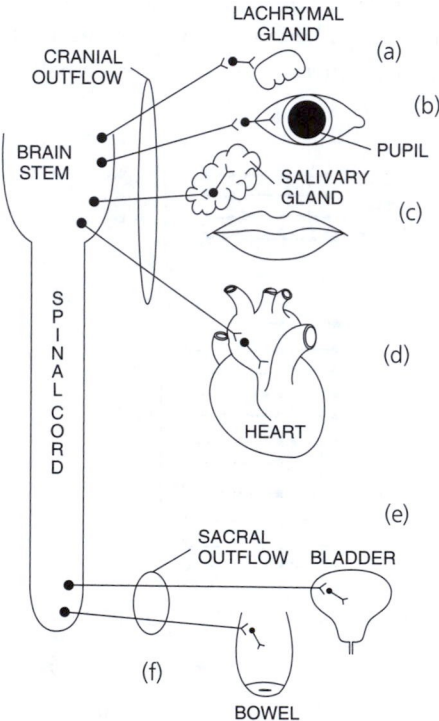

FIGURE 14.2 Antimuscarinic drug side effects. These are caused by drugs blocking the muscarinic receptors in the parasympathetic system, and therefore stopping acetylcholine (ACh) from binding. This prevents parasympathetic activity of the target organ. The effects of this parasympathetic blockage are as follows: (a) *dry eyes* are due to the lack of lachrymal gland activity (lachrymal glands normally produce fluid that lubricates the eyes); (b) *pupil dilation* and blurred vision are due to reduced parasympathetic control of the intraocular eye muscles affecting the pupil size and the lens; (c) *dry mouth* is due to changes in the salivary gland activity caused by loss of parasympathetic stimulation; (d) *palpitations* may occur if the parasympathetic (vagus nerve, cranial nerve X) input is reduced to the heart and the sympathetic input takes over, increasing the heart rate and force of contraction; (e) *urine retention* happens when the parasympathetic bladder-emptying mechanism is lost and the bladder fills with urine; (f) *constipation* is similarly due to loss of the parasympathetic bowel-emptying mechanism and the sympathetic mechanism takes over, retaining the bowel content.

Dilated pupils

Dilated pupils allow bright light to enter the eye and this can cause adverse effects to the retina. Pupil constriction is activated by the parasympathetic nervous system, and drugs blocking the muscarinic receptors prevent this parasympathetic pupillary constriction, with sympathetic dilation taking over control of pupil size and causing wide pupillary dilation.

Blurred vision

Atropine is a **cycloplegic drug** (i.e. it paralyses the **ciliary muscles** of the eye). There are other drugs that do this, e.g. cyclopentolate, homatropine and scopolamine, and these are used in ophthalmic medicine to dilate the pupil of the eye during examination (i.e. they are called **mydriatics**; mydriasis = pupil dilation). They work by blocking muscarinic receptors (i.e. they are muscarinic antagonists), which prevents parasympathetic activity on the muscles of the pupil and allows sympathetic activity to dilate the pupil of the eye (see dilated pupils, p. 218). **Cycloplegia** means paralysis of the ciliary muscles, which are the muscles responsible for changing the shape of the lens for the purpose of accommodation (i.e. focusing on objects). With the muscles paralysed, the lens adopts a relaxed shape with corresponding loss of accommodation. This is done for the purpose of further visual tests and as part of the treatment for uveitis (an inflammatory disease of the eye). The side effect of these intraocular changes of the lens shape is blurred vision. Since these drugs are given locally (i.e. directly into the eye), they have little effect systemically.

Urine retention and constipation

Urine retention is a state of being unable to pass urine, and the urine accumulates in the bladder to cause an acute emergency, requiring urgent treatment in the form of catheter drainage. Emptying the bladder (and the bowels) is a function of the parasympathetic nervous system (Figure 14.1) and muscarinic blockade by drugs reduces or even stops bladder and bowel emptying (i.e. constipation, see Figure 8.1, p. 134 and Figure 14.2).

Dry mouth

A dry mouth is due to the reduction of salivary gland stimulation by the parasympathetic nervous system. This system normally causes the glands to produce a watery type of saliva (the sympathetic system causes a thicker form of saliva). Drugs that block the parasympathetic muscarinic receptors cause a reduction of the salivary gland's ability to produce watery saliva. This loss of watery saliva results in a dry mouth, and, if not corrected, this ultimately leads to a dirty mouth and all the complications this creates (see p. 85).

Dry eyes

A similar situation occurs with the **lachrymal glands,** i.e. the glands that produce lachrymal fluid that bathes the eyes. Antimuscarinic side effects include **dry eyes** because the drug blocks the parasympathetic activity of these glands. Dry eyes can result in corneal ulceration and potential blindness if they are not lubricated often.

Palpitations

Palpitations are caused by muscarinic blocking drugs reducing the parasympathetic nerve branch to the heart. This is the vagus nerve, which normally slows the heart rate down, and the drugs reduce this vagus nerve activity, thus allowing the sympathetic system to speed up the heart rate and increase the force of contraction. These increases in cardiac parameters sometimes result in the patient experiencing beating or fluttering of the heart.

Extra-pyramidal effects

The **extra-pyramidal system** controls skeletal (voluntary) muscle activity subconsciously. It involves the **basal ganglia**, five nuclei located deep in the brain. Two of these nuclei, the **putamen** and **caudate nucleus**, make up the **corpus striatum**. Between the corpus striatum and a third area, the **substantia nigra**, is a neuronal pathway that uses **dopamine** as the neurotransmitter (i.e. it is **dopaminergic**). This is the **nigrostriatal pathway** (*nigro* = starts in the substantia nigra; *striatal* = ends in the corpus striatum) (Figure 14.3).

Being dopaminergic, it uses dopamine receptors in the corpus striatum, and therefore the pathway is susceptible to blockage by **dopamine antagonist** drugs (dopamine receptor

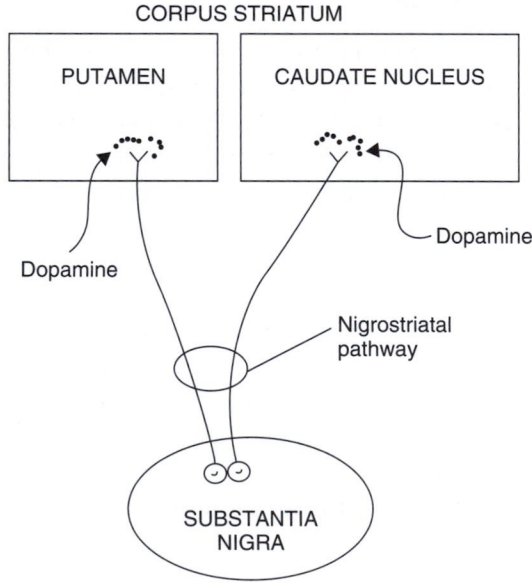

FIGURE 14.3 The nigrostriatal pathway. This starts in the substantia nigra and passes to the corpus striatum (an amalgamation of the putamen and caudate nucleus). It uses dopamine as the neurotransmitter at the synapses.

blocking drugs, e.g. the antipsychotics). The extra-pyramidal side effects from these drugs include tremor and rigidity.

Tremor and rigidity

Tremor is an involuntary, rhythmic repeated muscle movement (shaking), often seen in the limbs, especially the upper limbs, which then shake backwards and forwards. Fine tremor of the hands and fingers is also seen. **Rigidity** means stiff muscles with corresponding loss of movement, and is due to excessive **muscle tone**. Drugs blocking the dopamine receptors in the corpus striatum reduce the activity of the nigrostriatal pathway, and the loss of function of this pathway is the cause of these side effects. They are often referred to as **Parkinsonism** because they look like the symptoms of **Parkinson's disease (PD)**, but, unlike the disease, Parkinsonism can be mostly reversed if the drug dosage is reduced or the medication removed. The exception is **tardive dyskinesia**, a problem of uncontrollable, involuntary movements of the face, eyes, mouth, jaw, tongue and lips. It is seen in long-term use of dopamine antagonists (antipsychotic) drugs (i.e. *tardive* = very slow onset, 20 years or more). The long-term use of these drugs can cause permanent changes to the nigrostriatal pathway. The evidence points towards a state of hypersensitivity of the D2 dopamine receptor in the nigrostriatal pathway, although this remains to be confirmed.

Other possible Parkinsonism drug side effects include the following (*kinesia* = movement; *tonia* = muscle tone):

- **Akinesia**, inability to start movements, e.g. inability to rise from a chair or hesitation before walking. It appears to be due to low cell activity in dopamine pathways related to movement, i.e. the basal ganglia.
- **Akathisia**, motor restlessness, e.g. inability to sit still, seen mostly as a side effect of the antipsychotic drugs but sometimes seen in Parkinson's disease, possibly again as a side effect of the drugs used to treat the disease. In akathisia, the brain shows higher than normal levels of noradrenaline, and this in turn may be due to dysfunction of the N-methyl-D-aspartic acid (NMDA) glutamate receptors in the brain. Noradrenaline has an alerting effect on the brain, i.e. it excites the brain into action and motor restlessness appears to be the result of over-activity of either the motor cortex or the basal ganglia. Noradrenaline itself is regulated to some extent by glutamate acting on the NMDA receptor.
- **Dyskinesia** is a reduction of voluntary movements, which are difficult to perform or distorted. This is often combined with some abnormal spontaneous involuntary movements such as chorea (regular involuntary movements of head, neck and trunk). It can be a side effect of antipsychotic drugs or levodopa (i.e. drugs affecting the basal ganglia).
- **Bradykinesia** is slowness of movements throughout the full range of movement. It is a key feature of Parkinson's disease but rarely seen in Parkinsonism drug side effects.
- **Dystonia** is a wide range of dysfunction of muscle activity and muscle co-ordination problems causing postural abnormalities, muscle spasms (caused by involuntary movements) and muscle pain. It can be due to drug side effects (notably the antipsychotic drugs), but is also seen in various disorders where drugs are clearly not the cause.

- **Ataxia** is abnormal gait (gait = the way one walks) induced by a gross lack of muscle co-ordination. It involves any brain area that is responsible for involuntary muscle co-ordination, such as the cerebellum. As a drug side effect it is seen mainly as a result of drugs that have a depressive effect on the brain. Alcohol intoxication is a major cause of ataxia, but it can occur with the anticonvulsant drugs, cannabis, lithium and a range of illicit drugs. Any drug that is an NMDA glutamate receptor antagonist can cause ataxia.

Other CNS side effects

Fatigue

Fatigue (lethargy or exhaustion) is a profound feeling of tiredness and lacking energy (weakness). A range of different drugs are known to cause fatigue, in particular, beta-blockers and cancer chemotherapy (causing **cancer fatigue syndrome, CFS**). The mechanism by which drugs cause fatigue is elusive, and many factors appear to be involved. Chief among these factors is a drug-induced **anaemia**, a reduction in the oxygen-carrying capability of the blood caused by the effects of the drugs reducing the red blood cell numbers produced by the bone marrow. Other factors involve drug-related changes in hormones and cytokine production, and the direct effect of drugs on some brain areas. The brain areas affected appear to be parts of the cerebrum (the prefrontal and temporal cortex), the anterior cingulate and cerebellum. The evidence points to an abnormality with the use of fatty acids as an energy source leading to low neurotransmitter production (Kuratsune *et al.* 2002).

Tinnitus

Tinnitus is the presence of a constant sound in the ears, often a ringing sound but it can be a buzzing or some other sound. It may be very quiet, and therefore largely ignored, or loud, causing some distress. Some days it can be worse than others. It occurs both as a symptom of disease or injury, or as a drug side effect, notably the NSAI drugs (e.g. aspirin). There is now some movement towards accepting tinnitus as a disorder in its own right. A host of theories concerning the cause of tinnitus have been proposed, both those concerning the ear itself, and others concerning the auditory pathways of the brain. However, there remains little in the way of hard facts to support these theories. Consequently the mechanism behind tinnitus, particularly drug-induced tinnitus, is poorly understood.

Insomnia, drowsiness and nightmares

Insomnia is being unable to sleep. Sleep falls into two phases: **REM (rapid eye movement)**, which is shallow sleep linked to dreaming, and **NREM (non-rapid eye movement)**, which is deeper sleep. These two phases alternate throughout the night, starting and ending with REM (Figure 14.4).

Apart from insomnia, drugs can also affect this pattern of REM and NREM sleep. There are many physiological, psychological (emotional) and environmental causes, but there are

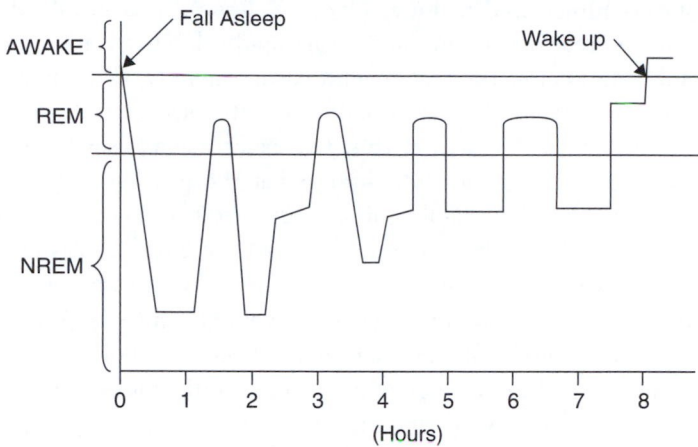

FIGURE 14.4 The normal REM–NREM sleep pattern for a young adult. Throughout the night, the normal sleep pattern alternates between REM (rapid eye movement) and NREM (non-rapid eye movement) sleep. REM occurs briefly first and then switches repeatedly with NREM. REM increasing gradually as NREM reduces during the night, and the individual wakes from REM.

also many drugs that list insomnia as a side effect (often referred to as **secondary insomnia,** i.e. secondary to taking the drugs). Some of the important drugs that cause insomnia are:

- **Psychoactive stimulants** (e.g. cocaine, caffeine, amphetamines and nicotine). Amphetamines and cocaine make it harder to get to sleep and cause shallow sleep rather than deep sleep. They do this by increasing dopamine accumulation in the brain, and high dopamine levels in turn causes brain excitement and over-activity, which is contrary to conditions needed for sleep. Caffeine blocks the brain receptors that are present for the substance **adenosine** (i.e. caffeine is an adenosine receptor antagonist). Adenosine normally slows down neuronal activity and induces sleep. By blocking these receptors, caffeine prevents adenosine activity, and the individual then stays awake.

- Some **anticonvulsants** (anti-epileptic drugs), notably the older medications, are reported to cause sleep pattern disturbances, including insomnia, with lengthening of the deepest levels of NREM sleep and reduced REM sleep. The reason is unclear. The newer medications do not appear to cause the same disturbances to sleep patterns.

- **Beta-blockers** are drugs used for treating high blood pressure. They are **beta-adrenergic receptor antagonists** that block the action of noradrenaline on these cardiac sympathetic receptors and thus reduce the force of ventricular contraction. Noradrenaline is the neurotransmitter of the terminal synapse of the sympathetic nervous system (see Figure 14.1). As a side effect, these drugs (especially the lipophilic, or fat-soluble, drugs) reduce the amount of REM sleep and cause night-time waking.

- Some **statins** (drugs used to lower blood cholesterol), especially the lipid-soluble forms, are reported to cause insomnia. The lipid solubility is important because the lipid-soluble drugs cross the blood–brain barrier more easily than the water-soluble drugs. They also affect the neurons more easily because cells have lipid membranes and myelin sheaths. Apart from this, the exact mechanism by which fat-soluble statins cause insomnia is not fully known but the problem appears to be reduced by switching to the water-soluble drugs. While statins have successfully prevented cardiac coronary disease by long-term reduction of blood cholesterol, there is now growing evidence to show that these drugs do cause a wide range of side effects. These including depletion of **ubiquinone** (or **coenzyme Q_{10}** or **CoQ_{10}**), which is a component of the energy production mechanism in the cell. A depletion of CoQ_{10} can lead to serious muscle and cardiovascular problems. Clearly, taking statins on a long-term basis must be considered very carefully.

Drowsiness is often a side effect of pain-relieving drugs, notably the **opioid analgesics**. Opioid drugs bind to and activate the mu (μ) brain receptor (see also loss of appetite, p. 252) which is inhibitory (i.e. it tends to reduce neuronal function). Mu receptors appear to be concentrated in the brain stem, where activation can cause suppression of various brain stem activities. The brain stem contains the **reticular activation system (RAS)**, which is very much involved in the sleep–wake cycle, i.e. cycling between the state of being awake and being asleep. It is a reasonable supposition that opioid drug activity on the brain stem mu receptors may suppress RAS function and cause drowsiness.

Other drugs causing drowsiness include the **anxiolytic** drugs (anti-anxiety drugs, mostly the **benzodiazipines**), alcohol, the barbiturates, and the antihistamines. The benzodiazipines, barbiturates and alcohol work by binding to a particular **gamma-aminobutyric acid (GABA)** receptor called **$GABA_A$**. When activated by binding GABA, the receptor opens an inhibitory chloride ionic channel (Cl^-), which causes suppression of brain impulses (**action potentials**) across that synapse. This sedates the brain activity, much as the brake in a car suppresses speed. Benzodiazipines, barbiturates and alcohol work on these receptors by promoting the GABA activity on this receptor, sedating the brain and causing drowsiness.

Antihistamines are drugs given to reduce the effects of an allergic reaction where histamine has been released from mast cells (see p. 268). They are **H1 receptor antagonists** (i.e. they block the H1 histamine receptor) and this reduces inflammation. However, this desired effect is mediated mainly through the *peripheral* H1 receptors (i.e. those in body tissues). But there are also *central* H1 receptors in the central nervous system (CNS), i.e. in the brain, and these drugs (particularly the older generation of antihistamines) cross the blood–brain barrier and block brain H1 receptors. This causes disruption to neurotransmission (nerve conduction) in the cerebral cortex, involving blockage of sodium channels and leading to a degree of sedation (drowsiness).

Nightmares are unpleasant and often frightening dreams, which can be caused by some medications, mostly the dopamine agonists, hypnotics, beta-blockers and amphetamines. The mechanism is largely unknown, but with amphetamines and the dopamine agonists it appears to be linked to the excess dopaminergic activity on dopamine receptors that these drugs cause.

Dizziness, vertigo, hypotension and fainting

Dizziness is a difficulty with body stability (i.e. disturbed balance or equilibrium) and a feeling of being giddy. **Vertigo** is a feeling of motion when nothing is moving; either the sufferer is feeling they are moving in a non-moving environment or they have a sensation that their environment is moving when it is not. Vertigo can be often accompanied by feelings of nausea and vomiting, and sometimes a wide range of other symptoms.

Hypotension is low blood pressure, and any drugs that cause a drop in blood pressure, e.g. **vasodilators**, are capable of causing dizziness and **fainting** (also called **syncope**). The three symptoms are linked such that a drop in blood pressure causes reduced blood flow to the brain, and this then causes dizziness and ultimately fainting. A drug-induced fall in blood pressure is the result of drugs causing **vasodilation**, i.e. dilating the **peripheral arterioles**, which then lowers the **peripheral resistance** and reduces the blood pressure (see also p. 52):

$$\text{Cardiac output (CO)} \times \text{peripheral resistance (PR)} = \text{blood pressure (BP)}$$

Therefore:

$$\text{CO} \times \text{reduced PR} (\downarrow) = \text{reduced BP} (\downarrow)$$

A similar situation can occur with drugs that affect the heart by reducing its output from the ventricles, i.e. the cardiac output (CO):

$$(\downarrow) \text{CO} \times \text{PR} = \text{reduced BP} (\downarrow)$$

These drugs are those such as **beta-blockers** that slow the heart rate and reduce the force of contraction.

The other way drugs can cause dizziness is through interference with the **vestibular** (i.e. balance) mechanism (see Figure 8.3, p. 139). This involves the **vestibular apparatus** of both ears, i.e. the **semi-circular canals**, which detect changes in movement and body position. The eyes give information on position and movement in relation to the environment around us. The sensory nerves from joints and tendons (called **proprioception**) tell the brain the position and movement of limbs. Finally, skin pressure detectors (nerve endings, see Table 9.1, p. 150) inform the brain about limb and body position in relation to gravity.

Vertigo is the result of conflicting information about movement sent to the brain at the same time by any of these position and balance sensory systems. If, for example, information about movement comes from the eyes and the vestibular apparatus, and arrives at the brain simultaneously, but the two bits of information do not match up (i.e. they give the brain conflicting information), vertigo is the result. The term vertigo is often used incorrectly, by being muddled with a fear of heights (which is **acrophobia**). Certainly looking down from a height can trigger a sensation of movement causing vertigo, but vertigo can also be triggered at any height, even at ground level. This would be the case when drug side effects trigger vertigo.

The **vestibulo-ocular reflex (VOR)** is a good example of how vestibular (balance) and ocular (visual) information work together and how disturbance of this system can cause vertigo (Figure 14.5).

The VOR allows for fixation of the gaze on an object during periods of head movement. The semi-circular canals detect rotational movement of the head and convert the movement into nerve impulses, which are then sent via the eighth cranial (**vestibulocochlear**) nerve to the **vestibular nuclei** of the brain stem (neuron 1, Figure 14.5). From here the pathways cross before passing out to the nuclei of the eye muscles (neuron 2) via the third (oculomotor) and sixth (abducens) cranial nerves (neuron 3). The VOR works in response to vertical head movements as well as horizontal. The eyes move in the same manner as the head but in the opposite direction in order to maintain the gaze on the object despite the head movements. This is a head movement compensatory mechanism. Vertigo can be caused by disturbance of the neurotransmitters that occur in the synapses between the three-neuronal system of the VOR, a disturbance that could be caused by drugs. These neurotransmitters include glutamate, acetylcholine, GABA, dopamine, noradrenaline and histamine.

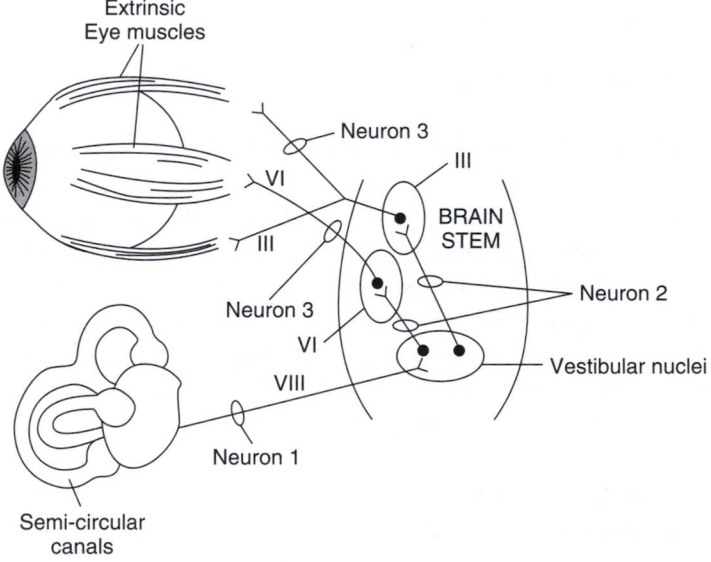

FIGURE 14.5 The vestibulo-ocular reflex (VOR). Neuron 1 runs from the semi-circular canals of the vestibular apparatus, taking information about head movements to the vestibular nuclei of the brain stem. Neuron 2 takes the information to the brain stem nuclei that control the external eye muscles, i.e. the nuclei of cranial nerves III and VI. Neuron 3 runs from the brain stem nuclei to the eye muscles. The purpose is to allow the eyes to sustain a fixed gaze on an object while the head turns. Some drugs can affect this system and cause vertigo.

Psychosis

Drug-induced psychosis is a growing problem because the incidence of drug addiction involving psycho-active drugs is increasing. Any drug that stimulates dopamine receptors in the brain is a potential cause of acute psychoses. Cocaine ('cocaine psychosis'), amphetamines and cannabis ('cannabis psychosis') are drugs which regularly cause psychotic episodes. These drugs are part of the reason why more than 80% of hospital admissions for acute psychosis each year in the UK are drug-induced. The dopamine receptors (especially D2 and D3) in the mesocortical pathways of the brain become over-stimulated and cause hallucinations, delusions, thought disorder and mania. Cannabis is well known for causing a high degree of paranoia (Blows 2011).

Headaches

Drug-related headaches can occur as a side effect, or as a feature of chronic drug over-use (i.e. long-term daily use of normal-dose analgesia), or even as a result of drug withdrawal (e.g. alcohol).

A very large number of drugs list headache as one of the side effects, but those medications that increase blood flow to the brain (**vasodilators**) and the amphetamines are especially known to cause this problem. The mechanism behind why a raised blood flow to the brain following drug-induced vasodilation of the cerebral vascular system causes throbbing headaches is not fully understood. It may be due to a rise in intracranial pressure, since normal cerebral blood flow contributes about 10% of the intracranial pressure, and vasodilation is likely to increase this percentage. The throbbing (pulsatile) nature of the headache indicates the involvement of arterial blood flow. **Glyceryl trinitrate** is a vasodilator drug used in treating the cardiac disorder called **angina**, and has headaches as a main side effect. The initial (primary) headache can be immediate or soon after administration and tends to be relatively mild with no other symptoms associated. A secondary headache is delayed and more severe, with symptoms of nausea, vomiting and **photophobia** (a dislike of light). **Nitric oxide (NO)** is the active metabolic product (called a **metabolite**) derived from glyceryl trinitrate and is the cause of the vasodilation that leads to the initial headache. The delayed secondary headaches are caused by the release of other chemical mediators, including the neurotransmitter glutamate (Bagdy *et al.* 2010).

Chronic daily use of normal-dose analgesia can cause rebound headaches (known as **medication overuse headaches, MOHs**). The problem occurs with other drug types as well, notably the **opioids** and the **triptans** (i.e. drugs used to treat migraine). The headache causes the patient to take the analgesic, but when the drug wears off, the headache returns and the patient then repeats the drug. If this continues over a period of days or weeks, a state occurs where the headache will automatically return at any time the drug is withdrawn. The reason for this is not fully understood but does appear to involve a genetic predisposition and changes in receptor and enzyme physiology in the brain.

Substance withdrawal headaches are known to occur if a substance, e.g. a medication or alcohol, is taken for longer than three months then stopped. Soon after stopping, the headaches begin, but if the patient can remain off the substance long enough (usually no longer than three months), the headaches will subside. The problem is due to tolerance, where the brain has got used to the presence of the substance and suddenly finds it is missing. These substances include opioid drugs, caffeine, alcohol and oestrogen medications.

Skin side effects

Drug side effects that involve the skin are usually the first to be seen and identified when side effects occur. They are also the ones that occur quickest, often because they are the result of rapid immune reactions, e.g. rashes.

Rashes

As a drug side effect, redness (erythema) and rashes begin most commonly within the first ten days of starting the drug, and often within hours depending on the level of sensitivity to the drug (see also Table 9.2, p. 154). Penicillins and sulfonamides are a common cause of rashes. The mechanism involves one of four types of immune reaction (see p. 268) causing vasodilation (redness), skin eruptions (rashes) and local skin oedema (swelling) (Lee and Thomson 2006). This is an immune drug allergy, and this topic is discussed further under **drug allergies** (see p. 267).

In addition, there are non-immune causes of skin rashes, including drugs such as the NSAIs (see p. 200) that directly (i.e. not through the immune system) release histamine from mast cells (see p. 268).

Hair loss

Alopecia (hair loss) is a well-known side effect of a number of drugs, especially anti-cancer drugs (known as **chemotherapy**). Hair grows from rapidly reproducing cells in the skin follicles. Anti-cancer drugs kill rapidly reproducing cells; therefore these hair follicle cells are vulnerable to these drugs.

Hair growth follows two phases; the **anagen phase** (3–4 years long) is the period of hair growth, followed by the **telogen phase** (about 3 months long) when hair growth stops and the hair 'rests'. At the end of the telogen phase the hair falls out and the cycle starts again. Drugs can cause one of two types of alopecia. **Telogen effluvium** (the most common form of drug-induced hair loss) is where the hair goes quickly into the telogen phase and falls out early (about 100–150 hairs lost per day). **Anagen effluvium** (the main cause of alopecia in chemotherapy) is hair loss during the hair growth phase. Here, the drugs destroy or disrupt the fast reproduction of hair follicle cells. It occurs quicker than telogen effluvium, and it can be very severe, causing total hair loss across the body.

Interesting other drug side effects

A web page showing some interesting drug side effects is available at: http://listverse.com/2011/02/03/10-bizarre-side-effects-to-common-medicines/ (accessed October 2011).

Drug interactions

Adverse drug interactions may occur when two or more drugs are taken together. The interaction involves one drug impeding or enhancing the action of another (Rodrigues 2008). Many oral medications can be taken safely together, but if any interactions do happen, they can sometimes be harmful, and even fatal. The elderly are at greater risk of this problem because they are more likely to be prescribed multiple medication (called **polypharmacy**), and because their metabolic and excretory pathways are less efficient due to the ageing process (Seymour and Routledge 1998). About 20% of the UK population, aged 60 years or older, consume 56% of all the dispensed medication, and the elderly population is growing in numbers. There are recommendations that the over-60 population should not be prescribed more than three medications at any one time because of the risk to health from drug interactions, but this is not always possible. Each additional drug added to the mix increases the risk of an interaction. And it is not just prescribed medication that is involved. A mix of 'over-the-counter' self-medication, or several illicit drugs used together during addiction, can cause an interaction.

And interactions can even occur when medication is taken by those who smoke, since nicotine is, after all, a drug. Smoking induces metabolic enzymes (see p. 266) and this interferes with the metabolic process of other drugs (see pharmacokinetic interactions, below). Nicotine also has pharmacodynamic interactions (see p. 267) with a wide range of drugs, and this causes changes with the activity and efficacy of those drugs.

Pharmacokinetic interactions

During **absorption**, some oral drugs may compete for uptake into the blood from the digestive tract. If one drug is absorbed first, this may block the absorption of another drug, causing it to be delayed in the gut. When this happens, the therapeutic effect of the delayed drug is reduced and it may be eliminated from the bowel before being fully absorbed. Alternatively, some drugs bind with specific foods, which then delays or prevents the drug's absorption, and those foods must be avoided when taking the drug. An example is the antibiotic tetracycline, which binds to calcium, and so the drug must not be taken with calcium-rich foods such as milk.

During **distribution**, drugs in circulation bind to blood proteins. Some drug combinations result in drugs competing for the same binding sites on the proteins. This competition causes some drugs to displace others for protein binding and this changes the activity level (the **bioavailability**) of the displaced drugs.

During **metabolism**, multiple drugs may compete for the various enzyme systems (i.e. multiple enzymes working together) that carry out the metabolic process, and can alter the enzyme activity (Scully 2008; Zhu and Humphreys 2008). Most drug metabolism takes place in the liver, and enzyme systems in the liver vary the metabolic process depending on which drugs are present. For example, some drugs increase enzyme activity (called **enzyme induction**) or decrease enzyme activity (called **enzyme inhibition**), and this may affect the metabolism of other drugs using those same enzyme systems. As a result, these other drugs may be delayed or accelerated in their metabolism. Delayed metabolism of a drug increases that drug's concentration in the blood, and this then risks reaching toxic levels. Metabolic interactions are particularly important mainly because one liver enzyme system, called the cytochrome P450 oxidases (CYP), is involved in the metabolism of the majority of drugs, and therefore is prone to enzyme induction or inhibition. Alcohol is metabolised by this enzyme system and also causes induction of some P450 enzymes, therefore disturbing the metabolism of any drugs administered at the same time. Usually the alcohol competes with and displaces the drug, which is therefore delayed in its metabolism. This delay causes the drug to lengthen its period of activity (as demonstrated by an increased drug **half-life**, see Figure 14.6), and this prolongs and increases the drug's activity.

Chronic alcoholism and smoking cause the induction of specific P450 enzymes to remain high. This will speed up the drug metabolism faster than normally expected whenever the drug is administered during periods when no alcohol or nicotine is present in the system.

Smoking causes a very large range of undesirable chemicals to enter the circulation, among which the **polycyclic aromatic hydrocarbons** are powerful inducers of some P450 enzymes. This has a profound effect on drug metabolism, a case of smoking speeding up the metabolism and therefore the clearance of drugs quickly, shortening the drug's therapeutic life.

During **elimination**, some drugs may cause other drugs to be eliminated faster or slower than they should be. Those eliminated too slowly will accumulate in the circulation and

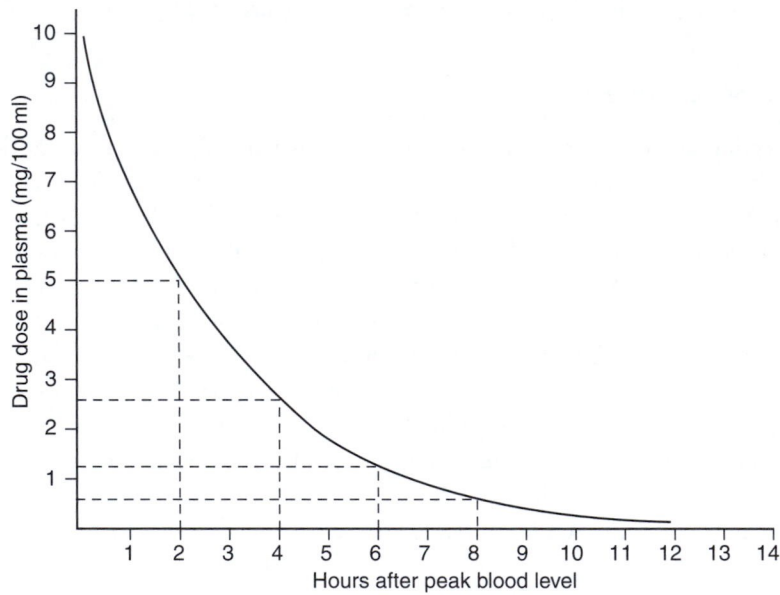

FIGURE 14.6 The half-life of a drug. This graph shows the elimination pattern of a drug (call it drug X, with a half-life of 2 hours) from circulation. From peak plasma concentration (in this case 10 mg/100 ml), the first two hours sees an excretion of half the original concentration (down to 5 mg/100 ml). The second two-hour period sees an excretion of half this new value, i.e. half the 5 mg/ml (down to 2.5 mg/ml). This pattern is repeated every further two hours, i.e. removing half the concentration of the drug found at the start of that period, until the drug concentration is virtually zero. Some drugs have short half-lives, others have longer half-lives.

may reach toxic levels. An example is the drug digoxin, which is delayed in its excretion by the presence of a range of other drugs, which must then be avoided to prevent digoxin toxicity.

Pharmacodynamic interactions

Pharmacodynamic interactions occur when two or more drugs administered together interfere with each other's mode of action, i.e. they alter in some way the mechanism by which one or both drugs carry out their function. This can happen in several ways, although receptors are usually the principal site for interactions to occur.

Receptors on cell surfaces are the site where many drugs act, and several drugs administered together may become competitive at the same receptor site (Figure 14.7). This means that one drug can easily affect the activity of another by preventing its binding. If two **agonists** (i.e. drugs that stimulate or activate a receptor type) are given at the same time, this may increase the normal expected activity, i.e. it will cause an *additive* effect, and that can lead to toxicity. Similarly, two **antagonists** (i.e. drugs that block receptors) given at the same time could reduce the receptor function to dangerously low levels. An agonist and antagonist for the same receptor, when given together, would basically cancel each other out with little therapeutic value.

Drug allergies

Allergies occur when a foreign substance (called an **antigen**) enters the body and sets up an immune response. Typically, drugs may react with proteins of the immune system (called

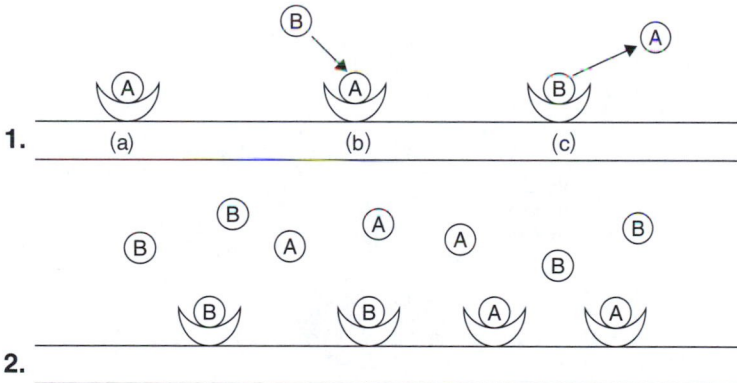

FIGURE 14.7 Pharmacodynamic drug interaction between two drugs. Drugs A and B are shown binding to the same cell surface receptors. 1. (a) Drug A has bound to the receptor. (b) Drug B is competing with drug A for the receptor. (c) Drug B has displaced drug A and now occupies the receptor. This means that drug B affects the function of drug A. 2. Both drugs A and B bind to the same receptors. When both occur together, some of each will bind, affecting the total function of both drugs. If the two drugs have opposing effects on the receptors, they may cancel out each other's effect.

antibodies, or **immunoglobulins, Ig**). This is a Type I response (see below), but equally there are three other drug allergic responses possible, Type II, Type III and Type IV (see below). Drugs become the antigen in all these immune reactions. The allergic response occurs each time the drug enters the body and the reaction triggers several chemical chain reactions, including histamine release, causing inflammation.

The four types of possible allergic responses that happen after the administration of medication are:

- **Type I** reaction is an acute response (i.e. rapid onset) causing skin rash, **urticaria** (inflamed patches of skin with red, raised, itchy bumps; also called **hives**), tissue swelling (due to local oedema, see p. 83), respiratory difficulties (due to bronchoconstriction), and even **anaphylaxis** (i.e. a severe shock) caused by extensive peripheral vasodilation leading to a loss of peripheral resistance and therefore collapse of blood pressure (see Chapter 3 and p. 261). Anaphylaxis is potentially fatal if not treated urgently. Type I reactions are IgE-mediated, meaning that the drug (the antigen) has caused an increase in the production of the antibody IgE that is specific to the drug's chemical properties. IgE binds to cells in the tissues called mast cells. **Mast cells** are specialised cells because they house **histamine**, and, when released, the histamine causes local inflammation. When the drug is introduced into the body, it binds to the IgE on mast cells in a cross-linked manner (Figure 14.8). Mast cells then release their histamine and inflammation occurs. Type I reactions are the fastest type of drug allergy, and include those to any medication containing a protein (acting as the antigen) such as insulin.

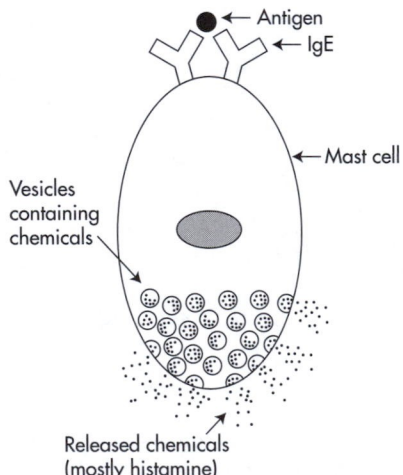

FIGURE **14.8** The release of histamine from mast cells by an immune response. The antibody IgE binds to the mast cell surface and cross-links an antigen (a foreign substance from outside the body, which can be a drug). This cross-linkage causes release of vesicles containing chemicals, mostly histamine, a cause of inflammation (i.e. an inflammatory mediator).

- **Type II** reaction is a delayed response where drugs bind to and modify the body's cellular proteins, which then appear as cell surface antigens in the body and cause an immune reaction. The immune system responds to these modified cells through activation of B- cell lymphocytes, which then release antibodies (IgG) to attack the antigenic (drug- modified) proteins. This leads to activation of K cells (K = killer) that have a cytotoxic effect (i.e. they kill the cells that are bearing the antigens). It also triggers a chemical reaction in the **complement system**. This series of blood proteins, when activated, produces substances that result in the destruction of the cell by **lysis** (i.e. breaking up the cells). Drugs that can do this include some antibiotics such as penicillins, cephalosporins and sulfonamides.
- **Type III** reaction is where drugs in circulation (the antigens) form complexes of different sizes with the antibodies **IgM** or **IgG**. The drug antigen is usually present in much larger quantities than the antibodies. The large immune complexes formed can be cleared by **macrophages (phagocytic cells)**, but small complexes cannot be cleared from circulation (a condition called **serum sickness**). In this condition, the complexes cause problems with renal **nephrons (glomerulonephritis)** and with the tiny blood vessels (**vasculitis**) and cause joint pain (**arthralgia**). The salicylates (e.g. aspirin) and chlorpromazine can cause these reactions.
- **Type IV** reaction is a delayed hypersensitivity caused by drugs applied to the skin surface (as in a **contact dermatitis**) or injected subcutaneously into the skin (as in some skin tests), which then react with **T cells**. This is the most common type of drug reaction in skin reactions (e.g. rashes), including nearly all topically applied skin medications.

Key points

Drug side effects

- Drug side effects are unwanted adverse effects, which usually occur from a chemical mechanism separate from the desired effect of the drug.
- Many side effects are mild and transient, but others are very unpleasant and can be harmful.
- Gastrointestinal side effects, especially nausea and vomiting, are common with many drugs, especially oral medication.
- Central nervous system side effects are also common and occur in many different types depending on the brain area involved.

Drug interactions

- Drug interactions occur when two or more drugs are given together, and one drug then causes unwanted changes in the other drug.
- Pharmacokinetic interactions can occur during absorption, distribution, metabolism or excretion of the drugs.
- These interactions allow one drug to impede or enhance the activity of the other drug.

- Metabolic interactions may often involve one drug affecting the activation of liver enzyme systems, which then affects the metabolism of a second drug.
- Pharmacodynamic interactions mean that two or more drugs given simultaneously may block or enhance each other's function.
- Most pharmacodynamic interactions occur at cell surface receptors.

Drug allergies

- Drug allergies can be mild or serious, even fatal.
- Drugs sometimes are seen as antigens, i.e. they can cause an allergic response as a foreign substance entering the body.
- There are four allergic responses possible when drugs cause allergic reactions: Type I, Type II, Type III and Type IV.

References

Bagdy G., Riba P., Kecskemeti V., Chase D. and Juhasz G. (2010) Headache-type adverse effects of NO donors: vasodilation and beyond. *British Journal of Pharmacology*, **160**(1): 20–35.

Blows W. T. (2011) *The Biological Basis of Mental Health Nursing*, 2nd edition. Routledge, London.

Gottlieb S. (2001) Drug effects blamed for fifth of hospital deaths among elderly. *British Medical Journal*, **323**(7320): 1025.

Gutierrez D. (2010) Drug side effects blamed for 20 percent of hospital readmissions. *Natural News*, May 6.

Kuratsune H., Yamaguti K., Lindh G., Evengård B., Hagberg G., Matsumura K., Iwase M., Onoe H., Takahashi M., Machii T., Kanakura Y., Kitani T., Långström B. and Watanabe Y. (2002) Brain regions involved in fatigue sensation: reduced acetylcarnitine uptake into the brain. *NeuroImage*, **17**(3): 1256–1265.

Lee A. and Thomson J. (2006) Drug-induced skin reactions, in Lee A. (ed.) *Adverse Drug Reactions*, 2nd edition. Pharmaceutical Press, New York.

Makins R. and Ballinger A. (2003) Gastrointestinal side effects of drugs, *Expert Opinion on Drug Safety*, **2**(4): 421–429.

Rodrigues A. D. (2008) *Drug–Drug Interactions*. Informa Healthcare, London.

Scully C. (2008) Drug interactions. *Drug Metabolism Reviews*, **41**(3): 486–527.

Seymour R. M. and Routledge P. A. (1998) Important drug–drug interactions in the elderly. *Drugs & Aging*, **12**(6): 485–494.

Zhu M. and Humphreys W. G. (2008) Metabolism-mediated drug–drug interactions, in *Metabolism Clinical and Experimental*, Wiley-Blackwell, New York, pp. 113–136.

Index

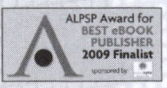